An Approach to
Occupational Therapy

An Approach to Occupational Therapy

Mary S. Jones
MCSP, SRP, FBAOT, SROT

Third Edition

Revised by

Peggy Jay
MBAOT, SROT

BUTTERWORTHS
LONDON - BOSTON
Sydney - Wellington - Durban - Toronto

The Butterworth Group

United Kingdom London	**Butterworth & Co (Publishers) Ltd** 88 Kingsway, WC2B 6AB
Australia Sydney	**Butterworths Pty Ltd** 586 Pacific Highway, Chatswood, NSW 2067 Also at Melbourne, Brisbane, Adelaide and Perth
South Africa Durban	**Butterworth & Co (South Africa) (Pty) Ltd** 152–154 Gale Street
New Zealand Wellington	**Butterworths of New Zealand Ltd** 26–28 Waring Taylor Street, 1
Canada Toronto	**Butterworth & Co (Canada) Ltd** 2265 Midland Avenue, Scarborough, Ontario, M1P 4S1
USA Boston	**Butterworth (Publishers) Inc** 19 Cummings Park, Woburn, Mass. 01801

First published 1960
Second edition 1964
Reprinted 1967
Third edition 1977

© Butterworth & Co (Publishers) Ltd 1977

ISBN 0 407 00053 4

British Library Cataloguing in Publication Data

Jones, Mary Senior
    An approach to occupational therapy. – 3rd ed
    1. Occupational therapy
    I. Title II. Jay, Peggy
    615'.8515   RM735   77–30007

    ISBN 0-407-00053-4

Typeset by Butterworths Litho Preparation Department
Made and printed by litho in Great Britain by
W. & J. Mackay Ltd., Chatham, Kent

Preface to the Third Edition

Mary Senior Jones (Molly to her colleagues) was one of the pioneer occupational therapists. Originally she trained as a physiotherapist at St Thomas' Hospital, London, and was later persuaded to take a shortened course in occupational therapy during the Second World War to widen the scope of treatment offered at the Rowley Bristow Hospital, Pyrford, where she was then working.

At Farnham Park she initiated many new ideas. She did not like her patients to be tied up to apparatus just in order to utilize a particular movement. She preferred them to use directly purposive movements carefully chosen to strengthen muscles, mobilize joints and increase stamina. To make this possible, particularly for those with lower limb injuries, she needed machines for her patients to work on. At that time there was almost no occupational therapy equipment available commercially. So she had to design and make her own. A bicycle fretsaw, bicycle file, foot-treadle drilling machine, ankle rotator, bowl lathes, wire-twisting machine, pronator-supinator drilling machine, bicycle-seat stools and overhead arm supports were all made to her specifications by her very able technician, Tom Dunn. She never patented her machines because she wanted them to be freely available to other people's patients, and consequently few occupational therapists now realize what she invented.

Another of her achievements was to create such a good atmosphere in her workshops that the patients' morale was invariably high. They worked hard at their carefully chosen activities and sometimes seemed to show improved function just by being there. Her personality was such that patients who had perhaps spent only a short time with her would come back to visit and report their progress, often many years later.

Molly Jones died in 1974. She had already asked me to produce the third edition of her book. When the first edition was published I was her assistant, and when the second edition came out she had retired and I had taken over as head occupational therapist at Farnham Park.

Bringing out a third edition has presented problems, since the original book was based on Molly Jones' experience in treating 4115 patients at Farnham Park over an eight-year period. Recent medical and surgical advances have brought changes in the types of conditions treated at Farnham Park and also in the stages of treatment at which patients are admitted. New materials for splint-making, and increasing emphasis on more formal assessment at all stages of treatment and on helping patients to return to employment have altered the work done in the department. I have tried to marry together those parts of the original book that are still current practice with new approaches developed by me or by my successor as head occupational therapist, Lynn Cheshire.

This book covers only certain aspects of occupational therapy, although these are described in considerable detail. It should be of interest to both practising occupational therapists and students who are concerned in treating patients in the physical field. It should also interest those doctors and others concerned with disabled people who have not experienced the contribution that occupational therapy can make in helping the disabled reach their maximum potential.

So much of Molly Jones' approach to occupational therapy is still impeccable and so many of her treatment techniques are still widely used. At this stage of the development of our profession, when there is perhaps too much emphasis on assessment at the expense of treatment techniques, it is hoped that this book may do something to redress the balance. Sound assessment is, of course, essential, but if it is not followed up or accompanied by appropriate treatment it may not be of much benefit to the patient.

PEGGY JAY

Author's Notes to First Edition

Theoretically, occupational therapy may be described as purposeful activity designed to stir the patient's creative instincts and through this channel to provide opportunities for therapeutic physical and mental exercise. The occupational therapist is expected to aid in the restoration of the patient to his normal place in society as quickly and efficiently as possible. The aims of treatment for each patient are indicated by the medical officer. It is left to the occupational therapist to discover and encourage the interest of the patient, and to teach, to supervise, and to guide the patient's activities so that these may have a beneficial effect. These aims require considerable knowledge of anatomy, kinesiology and psychology, with common sense, humour and a capacity for observation to temper and apply this knowledge. Simple crafts and activities are used as a basis for the effective occupation of patients with varying disabilities. Workers who are interested in their jobs are never satisfied by the basic knowledge which qualifies them to practise. In a profession such as occupational therapy the search for further knowledge must be continued by reading, listening, observation and experiment. As we learn, we find some satisfaction in the improvement of techniques of treatment, but still other vistas are revealed to tempt us on to further effort.

Practically it is inevitable that some specialization will develop. Patients who are so mentally deranged as to be irresponsible members of a free society are segregated for treatment from those whose disabilities are mainly physical. Yet no one can fail to note how closely physical disabilities are related to mental obliquity. Neglect of either aspect will intensify dysfunction of the individual as a whole. The restoration of the patient's attitude towards the responsibilities of life is of first importance.

In the physical field there are centres with various specializations such as the training of patients in the aids to daily living, the means of personal care and independence of locomotion. Here at Farnham Park we have specialized in the treatment of the short-term patient with the expectancy of a quick return to a normal life in a professional or industrial capacity. We have designed and made workshop machinery which demands exercise of increasing effort, dexterity and controlled movement. We have aimed to make machinery which does not look very different from that in common use. We have avoided the use of weights and pulleys which entail fixing the patient in such a way that much exertion is applied to a trivial task. We still plan improvements to make our lathes, saws and drills move more smoothly, and so encourage a rhythmic series of muscle contractions. The product of work is designed to be graduated in size, weight or elaboration so that increasing demands are made for muscular effort and mental concentration.

This survey is entitled *An Approach to Occupational Therapy* to emphasize the belief that the field of study is vast and that we have much to learn. The literature at our disposal is scanty, and our practice is often empiric and personal to a degree that may dishearten students in their early stages. For those of us who are older the possibilities of wider knowledge act as a stimulant.

The work of the 'rehabilitation team' is often quoted and some of the work consists of repairing the stable door after the horse has gone, as well as finding and reassuring the horse. In many aspects of medicine preventive work is being developed alongside curative work. This is true not only in research and practice of immunization against disease but also in the development of occupational hygiene as a part of industrial medicine. The therapeutic dietitian grows to realize that much disability would be prevented by the early inculcation of good habits of eating; the physiotherapist must often feel that the teaching of controlled movement in games would prevent casual trauma.

In the same way, as occupational therapists, our thoughts must spread from the corrective to the preventive fields of study. Perhaps in days to come occupational therapists may have wider opportunities for studying productive activities, and be able to make a contribution to preventive as well as therapeutic medicine.

Reference is made in this survey to the writings of some eminent authorities. Other sources of information which have been tapped are too numerous to mention. One author, Laurence Sterne, must not be omitted, for he wrote of Corporal Trim who had only one patient, Tristram Shandy's Uncle Toby. Corporal Trim persuaded Uncle Toby to activity whilst still in bed; for two years they made together a model of the fort at Namur where Uncle Toby had been wounded. Then he coaxed Uncle Toby to live in the country and to build a bigger and better model of the fort in the garden: 'Where your honour will not only get pleasure and good pastime but good air and exercise and good health and your honour's wound would be well in a month'. Here's to Corporal Trim and to his principles of reablement!

Now, in March 1960, these notes are written after some years of work on the survey of my practice of occupational therapy. Some emotion of nostalgia is aroused by the memories of experiments in reablement, but changes bring new hopes for the future. I belong to the generation which was brought up on Tennyson: 'The old order changeth yielding place to new and God fulfils himself in many ways, lest one good custom should corrupt the world.'

Farnham Park Rehabilitation Centre,   MARY S. JONES
Farnham Royal, Bucks,
March. 1960

Acknowledgements

Some years ago an anonymous donor gave one thousand pounds to what was then the Association of Occupational Therapists for research. Mrs M. S. Jones applied to the Council of the Association with a proposal to undertake, as a research project, a survey of occupational therapy used for patients at Farnham Park. Her proposal was accepted and so the first edition of this book came to be written.

Many people have been involved in the preparation of the third edition. The staff of the occupational therapy workshops at Farnham Park have given up time to help in updating the book, by providing new information and drawings, checking the typescript and helping with the preliminary typing. Occupational therapists from outside the Centre have helped by reading and commenting on sections which related to their particular treatment expertise. I thank them all for their help and encouragement.

Photographs and drawings have come from a variety of sources, some from patients. I would like to acknowledge and thank the photographic departments of the King Edward VII Hospital at Windsor, Wexham Park Hospital at Slough, the Canadian Red Cross Memorial Hospital at Taplow, and The London Hospital at Whitechapel, for their help. I also thank the British Association of Occupational Therapists for permission to reproduce photographs from their Journal.

Lastly and in particular, I would like to thank Lynn Cheshire, previously my deputy and now my successor as head occupational therapist at Farnham Park, for all her help and co-operation in bringing this new edition up to date.

PEGGY JAY

Contents

1

Occupational Therapy at Farnham Park

The patients

The patients accepted at Farnham Park Rehabilitation Centre must be ambulant and mobile, and able to dress and feed themselves with sometimes a little help from the nursing staff or other patients. The resident patients must be able to get upstairs to their bedrooms. Patients are mostly between the ages of 16 and 65 years, that is, of employable age, though a few above or below these age limits have been accepted for special reasons. Women as well as men are accepted for rehabilitation. The women form a group fluctuating in number, usually between 20 and 25 per cent of the total. Patients come from every imaginable walk in life and range from the highly educated and highly skilled to the illiterate and unskilled. They have been of many nationalities, some able to speak but little English and understand less. Naturally, a substantial proportion of patients are referred by consultants from local hospitals or from hospitals in London. But others come from hospitals much farther afield, for example Wales, the West Country, Scotland or Ireland. Readmissions include patients who come again, whether after further treatment for the original disability, or after an incident of illness or injury unrelated to their previous visits.

It is the custom of the head occupational therapist to see the new patients as a group before they begin treatment in the workshops. It is stressed that occupational therapy work is planned to fulfil the doctor's aims of treatment, be these aims a better range of movement in certain joints, more power in certain groups of muscles, better control of movement, or improved capacity to carry on through working hours. The patients are told that each one of them will be seen individually, so that the reason for choosing a particular type of work for his treatment can be explained. It is important that everyone should understand

1

why he is being asked to do such work, so that he can participate in his own treatment and take some responsibility for helping himself to get better. If at any time a patient does not understand the reason for an activity he must ask the head occupational therapist to explain it. During this preliminary group conversation, patients are asked to help in keeping the workshops tidy, to put away their own work and tools, and to help other patients who by reason of being on sticks or crutches cannot do so. Their help is also asked in the care of tools and equipment, so that these may last for the use of future patients. Those patients with skills are asked to help by handing on their knowledge.

It is found that this short explanation of the aims and method of occupational therapy, taking at the most 10 minutes, is well worth the time and trouble. Patients are found to settle down more quickly and with more confidence when they understand the rough outlines of our work as occupational therapists, than was the case in the early years when no such introduction was given. A friendly atmosphere and improved morale visibly develop as the patients appreciate that their talents will be valued, and that they themselves have something to contribute in the treatment of others whose plight may be more apparent than their own.

New patients are seen by the doctor on admission, examined and given their individual programme of treatment. Sample programmes, including the changes that may be made when the treatment is later upgraded, are shown in *Figures 1.1* and *1.2*. Regular clinics are held during the week so that patients can be seen by the doctor, either when the staff deems this necessary or at a patient's own request.

Three staff conferences are held each week, all at lunch time. One on Monday is attended by all the staff and is concerned with new patients, sessional patients and any urgent patient problems. The second, on Tuesday, is the resettlement conference attended by all the occupational therapists, the medical social worker, the speech therapist, one physiotherapist, one remedial gymnast and the DRO. This meeting considers those patients who are expected to have difficulty in returning to work or in managing for themselves at home. The final conference of the week, on Friday, lasts a little longer and continues through what would normally be the first treatment session in the afternoon. All the staff are present and all the 75—85 patients are briefly discussed. Occupational therapy students attend all conferences.

Three meetings a week may appear to take up a disproportionate amount of staff time but, being held during the lunch break and extending beyond this on one day only, the patients' treatment programme is hardly interrupted. A recent management survey concluded that by reviewing each patient every week with all staff present, good communication and a smooth-running programme were most efficiently achieved. This conference system gives all staff immediate direct communication with each other, thus reducing time-wasting conversations or written memos, which may not reach all those concerned or may be misconstrued as they are relayed.

FARNHAM PARK REHABILITATION CENTRE

OCCUPATIONAL THERAPY

Surname	First Names	Date of Birth	Hospital No.
PATIENT	JOHN MICHAEL	15·6·47	12345

Address		Civil State	Sex
43, High Street, Sometown, Someshire		M.	M.

Occupation and Firm	CATEGORY (I. P. D. P. or Sessional)
Maintenance Fitter Sometown Bearings Ltd.,	In Patient

DIAGNOSIS (L) Medial Meniscectomy

AIMS Build up quadriceps, mobilise knee. Assess for return to work.

Rx —

PROGRAMME

DATE	1·3·77	8·3·77	15·3·77			
9.0.	O.T.	Hydrotherapy	Pre-Work			
9.45.	Straight Legs	O.T.	Pre-Work			
11.00.	Physio	O.T.	O.T.			
11.45.	O.T.	Intermediate Legs	O.T.			
2.0.	Straight Legs	O.T.	O.T.			
2.40.	O.T.	Weight-training	Late Legs			
3.20	Physio	Intermediate Legs	Games			

DATE	
P.H.	Several accidents whilst playing football, with subsequent episodes of locking of the (L) Knee.
22·2·77	(L) Medial meniscectomy performed (Torn cartilage found)
O/E	(L) Knee: R.O.M:- 175°—120° Quads. ↓+. Effusion: minimal. Dry dressing; crêpe bandage; 2 elbow crutches. Sutures to be removed 3·3·77.

Figure 1.1. – Occupational therapy referral card

It is most interesting to observe that a patient may respond much better to treatment in one department than in another. Occasionally the patient who produces the worst symptoms in the doctor's clinic may be noted and reported as one who is active and symptom free

FARNHAM PARK REHABILITATION CENTRE

NAME .... PROGRAMME

TIME	1st Change	2nd Change	3rd Change
9.0 to 9.45 a.m.	Individual Walking	Individual Walking	O.T Workshop
9.45 to 10.30 a.m.	O.T. Workshops	O.T Workshops	Physiotherapy
TEA BREAK			
11.0 to 11.45 a.m.	Early Movements	Physiotherapy	O.T Workshop
11.45 to 12.30 p.m.	Early Movements	Dancing	O.T Workshop
LUNCHEON			
2.0 to 2.40 p.m.	Speech Therapy	Speech Therapy	Speech Therapy
2.40 to 3.20 p.m.	O.T Workshops	O.T Workshops	O.T Workshops
3.20 to 4.0 p.m.	(Rest)	O.T Workshops	Intermediate Legs

ALWAYS KEEP THIS PROGRAMME WITH YOU

Figure 1.2. – An individual programme for a hemiplegic patient

when his attention is diverted in work or play. There is always opportunity for private discussion with the medical officer when this is considered necessary but the staff conferences are felt to be essential in the development of the team spirit. Everyone knows that a patient's improvement is the result of treatment by a team.

It is necessary to set this picture, to make these points clear, before starting a discussion of occupational therapy, which is an integral part, but only a part, of rehabilitation at Farnham Park. It is true that all patients who come for the whole day's programme of treatment come for occupational therapy, and that not all may be considered to need hydrotherapy, physiotherapy or group exercises. It is the medical officer's responsibility to place the emphasis of treatment where it is of most value to the individual patient. It is the duty of the staff to enlist the co-operation of the patient, as a member of the rehabilitation team.

The average stay for rehabilitation is between four and six weeks but some patients have only needed a week to relearn a particular movement, whilst others have needed 10 months. The programme of the average patient's day has been changed from time to time. On the whole the trend has been to increase the number of patients and the hours they spend in the occupational therapy workshops. For these reasons, the possibility of short stay and the number of patients treated together, the choice of work made available in workshop and garden has been gradually evolved on certain lines. It has been found practical to keep the types of work to simple projects which can be finished in a reasonably short period to a satisfactory standard. This scheme not only ensures that a patient will be able to finish a job before discharge, but makes it possible to plan a more progressive programme of work for each individual that becomes more demanding of both physical energy and mental effort. Progressive demands must be compatible with the individual's rate of recovery. Occupational therapy can sometimes be used as a group treatment but in a rehabilitation centre like Farnham Park, where patients with widely differing disabilities come for treatment, it has been found necessary to develop occupational therapy on individual lines.

The workshops

The occupational therapy workshops at Farnham Park are housed in two long huts which were originally put up to provide temporary accommodation for a war relief organization during the Second World War. They are joined by a short section built rather like a greenhouse. Over the years two small brick additions have been built on by our patients under the supervision of a technical instructor. One of these is a welding bay and the other a quiet room for patients working on assessment tests. The building bears little resemblance to anything that would be considered suitable when planning a new custom-built occupational therapy department. Yet very good facilities for treatment have been developed here and many visitors have remarked in a despairing tone of voice, 'But you have everything at hand'.

The facilities for occupational therapy have evolved gradually and the layout of work areas, benches, machines and equipment has changed many times since the department opened in 1947. This rearrangement has been generated first by increased numbers of patients, much later by increased numbers of staff, and also by changing patient needs, the acquisition of new machinery and the development of new occupational therapy techniques. Plans of the workshops and of the other facilities

6

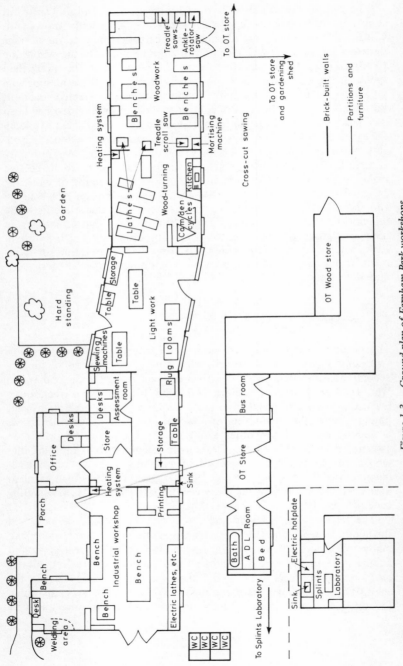

Figure 1.3. – Ground plan of Farnham Park workshops

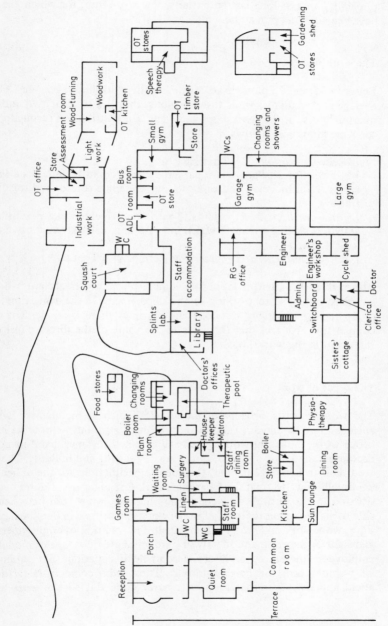

Figure 1.4. – Plan of Farnham Park Rehabilitation Centre

at Farnham Park are shown in *Figures 1.3* and *1.4*. There is now a possibility that at long last an entirely new workshop, for which plans have been drawn up, may be built.

The workload

Between 75 and 85 patients are treated in the workshops every day. On average each patient spends three sessions, that is a total of two and a quarter hours, in the workshops each day. The distribution throughout the workshops is as follows:

> *Woodwork section:* 5–18 patients.
> *Wood-turning section:* 6–20 patients. These could include 9 on the lathes, 2 on bicycles, and one each on the ankle rotator and treadle fretsaw.
> *Light workshop:* 3–8 patients. These could include one practising activities of daily living (ADL) and another being given a psychological test.
> *Industrial outwork and engineering section:* 4–10 patients.

Although each patient is given individually prescribed treatment, when so many patients are working in the department at the same time, a group feeling inevitably develops and at times there is an element of competition. We feel that this adds to the value of the direct physical treatment in the workshops.

The types of work

The work consists broadly of indoor work such as metalwork, light engineering, woodwork and wood-turning, printing, stool-seating, office work, industrial work, rug-weaving, remedial games, painting and decorating, and, out-of-doors, gardening, log-sawing and building. These are found to be congenial and therapeutic occupations for the patients we usually have to treat. Had Farnham Park Rehabilitation Centre been situated in the pottery districts of the Midlands, we should have been able to make good use of the traditional work of that area. In Buckinghamshire, woodwork and wood-turning are in the tradition of employment, and light engineering and metalwork are amongst the scope of modern employees; therefore, both are acceptable occupations for patients who come from the neighbourhood. Those who come from farther afield and may aver that they have never done this sort of work are influenced by the local people and accept it as a reasonable proposition. Patients have been encouraged to make their own designs if they want to make anything for their own homes. So long as the physical activity has been directed to carrying out the aims of treatment, the result of implementing an original design for any article has been found to satisfy and absorb the attention. The engineering section has been developed largely for making new equipment for the workshops, or repairing and altering old equipment. Sometimes a patient may bring in parts of a motor bicycle, the 'engine of his own destruction', for repair, or he may make parts of a carrier for his luggage or tools, bringing in his own materials. Within the scope of the workshops, he may choose his work, so long as he benefits from the activities involved and appreciates that this is the basis of his choice.

Working space

The Department of Health and Social Security (1974), when referring to heavy workshop facilities for patients, gives 'a recommended space allowance of 6.5 m^2 (71.5 ft^2) per place. Benches for light engineering work should be a minimum of 1.2 m (4 ft) apart, carpenters' benches 1.8 m (6 ft) apart and the width of centre gangways should not be less than 1.8 m'. Regrettably, in our present workshops we have only one-third of the space we really require.

In the early days the woodwork benches were arranged at right angles to the wall. Our workshops are really too narrow for an ideal arrangement, but we have found that putting the benches lengthwise, parallel to the walls, has been advantageous. Patients are apt to stack their unfinished work against the walls. In fact we have nowhere else to put it. Benches should therefore be drawn out from the wall to at least 1.5 m (5 ft). Sedentary patients, especially those requiring specialized seating, are encouraged to sit in this space, leaving the middle alley way between benches free for those who can move about and straighten up, to allow for freer flow of walking down the centre. This is especially important when a batch of visitors has to be shown through, and the minimal disturbance of working patients is desired.

Lighting

Good lighting in a workshop is an essential for the encouragement of good posture. The Department of Health and Social Security (1974) recommends an average illuminance of 300 lux for workshop areas for patients, with a limiting glare index of 22; it is also recommended that levels of illuminance should be at 0.85 m (2 ft 9½ in) above floor level.

It is suggested that after an illness during which there is general deterioration of muscle tone, the muscles of the eyes will also be affected. The lighting in an occupational therapy workshop should therefore be of a better standard than that judged necessary for working conditions of fit people. If a patient strains to see properly he will be inclined to stoop and peer over his work.

On some occasions, too, we have had patients who have lost the sight of one eye. They have to learn to use monocular vision instead of stereoscopic. They must learn to judge the size of objects by observing the depth and area of shadow cast by projecting parts. The absence of shadows is always quoted as an advantage by some who like strip lighting. The absence of shadows is definitely a disadvantage to the one-eyed patient.

The splint laboratory

It has been found essential to have adequate facilities for thermoplastic splinting; they should be housed in one area, well away from the dust of the workshops, where there is sufficient room both for the equipment needed and for storage of materials. Our splint-making has become more effective and more cost efficient since a properly equipped unit was installed. Previously we had to heat plastic sheeting in or over the kitchen stove, deal with metal parts in the engineering section and with straps in the light workshops. Further details of the splint laboratory are given on pages 243–245.

The back of a bus

We had heard of and seen, in other rehabilitation set-ups, that the back of a bus was useful as a practice piece for patients to learn how to step on and off our commonest form of public transport. We had heard, and found it true, that the London Passenger Transport Board would be helpful. They provided us with plans and a lot of fittings and materials from disused buses for this project which took about six months to complete.

Our first problem was to find a place at Farnham Park suitable for this edifice. Our administrator found this. It was part of the old stables, originally a calf stall. During our early years it had been used to store the solid fuel for the central heating boilers. Now that new boilers using oil fuel had been installed, this area of the outbuildings was free and it was conveniently next door to one of the small gymnasia. The roof and walls were sound but otherwise the place was in a poor state with an uneven earth floor, a disintegrating window and various beams which may have originally carried feeding racks, but would be much in the way of the bus.

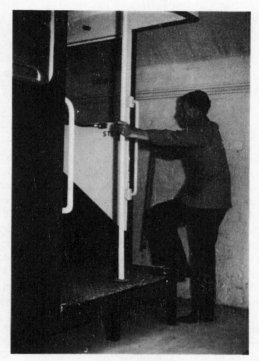

Figure 1.5. — Reconstructed back of a bus

A grant was made by what was then the Hospital Management Committee which served to pay for cementing the floor and for extra wood and paint. The floor was made level with the floor of the small gymnasium in the hope that some time in the future there would be a door between this and the bus room.

Then the occupational therapy workshop team got busy. We were lucky in having a civil engineer and a draughtsman as patients and their interests were easily engaged in the constructional problems of erecting the back of the bus. All the time the bus was being built we never had a professionally trained carpenter as a patient but there were a number who had done a bit of woodwork and had good standards of work and so were of great help. The main bones of the bus were erected before we had a suitable patient to scrape down the walls and ceiling of the room; this had to be done before the room could be colour washed or the bus painted. Meanwhile our technician cut, fitted and welded the metal strips for edges of steps. He and our maintenance man found an old window somewhere, cut out and enlarged the window space to fit, and removed the unwanted beams. After the first interior decorations had been done by patients, they helped to paint the bus itself in the appropriate colours. The technician excelled himself in painting a realistic wheel and tyre and the traditional notices. About this time, notices began to appear on the windows asking for applications for the post of conductress or 'clippie'. The finishing touch was the installation of a bell which really rang. For this we received various gifts, including the transformer to break down the current, and the bell itself. Patients could now become used to ringing the bell when necessary before attempting the descent to the road. The London Passenger Transport Board provided us with many accessories, including handrails and a used ticket-box. We even have three or four steps ascending to the imaginary top compartment, and two seats inside parallel to the door with their correct foot-rests.

A small platform, the height of an average pavement, is provided. This is not fixed to the floor but can be moved to different distances and angles from the bus platform. Not all buses stop beside or parallel to the edge of the pavement, and it is useful to practise stepping on to the platform from gradually more awkward starting positions.

The remedial gymnasts, physiotherapists and occupational therapists take the patients for practice on the stationary bus. When patients are accounted proficient the occupational therapy staff or students take them out for short shopping expeditions. Then the patient can practise the real adventure in public and gain confidence in more ways than one.

No plan of the back of the bus is given as the writer is sure that the London and other transport concerns would be as helpful to others in this country as they were to us. For overseas countries it would obviously be necessary to get plans of the public transport in common use.

As a project of work, building the back of a bus proved most useful in providing many activities for patients with various disabilities. The early planning was interesting for those who needed general activities but could do only minimal walking. Later the woodwork was carried out by patients with arm injuries and the final painting by those who needed practice in stooping low and reaching high, after spinal or abdominal conditions which had prevented such range in mobilization.

These last stages of painting involved the use of step ladders, an invaluable exercise for those who must regain balance and confidence for return to work at different heights from the ground.

Since its completion the back of the bus has proved useful to innumerable patients with stiff backs, hips, knees or ankles. They have been able to measure progress for themselves and encouraged to attain just that extra bit of mobility needed to get about independently. This practice can be carried out quietly and slowly before having to make the attempt in the outside world, where the scurry and bustle would make them nervous and unwilling to dare the adventure of using public transport.

The phrase 'to look like the back of a bus' is usually a derogatory description of an absent acquaintance, though it may carry a note of affection when followed by 'but'. Our bus needs no such qualification; it has a placid and friendly appearance whose stability encourages the faint-hearted to attempt the boarding operation.

The ADL unit

The first unit for activities of daily living was built in the middle of the workshops in 1960, alongside the wood-turning section. The kitchen part was subsequently glazed to the ceiling to keep out the noise and the wood dust. The bed and bath section had only a curtain, however, which could be drawn round for privacy but always got very dusty and dirty. The unit was used comparatively infrequently because many of the patients admitted to Farnham Park had no ADL problems. It was therefore felt that this curtained section of the workshops could be more profitably used for everyday activities, provided that some other place could be found for occasional ADL assessment and practice. An old coal cellar which had been converted to a female patients' changing room was very seldom used; as trousers for women became fashionable, these patients no longer required somewhere to change. This room was already heated and proved to be a warm, quiet and clean place for ADL assessment. It was fitted with a bed, an unplumbed bath and lavatory together with the usual rails, raised seats and dressing aids. The fact that it is away from the workshops, though only a short distance, has not presented problems, probably because a student can always be asked to stay with a patient during the therapist's brief absences.

The pursuit of tidiness

The ideals of tidiness and order in workshops are frequently recommended to occupational therapists. Their value must be relentlessly drummed into the ears of patients or students when the care of materials or tools is considered. The technical expert can barely endure the sight of tools handled with ignorance.

The best quality tools and materials are a necessary part of the function of occupational therapy. Their care in order and tidiness should be considered as a method of treatment of patients rather than a necessary chore of organization. Orderliness and tidiness are an essential background treatment to many who are referred for therapeutic help. There are patients with brain lesions, the result of trauma or disease, neoplasm or cerebrovascular incident. There are others with peptic dysfunction, spinal pain, and many others whose disabilities, though organic in origin, are increased by functional overlay. How then may these symptoms be treated by occupational therapy? The symptoms would appear various in intensity or causation of organic lesion, but patients all share one symptom. This is insecurity, a lack of orientation in the relation of themselves as human beings with their surroundings as objects which they can control to further their comfort.

The writer contends that orderliness and tidiness in occupational therapy workshops can play an important part in treatment. Taking the first group, where brain injuries various in origin have resulted in mental incapacities, orderliness is a necessary background to treatment. These patients have come to strange surroundings and they must learn to find their way about. At first they may just sit, in some relief at having found their way or been led in the company of others to the workshops. They have come perhaps straight from hospital where there is little responsibility or choice in the time or place of activities. If they have been home the anxious relatives may have been helpful, but had little time to give to the slow thoughts or intentions meandering through the muddled brain. In occupational therapy workshops they may sit and wait for work and tools. Their first step in gaining confidence may be found when they can remember what work they did yesterday and what tools and materials they may need again. The next advance will be observed when they can go for these with confidence that they will find them where they remember leaving them. Perhaps soon they will begin to observe the work of others and either desire to progress in imitation or feel that they can help someone, chairbound or on crutches, who is unable to carry his work to the bench. For these people familiarity with surroundings is essential, and orderliness and tidiness are necessary to breed this familiarity with confidence.

There are others with disabilities already quoted to whom the importance of orderliness may seem far-fetched. Functional overlay is a common term nowadays. It would appear to include a variety of symptoms which, though organic in origin, become exaggerated and inordinate in their demands of appreciation by the patient. They absorb so much of his attention that he has little use for the interests of life which stimulate others to neglect their disabilities. The doctor or the therapist may observe even some increase of symptoms which suddenly come to light when there is any talk of a return to work or ordinary life. It would appear that these people suffer from a lack of security in their normal background and are unwilling or unready to face the responsibilities of the outside world. They appear content to live as passengers supported by that impersonal body 'the State'. Some may have been advised wrongly. As London (1957) has said: 'This advice may come from workmates, which is to be regretted, from his trade union, which is to be deplored, or even from his solicitor, which is to be condemned'. The net result may be that the sense of responsibility suffers from disuse atrophy and 'benefits' are habitually accepted without considering that they are derived from taxes paid by their friends and relatives.

Even as muscles respond to activity, unless completely atrophied, the sense of responsibility may on occasion be treated by inculcating a respect for tools and materials originally furnished by the Health Service for therapeutic occupation. Those who have gone beyond recall in this direction have been in the minority and may for this reason be memorable. The constant care of tools and the using up of small pieces of material will create an atmosphere to which most patients will respond. If therapy is to make full use of its opportunities in occupation, then care, tidiness and orderliness must be directed towards the development of responsibilities. At first this may be in small things, such as washing out paint brushes instead of leaving them to harden or rot because the Health Service will provide a further supply. Many patients have improved beyond recognition in their approach to the workshops, tools and materials. Therapists cannot afford to neglect any opportunity which may help patients to return to normal life as responsible people.

The occupational therapy (OT) staff

The staff of this department at Farnham Park consists of a head occupational therapist, an assistant head, two other senior and one assistant occupational therapists and a technician. While the head occupational therapist has overall charge of the workshops, each of her five staff is in charge of one section. The four occupational therapists run the woodwork section, the wood-turning section, the light workshop and the ADL programme; this last includes not only personal and domestic activities of daily living but also problems of communication. The therapists alternate at intervals to gain further experience. The technician runs the industrial outwork and engineering section. Farnham Park has been in operation for 30 years, and in all that time it has never been necessary to have the help of a technician in running the woodwork and wood-turning sections, except for sharpening tools before a grinding machine was bought. Occupational therapists have found no difficulty in extending their woodworking skills to enable them to run such sections. Indeed, at one time a male occupational therapist, who had previously been a cabinet-maker, was doing his spell in the light workshop while the two female therapists were running the heavy workshops. A technician would not have the medical knowledge to supervise a post-meniscectomy patient with a knee that could 'blow up' without careful handling or a post-laminectomy patient who must work in spinal extension and only gradually start flexing.

The students

Seven students at a time come from four different occupational therapy training schools. Each is allocated to a section of the workshops, so that two sections have two students. They rotate every four weeks, each student working in three out of the five areas during 12 weeks' hospital practice at the Centre. Inevitably, they have ample opportunity of getting to know the other sections, too, as none of these operate in isolation. Although students always work under supervision and do not take direct responsibility for patients, they make a considerable contribution to the department and have enabled us to widen the scope of what is offered to patients. As well as working in the workshops, each student spends two days with the physiotherapists, two days with the remedial gymnasts and a day with the speech therapist, in order to gain a comprehensive picture of the treatment of patients. Lectures are given by all the occupational therapists, the speech therapist and the Centre's administrator. The students also attend the three staff conferences held each week, visit a local authority Day Centre, a Skill Centre and a local factory, and spend three or more mornings at a District General Hospital watching orthopaedic operations.

Follow-up of patients

For many years now, patients discharged from Farnham Park have been sent two progress report forms for completion, one three months and

FARNHAM PARK REHABILITATION CENTRE

CONFIDENTIAL.   *Date* _____

Name _____   Date of Discharge _____

Hospital Number _____   Diagnosis _____

Length of Stay _____   Employment _____

1.	Are you working?	Yes
		No
2.	Are you back at your original work?	Yes
	If "No" what are you doing?	No
3.	If answer to question 2 is "No" have you been re-trained by the Department of Employment Training Service Agency?	Yes
		No
4.	Are you earning more or less than you did before the onset of your disability?	More
		Less
		Same
5.	What is the general state of your health?	Improved
		Same
		Worse
6.	If you are not working, is the reason for unemployment due to	Disability?
		Lack of Jobs?
7.	If working are you content and happy in your work?	Yes
		No
8.	If answer to Question 7 is "No" is the reason for your discontentment due to	Disability?
		Unsuitable Jobs?
9.	Is your original disability	Improved?
		Same?
		Worse?
10.	How soon after being discharged from Farnham Park Rehabilitation Centre did you recommence employment or training?	

Figure 1.6. – Patient's Progress Report

the second six months after discharge. This follow-up system serves two purposes, to monitor the progress of the patient, and the efficacy of our treatment. If a patient's reply indicates that he has not maintained the level of competence reached before discharge, he can be asked to come back to see the medical director and, if necessary, be readmitted for a further spell of treatment. If, on the other hand, replies show that a high proportion of patients with a similar diagnosis are not doing well, or are having a long gap between being discharged as fit for work and actually starting work, perhaps the type of treatment being offered should be reconsidered and varied or the period of treatment lengthened.

REFERENCES

Department of Health and Social Security (1974). *Department of Rehabilitation — A Design Guide*. London; DHSS

London, P. S. (1957). 'Serious injuries of the hand.' *J. ind. Nurs.* **9**, 165

FURTHER READING

Health and Safety Executive (1975). *Health and Safety Executive Forms and Publications*. Government Publications Sectional List No. 18. London; HMSO

Health and Safety Executive (1976). *Lighting in Offices, Shops and Railway Premises*. London; HMSO

Ministry of Technology. Ergonomics for Industry Series: *Lighting of Work Places* (1966) and *Layout of Work Spaces* (1967). London; HMSO

The Illuminating Engineering Society (1958). *IES Code for Lighting in Buildings*. London; IES

2

Occupational Therapy Equipment

The study of ergonomics has become increasingly important for occupational therapists. They must have some understanding of the problems of seating, table and bench heights, heating and lighting. These are all environmental factors which influence a patient's work capacity and ability. A proportion of the chairs, stools, tables and benches should be adjustable in height, and the height should be expertly watched and constantly checked.

Chairs

The booklet *Seats for Workers in Factories, Offices and Shops* (Health and Safety Executive, 1970) has been found to give useful advice, and reference should be made also to *Seating in Industry* (Ministry of Technology, 1966). The back of a chair should give support to the dorsal and lumbar spine in its normal contours. The seat of a chair should be of a height which encourages bodyweight to be carried on the tuberosities of the ischia. The dimensions of the seat and its cushioning should give support without full pressure to the thigh. Height and dimensions and cushioning of the seat are here mentioned because the front edge of the seat should not give any pressure on the soft tissues at the top of the popliteal space. Such pressure may cause fatigue and discomfort in the normal person. For one recovering from trauma or illness this pressure would be deplorable in its effects.

It would appear that the most practical chairs for use in occupational therapy workshops are those with seats which can be raised or lowered and adjusted from 35.5 cm (14 in) to 69 cm (27 in) from the floor. These should be ideal for patients working on industrial outwork or woodwork where the bench may be higher than a normal table. The seat can be raised to a convenient height and the patient can sit with his feet supported on one or two rectangular wooden boxes.

19

For most purposes we would like to re-equip the workshops with adjustable chairs in three different ranges, and all with locking devices. Our present adjustable chairs have too big a range of adjustment. For those patients who work at a table, these chairs always seem to be too high and either the therapists are constantly adjusting them or the patient sits with legs dangling or, worse still, slumps in the chair so that his feet can touch the ground.

Adjustable chairs do not always have locking devices. A freely swivelling chair has some advantages; for example, a patient may find it easier to take up a sitting position close to a bench if he sits on the seat sideways and then swivels round to face the bench. More often, however, a chair which swivels is a hazard for some patients, for instance, those with disorders of balance due to a head injury, hemiplegia or a neurological condition. Such a patient is taught to put his hand behind him to feel for the chair seat before sitting down and, as he lowers his weight, this type of chair is likely to swivel round, with disastrous results.

A proportion of our rather old-fashioned adjustable chairs now have a column locking device that was suggested and fitted by the Tan-Sad chair manufacturers. This fixes the chair at the required height and also prevents the seats from swivelling whilst the patient is working. In the light workshops, where the patients sit round a table, sturdy wooden chairs of a standard height with foam rubber cushions have proved more suitable.

We have also been searching for suitable chairs for hemiplegic or arthritic patients who need arm-rests to steady themselves as they rise. These chairs should have low narrow backs to allow unhampered shoulder movement. The arm-rests should be low enough not to get in the way when the patient is working but high enough to give reasonable support when he rises. The chair must be stable, so that it will not tip sideways if the patient puts his full weight on only one of the arm-rests. The type of managerial chair often used in boardrooms seems ideal and is not necessarily expensive. We are at present trying out two different models.

Portable chair arms

A toilet aid frame, designed to fit round a lavatory to provide arm supports, can equally be used to provide arms round a chair. It is best to choose a model that does not have a reinforcing bar at the front but only at the back. A front bar could prevent the patient from bringing one or both feet back under his body to give a better thrust as he stands up. Portable chair arms will enable patients to raise themselves up to the erect position if their arms and hands are sound, even although their legs are weak, paretic or paralytic. The arms shown in *Figure 2.1* were made in the workshops from iron tube, 2.6 cm (1 in) in diameter, used for electric conduit. These were effective but much heavier for the

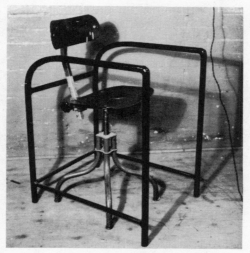

Figure 2.1. – Adjustable chair with portable chair arms made from conduit piping

therapist to move than the newer aluminium toilet aid. Two sets of portable chair arms were given to a girl with anterior poliomyelitis affecting both legs so that she had to be fitted with two full-length calipers. The calipers had a knee bending joint and both required locking in the extended position before she could walk with elbow crutches. She had one set of portable chair arms for home use and one for office use, so that she was able to go back to work as a clerk and be reasonably independent of help in getting up and walking.

Bicycle stools

Bicycle stools of various patterns have been made in the workshops. These seats have all been adjustable in heights ranging from 61 cm to 86 cm (24 in to 34 in). They are used with foot-power lathes when the patient is non-weight bearing, when the affected leg is slung under the lathe, and later when the patient is partially weight bearing with feet on the treadle. They are also used for patients with stiff hips who can sit more comfortably on a bicycle or motor bicycle seat than on a chair.

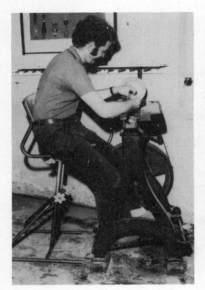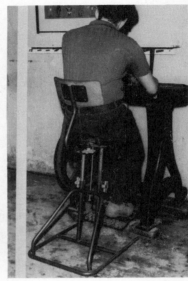

Figure 2.2. – Camden Multi-purpose Stool

An occupational therapist who worked at Farnham Park as a post-diploma student has now designed the Camden Multi-Purpose Stool (*Figure 2.2*). This is available commercially and is now used in the workshops instead of locally produced stools.

Foot-stools

Foot-stools with canvas slings have been made of various heights from 30.5 cm to 66 cm (12 in to 26 in). These are used by patients who are inclined to oedema of the feet or ankles. The stools have been made in the workshops of 38 mm (1½ in) wood or 1 cm ($^3/_8$ in) iron bar by patients interested in helping the workshops rather than making something for themselves. The canvas sling, approximately 38 cm (15 in) wide, has been found the most useful to give support from knee to heel.

Tables and benches

The working tables are usually 79 cm (31 in) high but for very small patients we have some tables 71 cm (28 in) high. The carpentry benches are adjustable in height, the 182 cm (6 ft) long benches by means of blocks (*see Figure 5.3*, page 131) and the 91 cm (3 ft) long benches by extension legs bolted through (*see Figure 5.2*, page 131). This gives a variation of height from 86 cm (2 ft 10 in) to 112 cm (3 ft 8 in). In practice these benches are seldom adjusted but arranged so that the woodwork section has two extra-high benches, two extra-low ones for sitting to work and the rest at normal height. Our smallest patient so far was 137 cm (4 ft 6 in) in height and our tallest 200.7 cm (6 ft 7 in). The latter was sent for rehabilitation for a spinal disability and forward flexion was forbidden. It will be appreciated that variation in seating and in height of working benches is very necessary.

Foot-treadle and hand-operated sewing machines

The simplest and most easily procurable of foot-powered machines is the sewing machine. The heel and toe movement involved is invaluable in teaching walking. The patient must be taught to use first one and then the other foot in the forward position. The rocking movement is essential in walking and should always be the first practised, unless this movement has been obliterated by arthrodesis. The foot-operated sewing machine has a disobliging habit of going into reverse if the rocking movement is not continued smoothly. It can be worked with a light and easy movement by a patient sitting in a chair. Articles which can be made with its help are too varied to enumerate and may include a dress for a patient or sand-bags for use in the gymnasium. It has often been observed that men like using a sewing machine as much as women do. Men have sometimes said that they had often wanted to use one but either their mothers or their wives had forbidden them to do so. It is easy to attach sloping blocks of wood under the feet to vary the range of movement.

When the sewing machine is worked by hand, the rotary wrist movement for the right hand involves elbow extension and flexion and a variety of shoulder movements. Unfortunately we have not been able to adapt our machine for a left-hand movement.

An electric sewing machine has been found useful for retraining co-ordination, for assessment of machinists who must return to this type of work, and also for rehabilitating housewives since many of them have electric machines. A further advantage is that it can be used with one hand. Ours is a heavy-duty machine capable of sewing through canvas, which means that it can be used for splint-making.

Foot-power looms

Foot-power looms are useful to teach a patient to lift the feet alter-nately. The pedals can also be tied to a height which the patient can only just reach by lifting his feet 15 cm (6 in) off the floor to exercise the hip, knee and foot flexors, and the work of pressing down each pedal will exercise the hip and knee extensors and the plantar flexors of the feet. As the patient is sitting at the loom the work is not very demanding, and the patient who is able to walk only a short distance can continue to lift and press on the foot alternately for an hour or more without fatigue. This has been found useful when treating patients who have had arthritis affecting the lower limbs, or an illness affecting the cardiac muscles. The treadling of the foot-pedal loom will serve as an introduction to stronger work on the bicycles. Pattern-weaving looms have six pedals, and by arranging that the patient must use the two outside pedals for getting the tabby sheds, regular movements of leg abduction must be performed.

Work on a foot-power loom calls for a combination of hand and foot movements which makes it valuable in the treatment of patients whose co-ordination has been seriously affected after cerebral or cerebellar lesions. Rhythmic work carried out at the patient's own pace on a machine which is stable will help to restore confidence. The immediate obviousness of a mistake, and the ease with which it can be repaired, will stir ambition to improve co-ordination and skill. Most types of looms can be so adapted that they will be found useful in the treatment of many types of disabilities.

The occupational therapist should beware of using adaptations which destroy the smooth rhythm and pleasure of weaving, or make it a heavy task with small results. The writer has seen a big man lifting a heavily weighted beam to change the shed on a scarf loom. The result of labour should be commensurate with the activity demanded.

Upright rug looms are useful in the treatment of patients with disabilities of the back. These can easily be heightened with adjustable legs bolted through the original frame. The springs on the beater can be replaced by others which are calibrated. (*See* page 97 and *Figure 5.7*, page 141).

Wire-twisting machine

The wire-twisting machine worked by pronation and supination of the forearm and gripping by the hand (*Figure 2.3*) was first designed and made up in the workshops at Farnham Park some years ago. It is now commercially available and has been well described in the booklet *The Thame Wire-Testing Machine* (Everett).

To develop pronation or supination of the forearm, the patient works with his hand gripping the handle of the machine which is fixed to a bench at a suitable height to ensure that the elbow is bent to

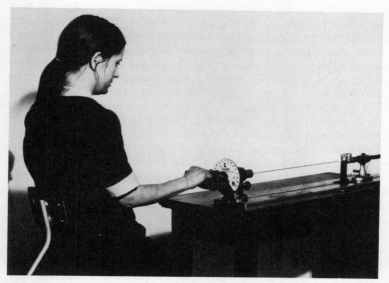

Figure 2.3. — Pronation and supination handle on the wire-twisting machine

a right angle and the arm kept close to the side. There is a reversible ratchet so that the same machine can be adapted for pronation or supination with either hand.

The machine can, of course, be used to exercise the biceps as illustrated by the following case. A patient who had torn some fibres of his biceps decided that he would never be able to bend his arm again. He was a man of fine physique but an attack of encephalitis in childhood had left him with very limited intelligence. He made many brushes on the wire-twisting machine and his biceps got plenty of exercise as a supinator, without any argument about bending his elbow which was supported in a sling. After 10 days or so he was invited to put his other hand on to the upper part of the working arm. He was childishly pleased to feel the muscle swell and harden, and soon he progressed to the cross-cut sawing of wood.

Another handle is held in a cylinder grip and is worked by either repeated flexion or extension of the wrist. A button at the end of the handle must be pressed first to release the handle and allow it to turn. This necessitates extension of the thumb followed by active opposition.

A long-armed handle is also available and is worked by a rotatory movement of the patient's arm and hand (*Figure 2.4*). It is used to increase range of movement in the shoulder and elbow, and adjustments can be made by altering the length of the handle arm or by seating the patient in different positions in relation to the machine.

The use of these handles on the wire-twisting machine requires a fair amount of power and it has been found that work of this variety should be used for short periods, beginning with five minutes and working up to half an hour. It may well be interspersed between other activities more generalized in character. The patient may easily become bored and so inclined to work carelessly, by moving the shoulder, shoulder girdle and even by flexion of the lumbar spine when the specialized movements of pronation, supination, or grip and dorsiflexion become very tiring and rather tedious.

A gauge is fixed to the machine and a pointer to the handle, so that the patient (and the occupational therapist) can take note of the range of movement achieved. Having a gauge to watch is a great help; the patient will proudly report that in making the latest brush the pointer has moved so many degrees 'without cheating'. As with much of the equipment made for occupational therapy, it was found better to encourage the development of the movement by depending on the patient's co-operation, and to gain this by explanation of the mechanism of movement in the various joints involved.

Twisted wire brushes are often used in the home. The variety of materials used to make them on the machine, soft hair or harsh bristles, and wire which is thin and pliable or thick and stiff, means that work with gradually progressive resistance can be provided whilst the desired movement is continually repeated. The loop end of the wire is held on a hook which is also spring-loaded to maintain tension as the wires shorten when they are twisted. A rod with a slot is used to prevent the wires twisting along their full length whilst the bristles are gradually fed in, inch by inch. When all the bristles are nipped between the wires in a loose spiral, the twisting process can be repeated.

Galvanized wire from 18 to 12 gauge is used, according to the patient's strength. Bristles or hair can be used depending on the type of brush needed. The twisted brush can be trimmed, bent or mounted on a handle to fulfil a multitude of purposes. For example, several brushes shaped into a small ball with the ends mounted on a rod and fixed pointing downwards over a wash basin will make it possible for the

27

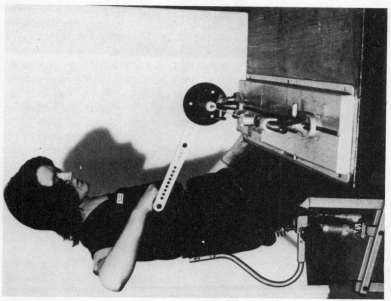

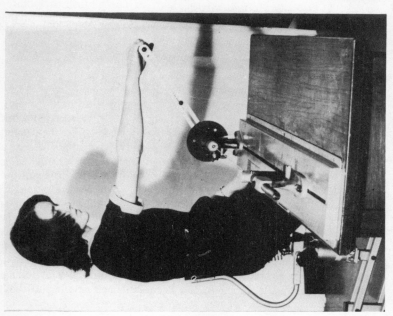

Figure 2.4. — Long handle on the wire-twisting machine

one-handed patient to scrub his fingers thoroughly without help. Small Christmas trees can be made from green bristles and trimmed to shape when the brush is finished. The short ends of cotton warp, trimmed off woven rugs, can be used to make washing-up or floor mops.

It may be added that this machine can also be used for making twisted flower supports (*Figure 2.5*). These can be made from the same sort of wire, annealed galvanized 18–12 gauge, and in various lengths. After twisting, the loop end of the wire is pinched or hammered together to

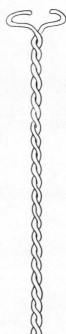

Figure 2.5. – Stem holder for tall flowers, made on the wire-twisting machine

form a spike which can easily be thrust into the ground. The open ends are separated, and bent to form a slightly overlapping circle to hold the stalk of a gladiolus, a carnation or other plant with slender stem and heavy flower. Sometimes disposing of large numbers of completed brushes can be a problem, but we have had no difficulty in selling flower supports by the dozen to the keen gardeners among staff and patients.

Printing machine

We were fortunate to be given a printing machine by an ex-patient. This stands on the floor and requires the use of both hands, and it has a foot-treadle which can be worked by either foot. This usually requires standing as the platen is too high from the floor to be operated in the sitting position, even on a high stool, by anyone who is under 178 cm (5 ft 10 in) in height. A second printing machine was acquired later, a conventional Adana table model. Many large firms are currently changing to more modern machines and therefore often have type and other printing equipment to give away.

Printing has been found a very useful addition to workshop machinery. It is used unadapted because we have so many other machines which have a much simpler end-product, and which can be so easily adapted to provide specific exercise for the upper and lower limbs. We therefore use printing as an activity in its own right, and it has proved particularly valuable in the treatment of highly intelligent patients, such as a former consultant in physical medicine who had become a hemiplegic and who found printing psychologically stimulating as well as physically therapeutic.

Bicycle fretsaw and filing machines

Bicycle fretsaw and filing machines were designed and made up in the occupational therapy workshops from angle iron. The Farnham Park bicycle saw and filing machine can be used by patients varying from 198 cm to 132 cm (6 ft 6 in to 4 ft 4 in) in height. Manufacturers have now copied the ideas of bicycle fretsaws pioneered at Farnham Park, and there are several on the market. The Camden Cycle is most like those originally used in our workshops, and the sanding attachment on that machine makes it unnecessary to have another machine as a bicycle file. We now also have an Oliver bicycle (*Figure 2.6*).

With all these bicycles, the height of the seat, distance from seat to working table, height of the working table and the length of each pedal crank can be adjusted individually to suit each patient's requirements. All these movable parts are marked so that a record can be kept of the patient's position, and improvement in range of movement can be noted and encouraged. The seat can be easily removed to allow the patient to walk on to the machine, and the seat can then be replaced behind him. This is necessary when the patient cannot lift a leg over the frame. The bicycle is adjusted to suit the range of movement of the impaired leg. The pedal crank on the unimpaired side is set to the same length in order to produce as smooth a rotary movement as possible. If one pedal is on a full length crank and the other on a much shorter one, the movement may be jerky and also the unimpaired leg will be encouraged to do most of the work. Both pedals are gradually adjusted to a longer crank as the mobility of the limb increases.

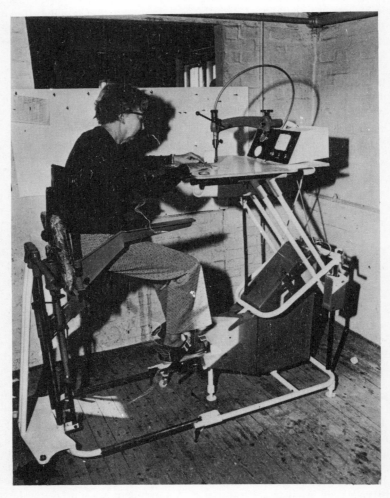

Figure 2.6. – The Oliver rehabilitation machine

The patient is instructed to avoid using lumbar flexion and pelvic rotation to assist hip and knee movement. The therapist must watch carefully and may need to stand behind the patient and manually steady the pelvis. The range of movement at hip and knee can be increased by small degrees when the pedal crank is lengthened and the seat is lowered and brought in nearer to the working table. This fine graduation makes bicycle machines very suitable in the treatment of patients with a limited range of flexion after prolonged immobilization. In some cases there is considerable muscle-shortening from scar tissue or from generalized contractures caused by disuse. The restretching of such tissues calls for particularly careful graduation, as sudden over-stretching may cause painful spasm in a muscle. The patients themselves appreciate the value of this type of movement, and after a manipulation under anaesthetic in the morning will present themselves at the workshops in the afternoon and ask to be allowed to work on the bicycles. Smoothness and rhythm of movement will do much to overcome spasm.

Since bicycling is carried out in the sitting position, it can be started when the patient is in the early stages of partial weight-bearing. Patients who have had a hip arthroplasty can usually start on this activity as soon as they are admitted for rehabilitation.

TABLE
Bicycle machine adjustment

Movement	Saddle position	Pedal crank
Hip extension	High and forward	Long
Hip flexion	Low and forward	Long
Minimal hip flexion	High and back	Short
Maximum hip range	Mid-height and forward	Long
Knee extension	High and back	Long
Knee flexion	Low and forward	Long
Minimal knee flexion	High and back	Short
Maximum knee range	Mid-height and forward	Long
Ankle dorsiflexion	Low and forward	Long
Ankle plantar flexion	High and back	Long

When a patient has one or more stiff joints, it is often difficult to avoid compensatory movements in other joints. This is partly because of mechanical reasons and partly due to habit. The patient must be

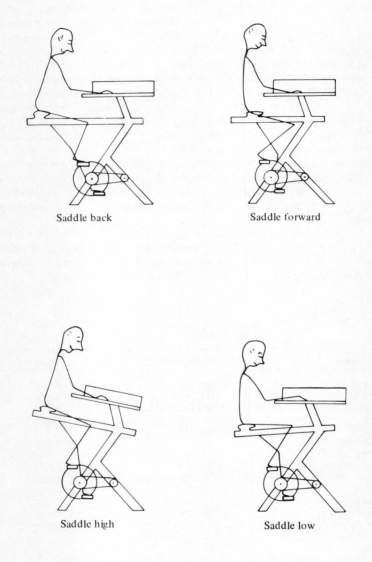

Saddle back

Saddle forward

Saddle high

Saddle low

Figure 2.7. – Variations in lower limb range of movement available on a bicycle

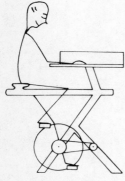

Pedal cranks long

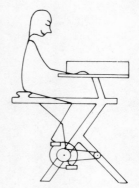

Pedal cranks short

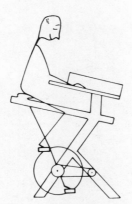

Max. knee extension—
saddle high, back, pedal
cranks long

Figure 2.7. (continued)

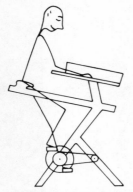

Min. hip and knee flex-
ion—saddle high, back
and pedal cranks short

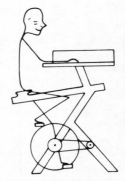

Max. knee and hip flex-
ion—saddle low, for-
ward, and pedal cranks
long

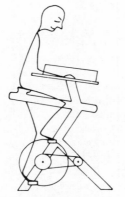

Max. hip extension—
high seat, forward and
pedal cranks long

Figure 2.7. (continued)

taught how to perform the movement correctly and the bicycle must be set up so that the required movement is possible (Table and *Figure 2.7*).

Methods of upgrading treatment on the bicycle machine include:

1. Increasing the thickness of wood to be cut, from thin plywood to thick wood.
2. Increasing the density of wood from deal to hardwood.
3. Changing the saw blade and cutting out metal, progressing from aluminium to copper or brass.
4. Increasing the length of time on the bicycle. On some machines this can be measured by the revolution-counter on the mileometer, which makes accurate grading possible and acts as an incentive for the patient.
5. Progressing from cutting shapes or curves which require gentle pressure in order to keep to the pattern, to straight cutting which can provide more resistance.
6. Using the braking system, if the bicycle has one.

The more sophisticated electronic bicycle machines can be used for a variety of different activities, many of which in themselves offer little resistance to the pedalling mechanism. The braking system must therefore be used to upgrade treatment.

The ankle-rotator saw

This is another machine that was first made and used at Farnham Park and is now commercially available. It is described in detail in a booklet *The Ankle-Rotator Machine* (Savage).

The ankle-rotator works on the principle designed to develop an active rotary movement of the foot. This calls principally for plantar flexion, eversion and dorsiflexion, or plantar flexion, inversion and dorsiflexion. The order of movement depends on the direction of the rotary movement, either clockwise or anticlockwise. The machines may be used by either foot in turn but not both together.

The normal person can cross the legs at thigh level and rotate the dangling foot freely at ankle-joint level. This can be done independently of other movements at knee or hip. With the added weight of a foot-plate attached to a wheel working the pulley belt of a saw, the muscle activity entailed is not only greater but spreads to other muscles moving joints higher in the leg. Hip rotation as well as knee flexion and extension are included to reinforce the effort of foot rotation. For many patients this is beneficial, but sometimes a patient must avoid letting the knee ill inwards when the foot is being worked in eversion. The ankle rotator is fitted with pads which can be clamped either side of the knee. These are intended to prevent unwanted compensatory movements of the hip and knee and to allow only isolated movement at the ankle joint.

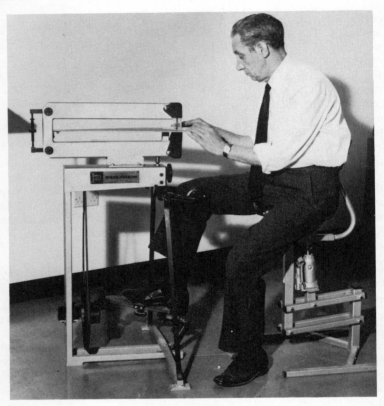

Figure 2.8. – Ankle-rotator machine

This machine has a useful but limited function. We now consider that it should not be used during the early stages of treatment. The design of the ankle-rotator is such that when the ankle goes through a limited range of movement the work is hard, and yet to make the movement easy enough for weak muscles the ankle must go through a large and unnatural range of movement. Any severe muscle weakness will affect the stability of the ankle joint, and putting the joint through this large range of movement will risk stretching the surrounding ligaments and damaging the joints.

There are other contraindications. It is not necessarily helpful to start treating an ankle by re-educating inversion and eversion. Plantar and dorsiflexion are usually the priorities in order to improve the pattern of walking. These movements can be better developed on other apparatus. The ankle-rotator should also be avoided for any patient with arthritic changes in the joint.

The ankle-rotator has proved useful in the later stages of treatment for those patients whose lower limbs are expected to recover full strength with no residual disability. It is particularly valuable in treating injuries to the foot since it strengthens and re-educates those muscles used in inversion and dorsiflexion. These movements are also responsible for improving and maintaining the muscular control of the longitudinal and transverse arches of the foot. There are few other pieces of occupational therapy apparatus which use these movements.

The ankle-rotator is also invaluable when the intention is to build up the muscles surrounding the ankle joint to greater than normal strength, as when treating patients who have had sports injuries. It can also be used to provide a generalized strengthening of the muscles of the lower limb, and is an excellent pre-skiing exercise.

Articles which can be made on bicycle fretsaw and filing machines and on the ankle-rotator saws

The bicycle and rotator saws can be used to cut wood or plywood from 3 mm to 25 mm ($^1/_8$ in to 1 in) thick, or thin metal such as 12 to 20 gauge sheet copper, brass, nickel or mild steel, by fitting the appropriate types of fretsaw blades. Plywood toys, pictures mounted to make jigsaw puzzles, and blocks to make up sets of alphabets or numerals for children's games or house names are popular. Brooches and plaques with county or club badges may be cut out of several metals and riveted together to build up the desired picture. Increased resistance can be provided by the use of thicker materials.

One patient worked out that it took him 1200 revolutions of his legs on the bicycle saw to cut a distance of 30.5 cm (12 in), using 3 mm ($^1/_8$ in) mild steel; he carried out this work in 15 minutes. He had had a comminuted fracture of the lateral tibial condyle five months previous to his admittance. During seven weeks of treatment his knee movement improved from a range of 170–100 degrees to one of 180–90 degrees. He returned to his previous employment as an insurance agent which involved a great deal of bicycling.

Foot-power lathes and accessories

The full range of a normal knee is from 180 to 70 degrees in an arc of 110 degrees but the treadle of a foot-power lathe moves through an arc of about 20 degrees only. The action of treadling a foot-power lathe therefore will not put the knee joint through its full range of normal movement, though the actual range depends to a certain extent on the worker's height and his length of leg. The lathe can be set on blocks and, in a person 167.5 cm (5 ft 6 in) tall with the lathe set up on 15.2 cm (6 in) blocks the range of movement is from 175 to 80 degrees. It is also possible to add foot-blocks to the treadle itself so that the patient will flex the knee more and work will be carried on in the inner range of movement. The Larvic lathe has an extensible foot-plate which effectively lengthens one side of the treadle of the lathe. This makes the patient flex the knee even more than when a block of wood is fixed to the treadle because the treadling foot is farther away from the lathe than the standing foot.

If the worker stands on a platform, the movement will be carried out in the inner range of movement, and full extension of the knee will be obtained at the bottom of the stroke. Care must be taken in this latter position that extension does not end in a jolt with hyperextension, which would be painful and cause spasm in the quadriceps. The best muscle contractions are usually obtained in the middle range of movement and this is certainly the range in which the patient is able to exert his maximum power on the wood-turning lathe.

The main value of these lathes is that they can be adapted to develop muscle power in the lower limb in varying stages of treatment, non-weight-bearing, partial weight-bearing and full weight-bearing, whilst the patient can practise and become proficient in the use of tools, and produce a complete article.

The patient who has an extension lag or an injury of the leg which prohibits weight-bearing can work sitting with that leg in a wide canvas sling which gives support from above·the knee to the heel (*Figure 2.9*). This method is contraindicated for a patient with an unsupported fractured femur lest stress be produced at the fracture site. The sling is attached to a hook on the back of the lathe and the patient can easily detach it himself, which prevents that feeling of being 'tied up' to the apparatus which nearly all people dislike. The patient then works the treadle with the uninjured leg. The muscles of the leg in the sling work as stabilizers of the pelvis, rhythmically in time with the action of the leg treadling. This maintains tone in the quadriceps and hamstrings, and exercises all the muscles round the hip. It has been said that small or static contractions are of particular value in maintaining the sliding

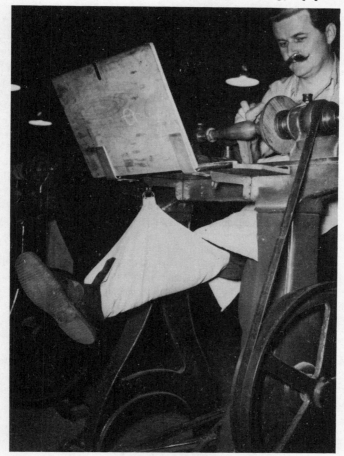

Figure 2.9. − Patient working with right leg slung on lathe, showing the arrangement of hooks added to the back of the lathe and the canvas sling which should extend from just proximal to the ankle to just proximal to the knee

action of fascia when a limb is immobilized during treatment after fracture.

The patient may sit on a chair of suitable height, or on a bicycle stool. The muscle contractions will be stronger if a bicycle stool is used because it is more difficult to balance the pelvis on the small base. This method is used in treating patients in the early days after a meniscectomy when knee flexion is not allowed, either because the stitches have not yet been removed, or because there is still some effusion in the joint. A patient whose leg becomes oedematous when a plaster-of-Paris splint is removed will also benefit from work entailing contractions of all muscles with the leg in elevation, especially if the leg is kept raised high for a resting period after work to assist the venous return by postural drainage.

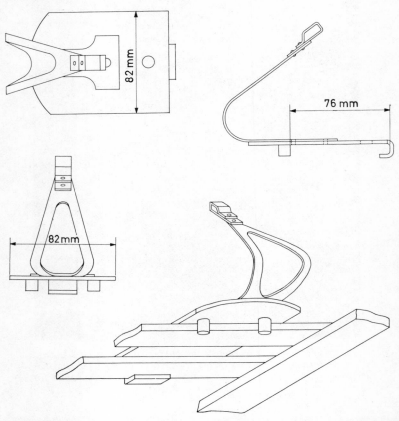

Figure 2.10. – Bicycle toe clip adjusted to fit on treadle of foot-power lathe. This clip can be covered with leather to avoid patients' shoes becoming scratched

When partial weight-bearing is permitted and knee flexion may be encouraged, the patient continues to sit on a chair or bicycle stool and puts both feet on the treadle. The good leg will do most of the treadling, but the other knee will be getting some passive flexion if the foot is kept in place on the treadle with a bicycle toe-clip (*Figure 2.10*). We have filled in the treadles of the lathes with iron slats 2.5 cm (1 in) wide and 2.5 cm (1 in) apart. The toe-clip can be moved progressively

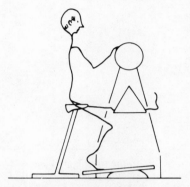

Patient working with the affected leg slung in order to obtain static quadriceps work. Patient treadles with the unaffected leg

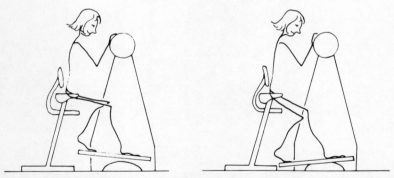

Patient working with both feet on the treadle, partially weight-bearing, with the affected leg nearer the back of the treadle, to avoid forced flexion of the injured knee. Treadle in up and down positions respectively

Figure 2.11 — Variations in lower limb range of movement obtainable on a wood-turning lathe

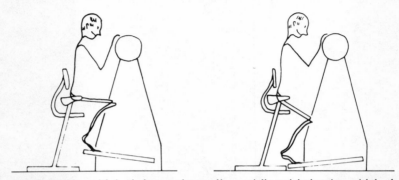

Patient working with both feet on the treadle, partially weight-bearing, with both legs in the same position for maximum flexion of hip and knee. Treadle in up and down positions respectively

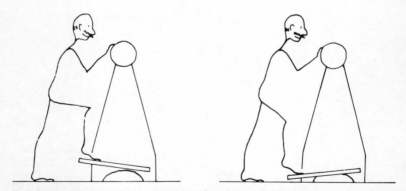

Patient working standing at lathe, fully weight-bearing, treadling with affected and unaffected legs alternately. Treadle in up and down positions respectively

Figure 2.11. (continued)

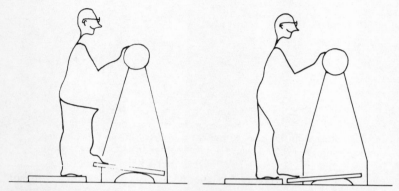

Patient works standing on a block, treadling with affected leg to produce more knee extension, and hip extension. Treadle in up and down positions respectively

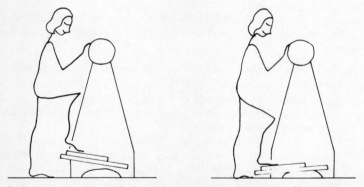

Patient works with a block on the treadle, treadling with affected leg, to produce more knee and hip flexion. Treadle in up and down positions respectively

Figure 2.11. (continued)

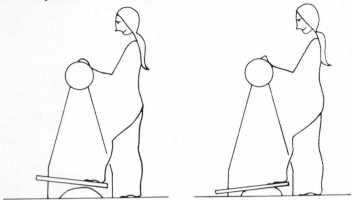

Patient working from the back of the lathe to obtain plantar flexion and dorsiflexion of the ankle. Treadle in up position for dorsiflexion, down position for plantar flexion, respectively

Figure 2.11. (continued)

nearer as the flexion of the knee improves. The patient will gradually use the quadriceps in stronger active contractions to get more power on the treadle of the lathe.

When the patient is allowed to take full weight-bearing the work can be carried out in the standing position. The patient is taught to use the legs alternately for standing and treadling, so that hamstrings and glutei get a fair share of exercise in turn with the hip flexors and quadriceps. The patient must be taught to brace back the knee of the standing leg. It is fortunate that a good firm stance makes for steady workmanship.

Methods of upgrading treatment on the wood-turning lathe include:

1. Increasing the diameter of the wood, progressing from a skittle or lamp stem to a lamp base or small bowl, to a salad bowl; the greater the diameter of the wood, the more resistance offered to each stroke of the treadle.
2. Using harder wood, progressing from sapele or beech to African hardwoods. (Soft wood is not suitable for turning because it tears.)
3. Progressing from two patients treadling together to one treadling alone.
4. Increasing the length of time spent on the lathe.
5. Using a larger gouge or chisel, so that more metal is in contact with the wood at each stroke.
6. Changing lathes. Some makes of lathe are harder to treadle than others.

Some lathes have weights which can be added to give more resistance but these make the work too hard for all but the fittest patient. We have found it best to upgrade by methods which clearly show the patient his progress, such as treadling unaided or turning a bigger bowl, rather than adding artificial resistance which can be discouraging.

The gearing system of the lathe can be altered by moving the driving belt. When the belt runs between the largest flywheel flange and the smallest pulley on the headstick, the wood will revolve more quickly, and slightly more effort will be required to treadle. This extra effort is minimal, however, and changing the gearing is not a useful way of upgrading the activity.

Bowl lathes

Conventional lathes had only a 10 cm (4 in) centre. This is not sufficient to turn a good salad bowl. Therefore we constructed in the workshops two lathes with 20 cm (8 in) centres. Neither of these have tailstocks. One is made to turn the outside of bowls, the other so that the inside of the bowl faces the worker (*Figure 2.12*). This is achieved by using a universal joint on the foot-treadle to permit the belt to remain in alignment with the headstock.

These two bowl lathes give considerable resistance when carrying a large piece of wood 30.5—38 cm (12—15 in) in diameter. Tools must be kept very sharp and the tool-rests are altered frequently to keep the edge of the tool supported firmly and close to the surface of the wood. Tool-rests of various curves must be made also so that they can be adjusted inside the circumference of the bowl as it is being cut out. The worker must be taught to hold the cutting tools very firmly on the tool-rest and at a level just above the centre of work as well as at an angle of 45 degrees. If all these precautions are not observed the cutting edge of the tool may slip down between the tool-rest and the wood, whilst the end of the long handle jerks. The writer once got a black eye when demonstrating how *not* to turn.

Some attention must also be paid to the position of the feet when treadling any foot-power lathe. When standing with the ankles together and the feet turned outwards, much of the weight falls through the medial side of the knee joint. In even a normal knee there is some side-play on the medial side of the joint and the knee can bend a little inwards. After an operation such as meniscectomy the danger of straining ligaments and capsule of the joint is obvious. The weight also falls through the medial longitudinal arch of the foot, which might do damage if the intrinsic muscles are weak after prolonged immobilization in plaster. The patient must therefore be watched and instructed to work standing with the feet parallel to ensure that the joints of knee and foot are mobilized in safety. With our inside bowl lathe the surface of the wood to be cut is directly facing the patient, so he operates the

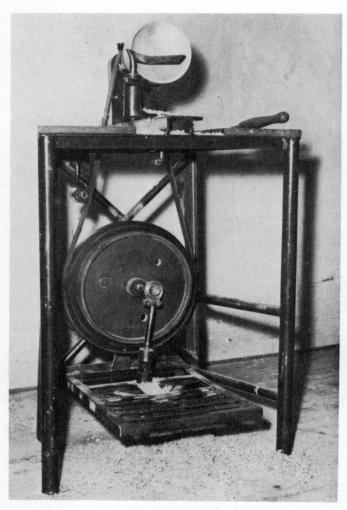

Figure 2.12. — Front view of bowl lathe, presenting inside of bowl to worker, showing arrangement of universal joint between treadle and flywheel, and use of jockey pulley to adjust tension of belt

treadle in the normal way. There is now another lathe on the market capable of taking a bowl, but the patient must either twist his body sideways to turn the inside of the bowl or stand sideways to the lathe and thus runs the risk of putting strain on his medial ligaments.

The scroll saw

The scroll saw (*Figure 2.13*) is an old-fashioned American saw worked by a foot-treadle which pulls on a strap working a bicycle free-wheel. It has been remade and given a heavier and more stable frame, but the principle of its machinery has not been changed. Its great advantage is

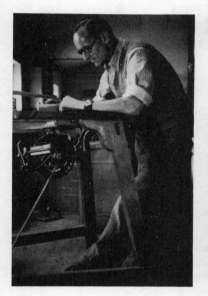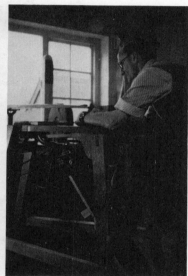

Figure 2.13. – The scroll saw

that it is best worked by a full stroke so that movement from flexion to extension at hip, knee and ankle can be developed. It is used with a coping-saw blade and will cut wood up to about 7.5 cm (3 in) thick to a circle ready for turning bases of table-lamps or bowls. It will take a junior hack-saw blade, and has been used to cut out 1.3 cm (½ in) mild steel to make saddle attachments for V-blocks.

The foot-treadle drilling machine

The foot-treadle drilling machine (*Figure 2.14*) is worked by the patient standing on one leg and treadling with the other. One hand pulls down the handle which presses the drill on the wood and the other hand holds the material in position for drilling. In this way

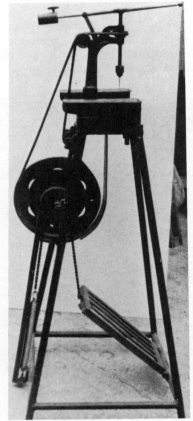

Figure 2.14. – The foot-treadle drilling machine

co-ordination of hand and foot is encouraged. It works equally well using either foot for treadling and either hand for holding the material in place. This machine is therefore suitable for patients with varying disabilities.

Stanley mitre saw

This piece of equipment can be set to enable a patient to saw wood at any chosen angle. This helps the patient with a hand injury or with inco-ordination or just with lack of skill to work to a much higher standard than would otherwise be possible. It also requires minimal supervision by the occupational therapist.

A patient with little movement in one hand can use this apparatus to saw with the other hand, even without a clamp, although a clamp may be used if required. The saw handle can be padded in the usual way if enlargement is needed. The bilateral saw handle (*see* page 390) can be attached for two-handed work.

Electric grinding machine

This is a machine designed for sharpening planes, chisels and gouges. It has attached jigs which can be set to the correct angle for each tool. It is oil cooled and therefore does not destroy the temper of the tool by over-heating, which can happen when using the grinder on the Myford lathe.

Myford 3½ in (9 cm) centre lathe

There are two centre lathes in the workshops. The second is more modern and has an automatic screw-cutting gear box. Both lathes have been of great use. The light, round-fingered grip on the turning handle has been invaluable for teaching position of the fingers when pressure on the palm is contraindicated, such as after plastic surgery on the palmar fascia necessitating its excision. The ability to balance and watch fast-moving machinery is often a stumbling block to the recovery of patients who have had middle or inner ear operations. If they can learn to tackle this small, fast-moving lathe one can be confident of their return to machine-work in factories. If one finds this capacity permanently impaired, time is saved in plans for resettlement. This lathe has also proved useful in bringing the outdoor worker to indoor work. For example, a patient who had had a mitral valvotomy, and was found to have incipient ankylosing spondylitis, had been accustomed to driving a bulldozer and doing other out-of-door work in the building trade. It took a little time, which he spent hoeing garden paths, for him to make friends with the occupational therapist, but when the rainy day occurred he had enough confidence in her to try turning handles for screwdrivers of various sizes. He became accustomed to working indoors and was ready to accept factory work on a capstan lathe.

Another patient, a centre lathe turner, had an accident at work. He had put his hand on the chuck to slow the lathe down more quickly. This is common practice although, of course, against factory regulations. He was very foolishly wearing a ring which caught on the chuck jaw and avulsed his finger. This was stitched back on and he was referred for treatment with his finger in fixed flexion. After serial splinting his finger was straightened out. He was frightened of using the lathe again but gradually regained his confidence with practice and eventually returned to work.

Myford lathes are used to make many small parts for machines used in the workshops. There is therefore usually work available when the occupational therapists want someone assessed for retraining or returning to work on a lathe either as a setter or an operator.

Milling machine

This machine is designed for cutting metal lengthwise either in grooves or steps or 'V''s. It is less often used than the lathe because most small parts that are made in the workshops are of the type that need turning rather than milling. It does, however, widen the scope of machinery and makes it possible to assess people who are returning to work or training either as setters or operators or setter operators.

Hand-worked bench-shaper

The hand bench-shaper is a useful piece of equipment in an occupational therapy workshop which sets out to make equipment for its own patients. It has helped to shape the plummer-blocks needed to hold the spindles of all the machines made in the workshops, as well as the V-blocks for vices to hold rod or bar metal for drilling holes in an even row.

It was originally designed for work with the right hand only but it was soon converted for use with either hand, and various grips on the handle were made for therapeutic exercise of the hand. It works on the push and pull principle and has provided work for flexion and extension of shoulder and elbow and the grip of the fingers.

Figure 2.15 shows one handle which can be used to encourage flexion of the terminal phalanx of either thumb or fingers depending on the position of the U-bar. The screw-and-nut fixation makes it adjustable to various sizes of hands or length of finger (Jones, 1955). On occasion it has been found that the over-enthusiastic patient is inclined to add leg movement, especially ankle flexion and extension

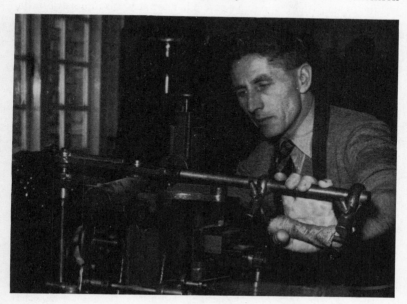

Figure 2.15. — Adaptation to bench shaper to encourage increase of span between thumb and index finger, and also flexion of terminal joint of the thumb

when swaying backwards and forwards, to assist function. However, this is a type of error which is very often encountered in occupational therapy workshops, where 'cheating' movement is often the result of ignorance and over-enthusiasm for results. Explanation of the aims of treatment will counteract the patient's temptation to speed up production at the expense of therapeutic benefit.

Welding plant

Oxyacetylene and arc-welding equipment are both used in the workshops. Because of the problems of storing oxygen cylinders safely, masking the bright light of the welding flame from passers-by and guarding against flying sparks, it was necessary to build a special welding bay on to the side of the workshops with a concrete floor and asbestos curtains. This provided a useful building project for the pre-work group of patients one summer.

Skill centres train patients in both oxyacetylene welding and arc welding. One patient who had a severe hand injury was interested in the former. He spent a few weeks learning the technique in the workshops with the technician and then visited by appointment the local Skill Centre, with an occupational therapist. The instructor took one look at the patient and said, 'You'll never be able to weld with a hand like that'. The occupational therapist persuaded him to let the patient demonstrate his ability. The instructor was amazed, the patient was accepted for training, completed this successfully and then found a job. Without a period of assessment and practice in the workshops this would never have happened.

REFERENCES

Everett, P. *The Thame Wire-Twisting Machine.* Nottingham; Nottingham Handcraft Company
Health and Safety Executive (1970). *Seats for Workers in Factories, Offices and Shops.* London; HMSO
Jones, M. S. (1955). 'Occupational therapy for the upper limb.' *Br. J. phys. Med.* 18, 119
Ministry of Technology. Ergonomics for Industry Series: *Seating in Industry.* London; HMSO
Savage, A. E. *The Ankle-Rotator Machine.* Nottingham; Nottingham Handcraft Company

FURTHER READING

Cheshire, L. *The Camden Cycle.* Nottingham; Nottingham Handcraft Company
Health and Safety Executive (1970). *Electric Arc Welding.* London; HMSO
Keane, W. and Creasey, M. E. *The Electronic Cycle.* Nottingham; Nottingham Handcraft Company
Lock, S. J. *The Larvic Rehabilitation Lathe Mark II.* Nottingham; Nottingham Handcraft Company
Mandal, A. C. *The Seated Man (Homo Sedens).* A. C. Mandal, Taarbaoek Strandvej 49, (DK) 2930 Klampenborg, Denmark
Ministry of Technology (1966). Ergonomics for Industry Series; *Design of Work for the Disabled.* London; HMSO
Oliver, E. *The Oliver Rehabilitation Machine (Bicycle Machine).* Nottingham; Nottingham Handcraft Company

3

Occupational Therapy Activities

The starting point and the pace of increase in activity must be compatible with both the specific treatment of the disability and the patient's general condition. Experience in occupational therapy for ambulant patients has convinced the writer of the value of studying the patient's posture in any activity which is designed to be therapeutic. Many patients have been sent for rehabilitation following disabilities affecting the abdomen, thorax, spine and pelvis which had required medical or surgical treatment in hospital. These patients have worked sitting at table, bench, loom or lathe, progressing to work in the standing position. They have worked indoors in the workshops, and out-of-doors in the garden. The choice of environment for their activities has depended on the weather and time of year, but most of all on the patients' tastes and interests. The muscles of the spine, thorax and abdomen are closely interdependent. Certain adaptations of equipment and position at work will lay more or less stress on the groups of muscles and joints affected by a specific disability. It has been found that in many ways it is easier to adapt the equipment than to change a grown person's tastes and interests, though on occasion these interests may need some searching out before they are discovered and engaged in productive work.

Often when a patient is admitted on a fine sunny day he says that his hobby is gardening. But by this he means that his hobby is his own garden, with all the varied types of work available. After a few days hoeing through rows of vegetables or sweeping up leaves in the more impersonal garden of an institution, the monotony of the work available and suitable as treatment will become boring. Also by that time the patient may feel more at home with the staff and able to pluck up courage to ask if he can come into the workshop and make something for himself. This preference is understandable, especially when he sees an attractive stool or coffee table that another patient may be taking home to his family.

WOODWORK

This is one of the most popular crafts that can be practised thera-peutically. A great variety of work is possible that will give opportunity for progressive development of physical strength and dexterity, as well as ingenuity and concentration. The materials used, from plywood to hardwood, with their varying resistances will make a progressive demand

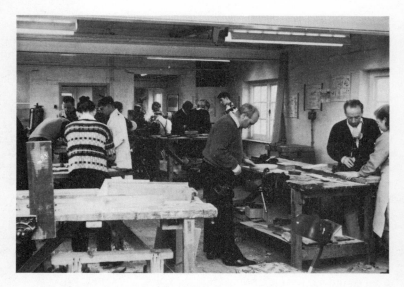

Figure 3.1. — The woodwork section of the workshops at Farnham Park

for effort. The requirements of sawing, planing, sanding and polishing depend on the size and type of the article being made. The height of a carpenter's bench can be altered with the addition of extensible legs or it can be blocked up to heights which will keep the patient working in a good upright position. It is an old wives' tale that a carpenter must work at the traditional height of 88 cm (2 ft 10 in). The elderly car-penter of 183 cm (6 ft) or more is usually round-shouldered, whilst his contemporary of 163 cm (5 ft 4 in) carries himself like a guardsman. Sawing, planing or polishing on a bench of the height which keeps the individual in an easy upright posture will develop the muscles of thorax, abdomen and spine and is invaluable in developing the postural reflexes.

Postural reflexes in their most effective state maintain the upward tilt of the pelvis, so that the intestines are more or less supported in the basin of the pelvis. In this position the intestines do not hang on the mesentery, where they are attached to the posterior abdominal wall. Abdominal muscles that are flabby and lacking in tone are frequently found in those patients who suffer from low backache of indeterminate origin.

Sawing

The postural reflexes that come into play with the free pushing movements of handsaw or plane stimulate the rhythmic contractions of spinal and intercostal muscles as synergists or stabilizers. The use of bodyweight in using these tools is led off by the head poised in a good viewing position. The index finger should be extended along the saw handle whilst the other fingers and thumb grip the handle. This pointing of the index finger does much to assist in sawing on the desired line. It has been observed that when a patient ignorant of woodwork is taught this grip, which is second nature to a carpenter, there is an improvement in confidence and skill which is reflected in improved postural tone. The skin on the anterior aspect of the index finger is richly supplied with sensory nerve endings. Extension of this finger means that maximum sensory feedback is gained by the use of the saw and also by the fact that the flexors are on the stretch. Postural tone in the whole of the upper limb is thus stimulated. It always seems natural to point in the direction in which one wants to proceed or towards an object which is a topic of conversation. Wagging of the index finger is often employed to emphasize admonishment or negation.

It may here be of interest to describe various positions of work in which a panel, rip, or single-handed cross-cut saw may be used, and refer to the various groups of postural muscles which will be brought into play with greater or lesser emphasis in one position than in another. These saws may be used on planks laid on two trestles, and if the sawyer is right handed he will usually bend up the right knee and use it to keep the end of the plank steady whilst he uses his left hand to hold the left edge of the plank. In this position there is almost full flexion of the left hip, and some flexion of the spine. Bodyweight is used to reinforce the right arm and shoulder muscles. These saws all cut on the 'push out' and a piece of hardwood 75 mm (3 in) thick gives considerable resistance. This half-kneeling, bent-back position certainly makes available more power than does the upright position, but it is not the best position of work for patients with disabilities affecting the spine, abdomen or thorax. For such patients it is necessary to put the plank upright in a vice on a bench so that the saw stroke is in the horizontal line. It is often a good thing to teach the patient to saw with an upward pushing stroke so that the saw blade goes through an arc of movement. The patient may stand or sit and still keep the back erect. As the saw cut proceeds down the plank it may be lifted higher in the vice to ensure that the upright position is maintained. The work of sawing done in this position is heavier on the spinal extensors than in the first position, as bodyweight and gravity do not assist in the same way.

On occasion it has been found useful to get a patient to saw sitting on the plank, with one leg on each side and both hands gripping the saw handle. The saw stroke is then carried out with a strong downward thrust of the hands and arms and the abdominal muscles work more strongly than in either of the first two positions.

The amount of power needed for sawing depends on the thickness and the type of wood used. It is therefore an extremely useful type of work for therapeutic purposes as it can be graded to suit the capacities of the patient. The better and more beautiful types of wood such as walnut, beech or oak provide much harder work, but they are used for more attractive articles than are soft woods such as deal.

Cross-cut sawing with a double-handled saw is carried out by two workers (*see Figure 3.15*, page 84). The cut is made by pulling the saw, not by pushing. It is essential that the work be done rhythmically. The two workers must try to balance each other in power and pace of pull, otherwise one might jerk the other into painful spasm. It is usual for each worker to hold the log on the sawhorse with one hand, and to use the other on the saw. One foot is usually used by each worker to steady the base of the sawhorse, the other for supporting bodyweight. The work involves a good deal of spinal rotation as well as use of the hand, arm and shoulder girdle. Little spinal flexion is required, as the hip, knee and ankle provide the forward and backward movements. Cross-cut sawing can be heavy work, depending on the diameter and texture of the logs. It is therefore very useful for the last stages of general toughening activities. The workers should be encouraged to change sides at intervals, so that various groups of muscles are used in full activity and mobility or in the static phases of holding.

Sawhorses of several heights should be made, from 117 cm (3 ft 10 in) to 86.5 cm (2 ft 10 in) to accommodate the varying heights of individuals. Sawhorses need to be bolted together securely so it is not practicable to make them adjustable in height. As they are usually left out-of-doors in all weathers some protective coating of paint, or its equivalent, is economic. The bolts holding them together should be well greased to prevent rust.

It is most essential that saws, like all tools, be kept sharp and well set. There is nothing more dispiriting than working with poorly kept tools.

Planing

The jack plane, unlike the saw, is held more at the side of the body, and both hands are used to keep it down on the wood. The use of the plane involves a fair amount of trunk rotation as well as bodyweight balanced from the ankles and knees. It is perhaps fortunate that both hands are required, and that many people will learn easily to plane using either hand on the handle or the front of the plane. It is possible thereby to share out the rotary movement of the trunk to both sides when necessary.

WOOD-TURNING

The nine lathes are Farnham Park are in constant use, many of them for the whole of the treatment day. The most satisfactory ones are the old-fashioned Union treadle lathes that were built as wood-turning machines. They are solid, sturdy and last for years with proper maintenance and replacement of parts from time to time. Because they are very efficient machines they run smoothly and work in the early stages can be made easy by using not very hard wood of small diameter and a narrow cutting tool. As the patient improves he can progress to making an article from harder wood of large diameter using a wider cutting tool. It is very easy to grade the work in this way and we have found no need to add artificial resistance to our lathes.

Wood-turning is an easily learnt skill. Most patients become proficient after about three hours work. They all make articles for themselves which they may buy to take home and this gives them excellent motivation. A patient trying to finish a salad bowl before he is discharged will exert himself to the maximum.

A wide variety of articles can be made on the wood-turning lathe. In addition to table-lamps, candlesticks and bowls, patients have made egg cups, skittles, children's wooden toys, pepper mills and even lace bobbins.

The therapeutic use of wood-turning is discussed in detail in the section describing the wood-turning lathes and their attachments, on page 38, and also on pages 160 and 234.

INDUSTRIAL OUTWORK

We have for many years made wooden rockers (*see Figure 6.8*, page 174) for application to leg plasters. These are used when the patient is allowed to start weight-bearing. They have been supplied to one London teaching hospital and two local hospitals. We have also made arm-slings (*see Figure 7.15*, page 238) for a local consultant using four different colours of webbing to differentiate between the three adult and the children's sizes. The hospitals were asked to pay for the materials and for any transportation costs. No remuneration has been given or expected by any patient doing this work.

It was then decided that following the pioneering work at Vauxhall Motors factory at Luton, and Austin Motors in Birmingham, where production-line work was adapted to provide remedial work as an integral part of rehabilitation, Farnham Park should have its own industrial section. So we bought a heavy-duty overhead drill and a fly-press, both second hand, to increase the scope of what we could offer to do for any local firm that would give us work. After that our first contract consisted of packing polythene gloves, eight into a folder and then 20 folders into a box. We never used the drill for production work and subsequently discovered that it is very much better to get a firm to supply any machines that were necessary for their outwork because they would then maintain them.

Packing polythene gloves provided useful hand movements and was good for assessing concentration and other attributes. But it was rather too clean a job for our workshops. We were always afraid of getting wood dust on the polythene.

Then a contract for assembling castors was obtained. This entailed the use of small hand-presses which could easily be adapted for specialized hand movements and also for specific leg exercise. They could also be used without adaptation for assessing concentration or manual dexterity.

Initially our attitude to industrial work was very purist. We felt that this was a therapeutic activity, that patients were doing this for exercise and should not be under pressure, and it would therefore be impossible and unethical to guarantee delivery dates. Our newly appointed tech-nician, who had come straight from industry, and who had the job of liaising with the local firms who supplied us, had doubts about the practicalities of working in this way. At that time we had two machines, and all went well until our doctors asked us to keep a young hemiplegic patient on one machine all day as part of his assessment for work. Because this patient's concentration was poor and his attention span was short, production output fell by nearly 50 per cent. As we had only just started working for this firm we felt that this was a crisis and so staff and students worked in relays in their lunch hour that week to bring production up to normal. This did us no harm because we were forced to learn what was involved in doing this kind of work.

Soon the number of machines increased and we no longer had production problems. The work accepted by the Centre was always well within the limits of our anticipated turnover so there was never any question of employing other than suitable patients. The factory lorry came once a week on Fridays, and the tempo of work increased towards the end of the week to produce as many completed boxes of castors as possible by the deadline. This was due to the patients' reaction to the situation, not to pressure from the staff, and it helped to create a factory atmosphere in the workshops which had, of itself, value in conditioning patients to a return to normal living. It was not unusual for women with hand injuries to ask to go on industrial outwork rather than conventional light activities such as stool-seating or mosaic because it was more like what they were used to. They took pride in their output and in earning money for the Centre. A much needed 3½ in (9 cm) Myford centre lathe was the first item purchased out of the industrial fund.

Occupational therapists and students often regard repetitive industrial work as tediously simple. We discovered that it was more difficult than we thought. The actual job was easy, but repeating this quickly and accurately for an hour at a time was another matter. We were ashamed to find that many patients were better at it than we were. They also enjoyed the work, chatting together in a group round the table, doing an efficient job with an element of competition and a good-looking end-product.

Hand-presses are used for light assembly work, and our contract was for putting together part of a castor of the type used for modern furniture. The figures on pages 60—68 show adaptations to machines which press a small metal ring, called a circlip, over the end of a white nylon socket. First the circlip is pushed inside the rim of a positioning hole on the platform of the machine by using a mandral, that is a solid cylinder of metal. The mandral is then put into the positioning hole, resting on a spring. The patient picks up a nylon socket, holds it on top of the mandral, pulls down the handle of the press so that the nylon socket presses on the mandral which in turn presses on the spring, forcing the circlip over the end of the nylon socket (*Figure 3.2*).

Another job entailed placing the stem of a hollow metal castor in a positioning hole, putting a small cap containing a circlip inside the rim of the stem, placing a larger cap over the top and pulling down the handle to press the cap into place (*Figure 3.3*).

These jobs are described to give an idea of the type of work that can be done on a hand-press. There are many, many variations of industrial work that can be done on these machines. They will all involve manual dexterity and pinch-grip in handling the components, and the press may be activated by a pull-down lever, kick action, or push

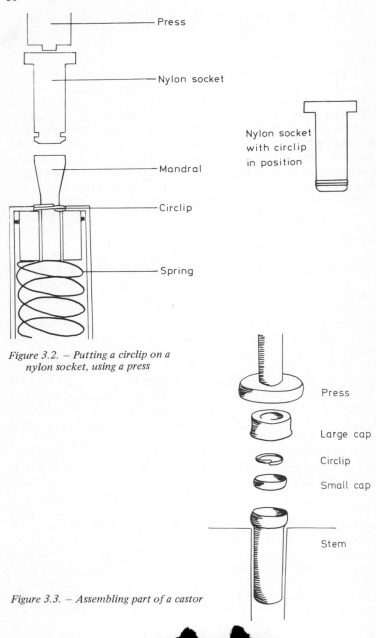

Press

Nylon socket

Nylon socket
with circlip
in position

Mandral

Circlip

Spring

*Figure 3.2. – Putting a circlip on a
nylon socket, using a press*

Press

Large cap

Circlip

Small cap

Stem

Figure 3.3. – Assembling part of a castor

action. These presses can very easily be adapted not only for different hand-grips but also to provide lower limb exercise. The conventional pull-down lever, although to the right of the press, can be used with either the right or the left hand.

The press handle is normally a long metal lever with a knob at the end, coloured red to lessen the likelihood of accidents. This knob can be unscrewed to allow a piece of Rubazote (foam rubber tubing) of suitable diameter to be inserted over the handle. This makes a more comfortable hand-grip and also an easier size of grip for someone with limited finger flexion.

Some patients pull the press down with a hook-grip in the initial stages of treatment when the hand is stiff and painful. It is not necessary to insist on a more conventional grip because once the hand improves the patient will usually automatically grip right round the handle.

Finger extensor adaptation

A motor bicycle handbrake is used to release a ratchet which unlocks the handle and allows it to be pulled down. The handbrake is held in the squeezed position while the press is operated. It is then released while the next circlip is put ready in position.

This adaptation makes the patient extend his fingers actively in order to span the distance between the motor bicycle handbrake and the press handle before squeezing them together. The handbrake has a spring and this adds slight resistance to the movement of flexion. Stronger springs can be substituted to increase this resistance. Extension of the fingers is not resisted nor would it be in a natural movement.

Finding work to provide finger extension in occupational therapy is not easy and this is a very good method. It also provides work in elevation for an oedematous hand. In the early stages of oedema it may be best to use the basic handle. Progression to the finger-extension handle, with the fingers alternately flexing and extending, will provide a pumping action which will help to aid venous return and disperse the oedema.

Wrist extension adaptation

An angled bar is fitted on to the press handle (*Figure 3.4*) in such a position that it is not possible to grip the handle to pull it down unless the wrist is in extension. This bar can be adjusted so that a greater or lesser degree of wrist extension is needed to make it possible to reach the handle.

This movement is valuable for many patients who have suffered hand injuries and who need to strengthen wrist extension, especially following radial nerve lesions, rheumatoid arthritis, burns, scar contractures and some crush injuries. When treatment is aimed at increasing

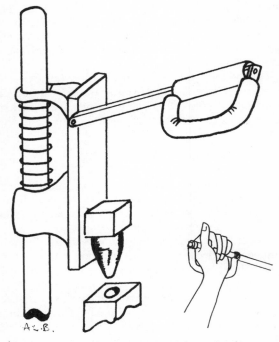

Figure 3.4. – Wrist extension adaptation to a hand-press

flexion of the fingers, it is important to facilitate this by using the wrist in extension. Extending the wrist automatically brings the fingers into slight flexion, and powerful finger flexion is only possible with the wrist in extension.

Bilateral overhead handle

With this adaptation (*Figure 3.5*), two hands can be used on the press at the same time to provide work for the spinal extensors, the elevators and depressors of the shoulder girdle, and for a wide range of scapular movement. This is largely static work for the spinal muscles because there is no flexion, extension or rotation of the spine.

This has been found useful for patients with low back pain who need a period of less active work during their treatment, and for patients with pain or stiffness in the neck, for example, following cervical spondylosis. It is useful for patients with cardiac and thoracic conditions when trying to increase the expansion of the rib cage, and also for patients with bilateral conditions such a rheumatoid arthritis. It has been found a very valuable method of exercising a frozen shoulder.

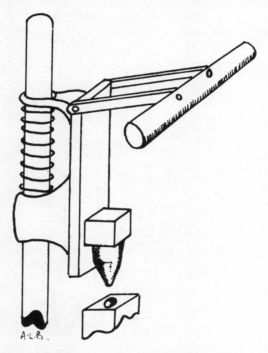

Figure 3.5. – Bilateral overhead handle on a hand-press

With both hands on the overhead lever it is not possible to tip the body sideways, and therefore even if the unaffected arm does most of the work, the frozen shoulder must go through the required range of movement.

When using the press for bilateral work, adjustment is made so that there is minimal clearance between the press and the nylon socket. The socket is placed in position and locates itself against the press, then both hands reach up to grasp the handles and pull them down to operate the press. The height of the handle can be adjusted by two lock-nuts on the machine, or by alteration of the height of the patient's seat.

Hemi-push adaptation

This handle (*Figure 3.6*) was designed to provide bilateral extension exercise for the upper limb when treating hemiplegic patients. It is described in more detail on page 383.

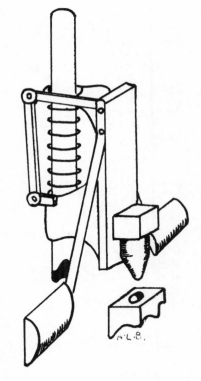

Figure 3.6. — Hemi-push handle to en-courage extension of the whole upper limb

Static quadriceps adaptation

This adaptation (*Figure 3.7*) is designed to be operated by the last few degrees of knee extension which lock the knee. It is mainly used with patients who have an extension lag, and provides one of the few ways of exercising vastus medialis in occupational therapy.

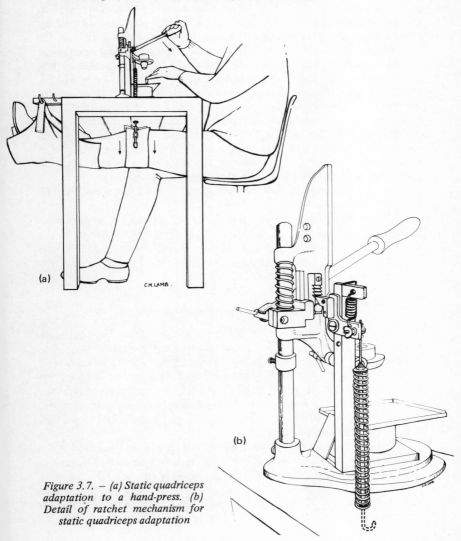

(a)

C.M.LAMB.

(b)

Figure 3.7. – (a) Static quadriceps adaptation to a hand-press. (b) Detail of ratchet mechanism for static quadriceps adaptation

A rod spring is let through a hole in the bench top and attached to a strap which goes under the patient's knee. At the top of the rod spring there is a lever which acts on a ratchet. The rod spring must be pulled down to release the ratchet so that the press can be operated.

The patient is seated on a chair, or a bicycle stool, at the bench. The leg to be exercised is supported by a sling which extends from the calf to beyond the heel. The strap which goes under the knee is attached to the hook above by a chain. The length of this strap is adjusted by moving the links of this chain. The patient must be slung with his leg horizontal, the ankle level with the knee. His position should be checked by asking him to extend his knee fully. If it is correct he will be just able to release the ratchet by pressing down as far as his knee will go. Contraction of the quadriceps, especially vastus medialis, is tested by palpation of the thigh 5 cm (2 in) proximal to the patella. If contraction is not occurring, the ankle sling is adjusted to hold the leg in a higher position. The patient will maintain this static quadriceps contraction for about 15 seconds, long enough to pull down the handle of the press. He then relaxes the muscles, and releases the ratchet, while he places another nylon socket on the press. He is told to repeat this pattern of activity until he feels fatigue in his quadriceps and then to rest. The usual period of work is half an hour.

The rod which runs down the centre of the spring is threaded. There is a nut at the top which can be tightened to compress the spring and so increase resistance. If the patient does not feel fatigue during his period of treatment the resistance should be increased.

Active quadriceps adaptation

This adaptation (*Figure 3.8*) is designed to strengthen the quadriceps muscle in the later stages of treatment when the patient is able to contract the quadriceps statically. The patient sits on a chair and operates the press by kicking forwards and upwards on a foot-press attached to a special lever under the bench. When the chair is in the correct position and at the correct height in relation to both the workbench and the length of the patient's leg, the press can only be operated if the knee goes into full extension.

It may be necessary to draw a chalk-line on the floor so that if the chair is inadvertently moved it can be correctly repositioned. This will also prevent the patient cheating by deliberately moving the chair to a position where the press can be operated without putting the leg into full extension. The degree of extension is also adjustable by a nut on the machine.

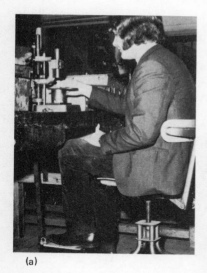

(a)

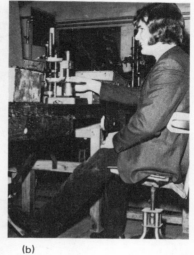

(b)

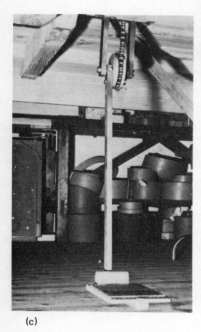

(c)

Figure 3.8.– (a) and (b) Active quad-riceps adaptation to a hand-press. (c) Detail of mechanism for active quadriceps adaptation

Plantar flexion adaptation

This is a footplate (*Figure 3.9*) on the floor under the bench which is directly linked to the press. The press is operated by a forward pivoting action of the footplate. The patient can sit on a chair with his knee

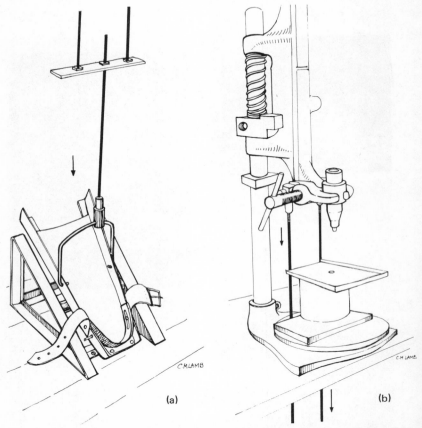

Figure 3.9. — (a) Footpiece of plantar flexion adaptation on a hand-press. (b) Detail of mechanism for plantar flexion adaptation

flexed or he can sit on a bicycle seat with his knee extended. The latter is a more valuable exercise because it involves the whole of the extensor mechanism of the leg in a similar pattern to that used in walking.

Fly-press

The fly-press (*Figure 3.10*) is a more powerful tool than a hand-press and it is therefore used for slightly different work. Typically a jig is fixed in position under the press. A piece of flat metal is placed on top of the jig and when the press is operated it forces the metal strip into the shape of the jig. Instead of being pulled down as with a hand-press,

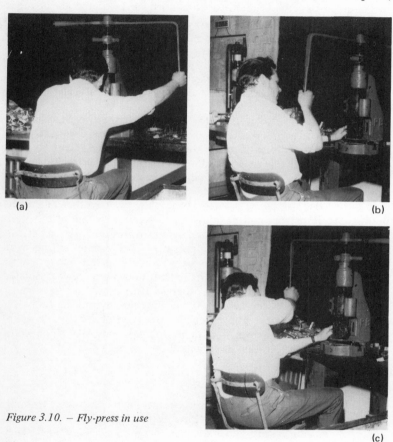

(a)

(b)

(c)

Figure 3.10. – Fly-press in use

the handle of the fly-press is swung in rotation from one side to the other. This is harder work than the hand-press and requires much more force.

A fly-press used in industry has a weighted ball on the opposite side to the handle. This helps to give momentum to the swing. Very often the press is set so that the handle does not only go from one side to the other but swings right round the press two or three times. This of course builds momentum and makes the final downward pressure much stronger. But it does mean that a heavy metal handle is swinging in a circle over the bench and this is dangerous in a workshop where there are disabled patients. Therefore work must be restricted to jobs that can be done by gently swinging the handle from one side to the other. This is no problem.

Work on the fly-press provides a useful range of movement for the shoulder and elbow. It is not possible to have a right- or a left-sided handle, but it is possible to work the press by starting with the right hand, changing hands when the handle reaches the middle and finishing with the left hand.

The fly-press is also suitable for some back conditions such as low back pain. It is a progression from using the bilateral overhead adaptation on the hand-press because the fly-press demands some rotation of the spine. Initially the patient will very gingerly press the handle from one hand to the other, keeping his spine as rigid as possible. As his confidence and his back muscles improve he will begin to speed up and swing the handle across from one side to the other all in one movement. Resistance can be added by tightening the ram of the press. The fly-press has a limited value compared with woodwork for patients with back conditions. It is impossible to alternate sitting with standing at the fly-press, whereas in woodwork he can move readily from a higher to a lower bench. The patient must be somewhat isolated when working the press because other patients must keep reasonably well clear, whereas woodwork with the general sharing of tools is a more sociable activity. The repetitive work on the fly-press is not totally engrossing whereas a patient doing woodwork can become so interested in the job that he forgets about his back.

Other types of industrial work

Various other bench jobs such as inspection, hand assembly, reaming, countersinking and filing flashes, have been undertaken from time to time. These add variety and have proved useful ancillary jobs. They require varying degrees of hand dexterity and can be used to assess, for example, concentration, but they cannot be adapted to provide any other remedial activities. If these types of work only had been available, and no hand-press work, it would not have been possible to develop such a large industrial section in the workshops.

It has been suggested that assembly work would also be of value in the woodwork section. For many years plaster rockers were made for various hospitals (*see* page 174) and these provided useful, simple work which could be done on a team basis. Some occupational therapy departments take on more elaborate woodworking jobs such as making tables, stools or benches for the local authority, schools or hospitals. We have always resisted these suggestions for several reasons. Most of these jobs entail making a fairly large number of joints, usually mortice and tenons. Making such joints entails relatively little movement, being mainly static work, and for the amateur woodworker such joints take a long time to complete and the work is not very interesting. Many of the patients doing woodwork have back problems and they need large movements against resistance, such as sawing and planing, which exercise their spinal muscles. They should be encouraged to make coffee tables or bookshelves out of wood that must be sawn and planed to size, and then assembled quite quickly, largely with glue and screws.

Woodwork is an activity that is attractive to most patients, especially if they are working on something they want to make for themselves. They become so involved that they forget the injured hand or shoulder or back and this is the first stage towards using the injured part normally. They are much less likely to develop this interest in something that they have been told they must do.

Keeping up standards in woodwork is much more difficult than standards in factory outwork. Carpentry is a skill whereas assembly work can be learned quite quickly. Patients have produced several quite strange-looking objects which they have taken home with great pride. But when woodwork has to be done to commercial standards the remedial aspect of the work can be lost, and patients can spend their treatment periods turning out a product rather than exercising specific groups of muscles or mobilizing certain joints.

Some occupational therapists welcome production woodwork because they are unsure of their own carpentry ability and they feel that if only a limited selection of items is produced, they can more easily learn how they are made and consequently how to teach the patients to make them. This is a quite unnecessary lack of confidence. Since Farnham Park opened in 1947 there has never been a technical instructor running either the woodwork section or the wood-turning section. There have been two male occupational therapists on the staff, but most of the time these sections have been run by female therapists who had no more than average, and in some cases far less than average, experience in carpentry. They all learnt sufficient do-it-yourself woodwork techniques to manage their section in a very short time. Many of the patients were eager and helpful in giving advice, and this not only assisted the therapists but contributed to the friendly atmosphere of the department and encouraged the patients to work together.

Industrial work as a medium for assessment

Most of the industrial work that has been done at Farnham Park over the last 10 years has come from the same firm and has consisted of the assembly of castors. Although there are several different designs in castors, and several different stages in their assembly, we have now learned most of them. The jobs we are sent rotate according to the firm's current requirements, but they do not change to something new and unfamiliar. Although no timings have been done on any of these jobs, we know from experience what to expect from a patient's performance.

The technical instructor who is in charge of this section has had considerable industrial experience and has a good understanding of the working norm. For 29 years he was in charge of a tool room and part of his job was the training of apprentices.

Industrial work has been used as a medium for assessing speed, concentration, accuracy and learning ability for simple processes. It gives a good indication of whether the patient is punctual and conscientious, and also his relationship with his fellow workers, when they are all sitting round a table together.

Running an industrial section covers many ancillary jobs besides the actual industrial process. Components and finished castors are stored in metal boxes. These have to be unloaded from the lorry on to a trolley and wheeled to the storeroom. They must be brought from the storeroom into the workshop as required. They must be lifted from the floor up to the worktables and down again. All this provides practice in lifting and carrying. It gives the technician and the occupational therapists an opportunity to assess how much a patient can lift and carry, and also whether he is doing this in the correct way. An industrial section can also be a noisy place and this makes it very suitable for helping to increase a patient's tolerance to noise.

Payment for industrial work

Individual patients have never been paid for doing industrial work. This was largely because it would have been very unfair to pay some patients attending the workshops and not others. The therapists needed the freedom to select whatever work would be most suitable for a patient's treatment without the complication of some patients wanting to do industrial work because of remuneration. Patients might even have been reluctant to attend the physiotherapy department or the remedial gymnasium because of the loss of earnings involved. Some individual patients might also have had problems with their level of earnings because this could have affected their sickness benefit.

The money that has been earned has gone into a special fund set up for the benefit of all the patients. This has enabled the Centre to carry out various improvements that would probably have been provided by the National Health Service at some future date, when the budget allowed, but which really needed doing as soon as possible. The front door at Farnham Park was large and impressive, and difficult for many patients to open and close. When it was left open a breeze swept through the hall and up the main staircase, lowering the temperature of the whole house. Keeping the door shut was a constant problem. Money from the industrial work fund enabled the administration to buy electrically operated, automatically opening doors.

The physiotherapy department was very small and quite inadequate for the numbers of patients attending for treatment. Plans were drawn up for knocking out one wall and doubling its size. This entailed installing additional heating and putting down new floorcovering over the whole area. The Health Service was unable to find sufficient money to finance this project, but when half the money was provided by the industrial work fund the Health Service was able to put up the rest.

All the patients when they first arrive at Farnham Park are told about the industrial work fund in an introductory talk. No one has ever objected to the system. It is not at all unusual for a patient to get great satisfaction from increasing his output, and to try and compute how much money he is contributing to the industrial work fund.

Supervision of industrial work

Although industrial work is usually very simple, some jobs are easier than others. Filing 'flash' off the edge of small plastic mouldings is a good example. Under the supervision of an experienced technical instructor our patients have done this job without any difficulties. At the same time the Occupational Therapy Work Centre in Slough ran short of industrial work and we sent them part of the job to help out. Although the patients there were manually no more handicapped than ours, and were keen to do the work, they were unable to file to a high enough standard. The Work Centre patients were supervised by occupational therapists who themselves found filing flashes difficult. Farnham

Park patients were supervised by a technician who was used to filing metal and who found filing flashes so much easier. His patients accepted his evaluation of the work and learnt to file accurately in a very short time.

Industrial work supervision is something that a technician with industrial experience can do better than an occupational therapist. He accepts assembly work as a worthwhile job and can bring something like a factory atmosphere into an occupational therapy workshop. An occupational therapist will have little or no factory experience. She is unlikely to enjoy production work and will almost inevitably find it difficult to make short-term patients work to a high enough standard for no monetary reward. Some years before employing a technician to set up the industrial work section at Farnham Park we had tried to introduce a small amount of industrial work under the supervision of an occupational therapist. It was a dismal failure. The work itself was ideal for the treatment of hand injuries but it was carelessly done and much of the therapist's time had to be spent on inspection and correction of faults. The patients resented working without pay, possibly because no scheme such as the industrial fund had been introduced. A deleterious pattern of thought arose in both occupational therapists and patients and this type of work was abandoned for the time being.

ENGINEERING AND METALWORK

The engineering section at Farnham Park is mainly used in the treatment of patients who are skilled in some branch of engineering and who are being assessed for return to work, or for patients who may be going to train in an engineering skill. Apart from simple exercises in welding, filing or turning, most of the work is concerned either with building new machines for the workshops or in repairing and servicing the old machines.

Patients interested in metalwork can use the hacksaw and the file to provide the same type of movement that woodwork tools give to the amateur or professional carpenter. The challenge of making new equipment for the occupational therapy workshops will interest those who like engineering. The problems may be rather different from those in general industry. In occupational therapy workshops equipment must be designed to demand or to exploit rather than to economize on certain human powers and capacities. In a workshop where there are patients with widely differing disabilities in various stages of recovery it is usually easy to call on a patient with mechanical knowledge and interest to help in the manufacture, setting up and maintenance of equipment.

Three technical instructors have worked at Farnham Park at different times since it opened. All were trained as either toolmakers or engineers and all have been invaluable in supervising such activities.

Wrought ironwork

This activity uses relatively soft 'school metal' strip which is easier to work than mild steel. All the equipment needed is attached to an extra-high bench. Patients work either standing or seated on a high bicycle stool. This high working position makes wrought ironwork more suitable than woodwork when bending over is contraindicated. It also provides the opportunity to exercise shoulder movement.

Wrought ironwork is used in the later stages of treatment for upper limb injuries, for building up strength and for toughening the palmar skin. It is a good bilateral activity for neurological conditions but if necessary can be done with one hand, except for the final assembly. It can be used to assess a patient's ability to follow written or verbal instruction, or the ability to design an individual project. Another use is to improve balance and increase standing tolerance, especially with a patient with post-head-injury ataxia or an above-knee amputation.

Wrought ironwork is popular with male patients, especially hemiplegics; it looks a reasonably heavy, masculine activity. It is also used for patients who dislike woodwork and feel happier working in metal. The finished articles usually look acceptable and are admired by other patients, even when not made very well. They are relatively inexpensive, since the metal is cheap, and small articles can be completed in a fairly short space of time.

OUTDOOR ACTIVITIES

There is the type of man, and more occasionally, woman, who will always prefer working out-of-doors at whatever there is available for him to do. It has been found an advantage to have some garden space round the workshops suitable on a fine day for sedentary work at a table, and with space for log-sawing, as well as for those actually engaged in gardening (*Figures 3.11* and *3.12*). Watching others engaged in work is often a useful incentive to increased activity.

Many patients may be trusted to stick to the type of work that will do them good. It is obvious, or will readily be appreciated when explained, that the crouching position of hand weeding is not going to help in the treatment of a patient with poor chest expansion or after a recent operation on spine or abdomen. The dictum that 'it is very nice to do good to the garden but it is essential to do good to the patient' may raise a laugh, but it will sometimes be remembered. There are others who may dare themselves, or genuinely forget, and try out work that is too heavy for their stage of recovery. Others again will find that

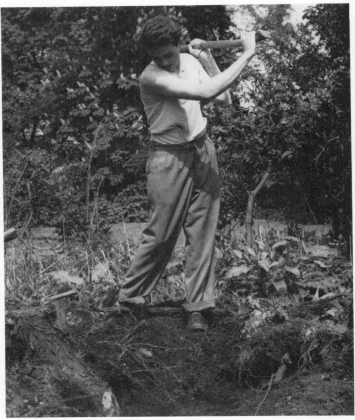

Figure 3.11. – Clearing rough ground using both hands. To encourage dorsiflexion of left hand, paretic after trauma affecting radial nerve

comparative solitude and freedom from supervision are a temptation to idleness. A nice 'sit-down' and a cigarette are not forms of occupation which fulfil the aims of treatment. With garden space round the work-shops the therapist will have some opportunity for observation and an assessment may be made of the working characteristics of the individual.

It may then be safe to encourage those who show common sense, reliability and a steady habit of work to carry on their activities in the more far-away regions of the garden where close and trained supervision is not practicable.

Draw hoe

Used to weed between rows of seedlings or vegetables. Light soil—light work, but may be wet underfoot.

Dutch hoe

Used to weed grass and the like out of gravel paths. Heavier work—drier underfoot.

Handle of hoe is long, 183—213 cm (6—7 ft) instead of usual 122—152 cm (4—5 ft). Blade is set at 160 degrees off the line of the handle. Made in the workshop in the metalworking section.

Movement—Pushing forward and pulling back in small jabs and using both arms. The patient is taught to do this standing partly sideways.

(a) Right foot forward, right hand forward on handle of hoe, pushing forward with twist movement of thorax to left.
Muscles emphasized—Right internal oblique; left external oblique; abdominals.

(b) Left foot forward, left hand forward on handle, pushing forward with twist movement of thorax to right.
Muscles emphasized—Left internal oblique; right external oblique; abdominals.

Both movements use intercostals and back extensors especially, as well as all muscles to some degree.

Garden rake

1. Used to rake up weeds, break up and smooth out soil dug for planting. Fairly heavy work.
2. Used to rake over gravel before rolling or after weeding. Heavy work.

Movement—Pulling backwards and needing longer strokes than the Dutch hoe.

The patient is taught to stand partly sideways, pulling backwards with twist movement of thorax.

Muscles emphasized—As in use of Dutch hoe, but pulling back to the left uses opposite muscles to pushing forward to the left. Handle of rake is long, 183 cm (6 ft) instead of usual 152 cm (5 ft). Rake head is set at 45 degrees off the line of the handle. Position helps the worker to keep more upright than when using handle of normal length and angle.

Light lawn rake

Made from welding bar, fan shaped. Handle 183 cm (6 ft) long, as for garden rake. Made in workshop metal- and woodworking sections.

Light fork

Three tines, 7.6 cm (3 in) across overall. Long handle, 76 cm (2 ft 6 in); this saves the patient from stooping. Made in workshop metal- and woodworking sections.

Hoeing, raking and sweeping

Hoeing and raking and sweeping up leaves (*Figure 3.12*) are always waiting to be done in every garden and they hold great satisfaction for the outdoor person. These jobs are all done standing, and by the use of hoes, rakes or bristle brooms with extra-long handles up to 183 cm (6 ft) the patient can work effectively with very little forward flexion of the spine. Both draw and Dutch hoes are used in cultivated soil between rows of vegetables or groups of flowering plants. It is only the surface weeds that are attacked and the top-soil that is broken up to a depth of about 5 cm (2 in), so that the Dutch and draw hoes can be used with a light, free movement not calling for much power. An increase in activity can be found with either tool if there are weeds growing up in gravel or cinder paths. This work can be done after a rainy spell when the roots of weeds are loosened by the rain whilst the paths will not be wet under foot. After wet weather the soil of the beds would be wet and cloggy to shoes and the tools, and unworkable for the benefit of the plants or the patients.

The garden rake is used to smooth over cultivated soil before planting, or to collect the weeds loosened by the hoes, and requires a longer pulling stroke. Rakes may be cut off at each end of the metal-toothed bar to about 18 cm (7 in) instead of 33 cm (13 in) in width to make their passage easy between groups of plants. The 91 cm (3 ft) wide wooden hay rake used for collecting leaves in the autumn requires considerably more strength for effective use. The bristle or twig broom is another tool that is ordinarily too short-handled, but can be adapted for therapeutic movement by fitting a long handle.

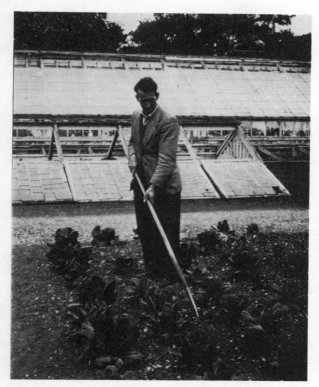

Figure 3.12. – Hoeing using a long-handled hoe to develop back and abdominal muscles

Work with the draw hoe or the rake is carried out with small pulling movements against the resistance of the earth, and pushing out the tool in between strokes to start again. There is greater activity in the rhomboids and the muscles that pull back the shoulders when using these tools than in work with the Dutch hoe. The Dutch hoe is used with small pushing-out movements against resistance and the return pull for the next stroke is lighter. This makes the demand for activity heavier on the pectorals and abdominal muscles than on the back. The twig broom, or besom, is used with wide sweeping strokes which require a fair range of rotary movement between the thorax and the hips and means fairly heavy work on the oblique and transverse muscles of the abdomen. These tools all require some power in the back muscles to keep the body upright, but more especially in the glutei as the body is usually held in a position of slight hip flexion.

The muscles of the hands, arms and shoulder girdle, of course, carry out holding, twisting and pushing of the tools, and the legs have to be capable of full weight-bearing and transporting the body on its way. It is of interest to note here that hoeing, raking and sweeping are particularly useful in the treatment of a patient who is unwilling to give up the support of a stick. Hoes, rakes and brooms appear to make available some visible support when a patient is apprehensive of balance or that a leg might suddenly give way.

The use of all these tools encourages rhythmic repetitive movement. The patient should be taught to stand rather sideways to the lie of the handle of hoe, rake or broom, with first, say, the right hand forward down the handle and the right foot forward. After a few minutes working in this position he should turn, putting the left hand and the left foot forward. In this way the oblique muscles of the abdomen and the intercostals will get their fair share of exercise, with the long extensors of the back, and fatigue and cramp will be avoided. The muscles of the hands, arms and shoulder girdle will be used actively and the muscles of the torso and legs will be called into play in small rhythmic contractions to act as stabilizers.

This work is admirably suited as exercise in the treatment of patients who are recovering from disabilities affecting the spine, abdomen and thorax and will help to restore their capacity to work in the standing position. It can be started gently and carried on for short periods at first, whilst another job in the workshops is kept as a 'reserve' occupation to be carried out sitting down if there is any sign of flagging in effort or enthusiasm. The garden round the workshops must be made into something like the gardens round our own homes; then the patients' pride in its upkeep and general appearance will visibly develop and the length of time they can work standing will be prolonged at their own desire. People who like gardening will appreciate how the activities will develop and increase naturally in the course of a few weeks.

Digging

Digging with either fork or spade entails stooping and lifting. This should only be allowed in the later phases of recovery. It will be useful when a patient is going back to a really heavy job and therefore needs prolonged treatment to develop the necessary musculature. It is always useful to teach a patient how to lift using his leg muscles and to spare the strain on muscles of the back and abdomen. But in digging one is always apt to lift with a twist to turn over the soil, and particular

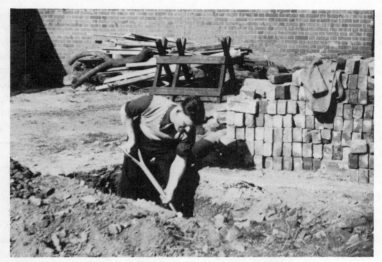

Figure 3.13. – Digging a trench to make a soak-away. A long caliper worn as a support after multiple leg fractures does not prevent full active work to improve general condition

caution must be used in teaching a safe and effective movement. The amount of flexion of the spine that is needed in deep digging makes it 'chancy' as an occupation when used widely for patients who have had spinal disorders (*Figure 3.13*).

Weeding

Some light cutting-out of weeds in a lawn or teasing up the soil with a small hand-fork can well be carried on even lying down, if the individual really wants to carry out this work for the good of a garden. Personal experience during recovery from compression fracture of mid-dorsal vertebrae proved that with a groundsheet, and a couple of cushions under the chest and the elbows, an adaptation of Klapp's crawling exercises may be used with quite good effect on the flower borders.

By using one elbow as a support, the other hand with the small fork can reach a surprising distance into the bed and the positions of hyperextension on alternate sides of arm and thorax provide very pleasant forms of exercise. This type of gardening may have a limited appeal to the conservatively minded patient but occasionally it is useful. After personal experiment it was used quite successfully as occupational therapy for a physiotherapist and for a nurse whose spinal and abdominal muscles were affected by poliomyelitis. Recently a patient with recurrent episodes of thrombophlebitis in the lower limb had the aims of treatment indicated as work with legs raised. The patient had few interests in handwork and was finding life planned on the institutional system rather trying. It was high summer, so instead of arranging work with the legs raised, work with the body lowered was suggested. Postural drainage in the horizontal position assisted physical recovery and the area of the garden lawn provided a small oasis which helped relaxation.

Hedge-clipping

Hedge-clipping might appear to be a useful activity to stretch up the trunk and exercise the extensor muscles of the back, but the demands made on the back muscles by this work have been found to be too strongly static. It is a strain for patients whose spinal and abdominal muscles are in poor fettle. It is a much more valuable type of work for hand injuries and stiff shoulders when the general condition is not much impaired.

Log-cutting

Three processes are used in the preparation of logs which are sold for firewood. These are described in the order in which the work must be done, not as a progression of treatment.

Beetle and wedge

This is the heaviest and most strenuous activity. It is only undertaken by strong patients who are at their final stage of rehabilitation and who are deemed medically fit. Large sections of tree-trunk are split up by driving in a wedge, using strong blows of the beetle (*Figure 3.14*). This has to be heaved in a large arc from behind the body, over the

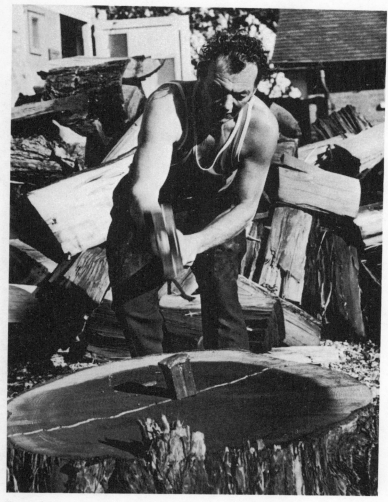

Figure 3.14. – Using a beetle and wedge in the final stages of treatment. This patient had low back pain and left sciatica following an accident at work. He returned to heavy labouring

head and on to the wedge in front of the patient. It is an excellent activity for back and lower limb injuries as a preparation for return to heavy work, and is also a good confidence-builder for the patient who mistrusts his fitness.

Cross-cut saw

This is used on smaller tree-trunks when a patient is capable of heavier work but should still not work with much flexion of the spine. The cross-cut saw (*Figure 3.15*), about 91 cm (3 ft) long with two handles, is worked by two patients, each working with a strong pulling movement with one hand whilst the other hand helps to steady the log on the log-stand. It is easy for even a right-handed worker to hold the upright post handle with the left hand, so that change-over can be made at intervals and each patient gets the strong pulling movement, with rotation of the thorax on each side alternately. This is a very valuable aid in developing mobility of the thorax. The bend forward naturally

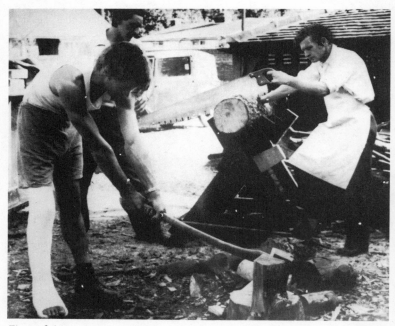

Figure 3.15. – Patient with long leg-plaster chopping wood. Both patients using the cross-cut saw have hand injuries which require activities to develop grasp of hand and full use of arm

takes place at the hips, and not in the spine, with full stroke of the saw. The usual type of log-stand is made rather too low to get a tall man working comfortably, so we use a higher stand which is 91 cm (3 ft) to the top notch of the crosspieces holding the logs in place.

Axe

After the wood has been sawn into manageable pieces, it is then chopped into firewood on the ground using an axe (*Figure 3.15*). Large swinging movements provide excellent heavy exercise for the spine and upper limbs. There is static contraction of the lower limb muscles combined with some hip flexion as the patient strikes the wood.

Patients can progress from cross-cut sawing to using the axe, and then to the beetle and wedge. Not only muscle but masculine ego benefit from log-cutting, and the combination can be a valuable boost to the patient who has suffered nagging backache for some months or years, and believed that he would never feel fit and energetic again.

VARIOUS BUILDING OPERATIONS

Levelling ground for building involves the use of some of the same tools as in gardening. Digging with a fork or spade may first be necessary, then raking over to level off the surface of the chosen site, and using a roller for packing down the soil, smooth and firm. The actual work

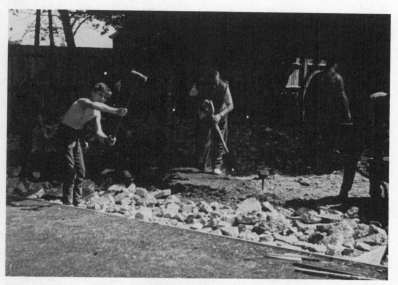

Figure 3.16. – A group of pre-work patients preparing the ground for a hard-standing area outside the workshops to be used for sedentary outdoor work in the summer

required will probably be much heavier, as the site may be uneven, hard and stony if it has not been previously cultivated. But preparing a site for a building project (*Figure 3.16*) provides work that is often suitable and interesting for the patient in the later stages of recovery who wishes to return to a heavy job outside, and nearly all out-of-door work is heavy.

Using the concrete-mixer

A motor-operated concrete-mixer (*Figure 3.17*) is used for larger projects. When there is a number of patients at the Centre requiring heavy work, a group project is often undertaken and concreting has proved a very satisfactory activity for this. It allows for a variety of

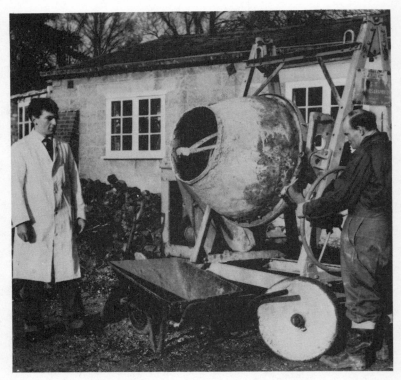

Figure 3.17. – The concrete mixer. A patient in the late stages of treatment supervised by an occupational therapist

processes, some very heavy and some less so, and each patient can participate at a suitable chosen level. For instance, the strongest patients can do the heavy shovelling and bucket-lifting, while less fit patients can level out the concrete on the site or operate the concrete-mixer. Projects have included a hard-standing area outside the workshops for sedentary outdoor work during the summer, and improvements to various paths around the Centre.

Cement-mixing

To make the foundations of a wall, cement must be mixed with suitable grades of gravel or sand, and with water. It is useful to have a small platform at ground level for this. An old door is often available that can

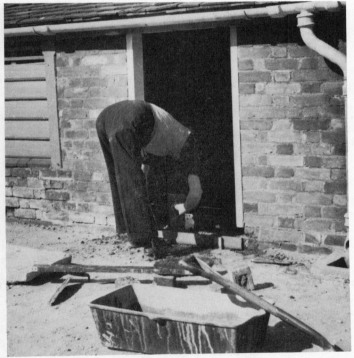

Figure 3.18. — Laying concrete at doorstep of woodstore. In spite of long walking caliper needed for support after multiple fractures of right leg, this patient can bend fully to work at ground level

be used or planks may be joined strongly together with back braces to make a good surface for shovelling together the required mixture. Patients cannot work for long at this type of activity and the programme of all forms of treatment is planned to give variety in activity. Cement once mixed must be used within an hour or two, otherwise it sets hard and cannot be used except to fill up holes in the ground—more economically done by raking surface stones into places where filling is necessary.

The foundation of a wall must first be laid. When the cement is spread out it must be levelled. A board with a straight edge must be provided and a 122—152 cm (4—5 ft) spirit level be available to test that the board is lying level at various angles across the site of the foundations. Small depressions may be filled with a trowel full of cement mixture and then relevelled. If a cement floor is being laid it is usual to finish it off with a rather liquid mixture of cement and water, using only fine sand, if any. A plasterer's float is often used for this operation. The pitch of a floor must be noted so that rainwater will drain out of, and not into, a building. The top of the floor must again be levelled with the board skimming off irregularities as needed.

Bricklaying

This requires additional tools: one trowel about 20—25 cm (8—10 in) long, for laying the cement on the bricks, and a small narrow trowel, 13—15 cm (5—6 in) long, for pointing the cement in between the bricks when the main job is finished. If the wall is built higher than shoulder level some simple form of scaffolding will be needed to allow the bricklayer to reach his work. Planks can be laid across a couple of saw benches, or two step ladders be used as supports for higher levels. It is essential to tie the planks on to the supports as a patient might shuffle along the boards, displace them, and so fall. A helper is usually needed to bring and hand up bricks and mixed concrete. Commercially a hod carrier is used, but for our scale of building an odd piece of board, 61 cm by 20 cm (2 ft by 8 in), preferably with rope handles, will carry all the bricks a patient can lift, and an old bucket will take the cement. A wheelbarrow has been used for transport of these materials and it is usual to lay a plank across ground that may be too rough for the wheelbarrow to run smoothly. A bricklayer also requires a heavy square-ended hammer and a bolster, that is, a 10 cm (4 in) broad chisel, as well as trowels. These he uses to trim off a brick to shape for fitting into corners. He also needs the long spirit level and two bricklayer's pins joined by some yards of cord, so that he may judge the straightness of his lines of bricks. If he is turning a corner to make an enclosure he needs also a square rather like a draughtsman's square, but bigger and heavier, which can be made in any woodworking shop. When the wall is finished the pointing trowel is used. Repointing is often a job needed on old walls to replace cement becoming friable and breaking away between lines of bricks. Pointing is not heavy work, and it can be carried out sitting on a box or stool when working at a low level. As the work gets higher, the patient will have to be able to stand. Apart from pointing, most of the work in building with bricks and cement is heavy but it can be graded up gradually by employing a number of patients together and limiting the period of the heavier part of the activities. It will usually be found that the bricklayer has a rest whilst his store of materials at hand is being replaced. The cement-mixer will pause a while, whilst another helper brings him a bucket of water. Gossip and discussion will inevitably fill up some of the time, and so will the performance of tricks, such as tossing a brick over and over in one hand, which is supposed to be the hallmark of the expert.

Trowels used by a bricklayer can also be used by a plasterer for smoothing over the inner side of a brick building. He will also need a 'float', a piece of wood with an oblong handle on one side, to smooth or 'float' off the surface the small irregularities with very liquid plaster; and a 'plasterer's hawk', also made of wood, about 30 cm (1 ft) square with a peg handle underneath to carry his mixed plaster. These tools can be made in any woodwork shop; in fact many plasterers prefer to make these themselves so that they can get just the right size and balance to suit their hands.

Painting

Painting and decorating may be carried on indoors or out-of-doors. If the surface has not been previously painted, it is usual to start by applying size which can be made from old well-boiled glue, thinned down to a suitable fluidity. Knots in wood may need several coats of this to prevent the resin in them leaking through and discolouring the finished paintwork. A surface that has been painted before will probably need cleaning off. Many patients will ask for a blowlamp to burn off old paint, but the occupational therapist must make sure that the patient is a responsible type of person who is either experienced or receptive of instruction in the use of a blowlamp. It can be a dangerous weapon in the hands of one who is ignorant or irresponsible. Accidents can happen quickly when supervision is withdrawn for a moment.

Various fluid mixtures are obtainable which will soften old paint so that it can be scraped off, just as efficiently as by a blowlamp, though perhaps not so rapidly. The final cleaning of the surface to be painted may be done with first coarse and then fine sandpaper. This last is one of the few processes in decorating that can be done efficiently with only one hand. The first undercoat of paint should be applied before any holes are filled with putty, and then another course of sandpapering will be needed on any uneven surfaces.

Though one hand only may be used, and the paint kettle stood on the floor or on a box, painting really requires the use of both hands, one to hold the paint kettle and the other to wield the brush. The obvious convenience of using both hands is a valuable incentive when the therapist wants to wean a patient from using a stick. One patient who had a cerebellar haemorrhage had taken a year to go through the stages of being bed-bound and chair-bound. He was still obstinately stick-bound when he came for treatment, and the stick seemed unnecessary. He was asked to do some painting which was presented as being urgently needed. He soon forsook his stick, first at work and later in walking. When he progressed to stand on one foot, treadle a lathe, and use chisels for wood-turning he was discharged. His farewell was notable. He had been a foreman bricklayer, and on leaving he begged the writer never to tell his friends that he'd been inveigled into painting. He recited a rhyme which gives the status of various building craftsmen:

> *The bricklayer has ham for lunch—*
> *The carpenter has cheese.*
> *God help the poor old painter man*
> *When the leaves fall off the trees.*

On several occasions patients at Farnham Park have worked brushing down old distemper off rough walls and ceilings before using fresh distemper. We have found it helpful to use rough wire brushes (such as those used to clean files) before the bass and soft sweeping brushes to get rid of loose distemper and dust. We have borrowed from the surgery old slings to tie round patients' heads to keep their hair clean, and surgical masks to tie round nose and mouth. Brown boiler suits have now been supplied to the department. The patients seemed to enjoy dressing up in all this paraphernalia, parading with brushes at the slope on their shoulders through the workshops as they marched off in formation to their 'dangerously dusty' job.

It would not be practicable to go into the detail of all the jobs in the building trade. The tools used have been described in some detail.

The amount of power required must be adjusted to the stage of the patient's recovery. One master builder, who knew all the processes of work to a considerable degree of skill, had had a coronary thrombosis.

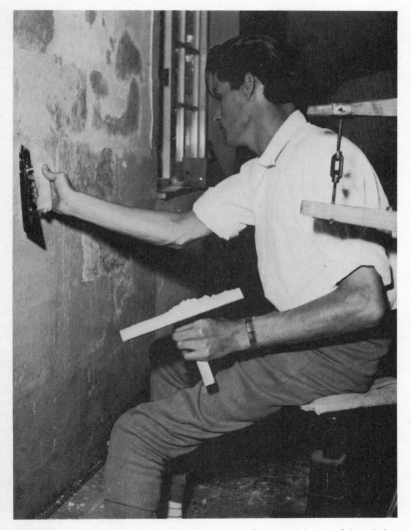

Figure 3.19. – Making good the workshop wall, an activity involving sitting, standing and kneeling. This patient had a below-knee amputation of the left leg, following fracture of the upper third of both tibiae

He plastered the inside walls of the office attached to the workshops. He worked slowly, but very efficiently, and enjoyed the practice of a skill he must have often supervised.

The muscle work involved in doing these activities is very generalized and therefore useful as treatment for the development of muscles anywhere in limbs or torso. Patients with very different disabilities can be variously employed but work in a group together. The rotary movements used are particularly good for spinal exercises, and flexion and extension of the spine can easily be modified as required. Abdominal muscles are toned up with the bending, stretching and twisting movements involved. The muscles of the upper and lower limbs will all be involved in chosen activities.

Before embarking on a building project, the writer would advise any occupational therapist to watch some constructional work. Such observation is nowadays made easy in many large cities in England, where building companies erect special 'viewing platforms' to satisfy the curiosity of the passer-by on what is happening behind a hoarding. It is a traditional joke in England that any hole in the road will be surrounded by onlookers. The student of the kinesiology used in the building trade is advised to join their band, and to study movement as well as enjoy seeing other people work, or have their tea, as the case may be.

PERSONAL ACTIVITIES OF DAILY LIVING

Many of the patients attending Farnham Park have already received ADL training in hospital. Those who do need help are most often hemiplegics, some of whom have not been to hospital, orthopaedic cases such as those with osteoarthritic hips, and patients with head injuries. Some hospitals are so concerned with the correct diagnosis of their patients' physical condition that they overlook their functional competence, and so the patients are not referred to occupational therapy.

Usually, ADL problems are overcome within the first week of treatment, unless the patient has perceptual problems. It is not unusual for a hemiplegic patient to claim that he can do everything for himself but, when questioned in detail, to say no, he could not possibly do this or that because he had had a stroke, as if the therapist were an idiot to suggest such a thing. Analysis of the problem is followed by tuition in the ADL section. An arrangement has been made with the nursing staff that patients with ADL problems may have breakfast in bed. This allows them to take their time in getting dressed either with some help or supervision by an occupational therapist or, later, alone. It also prevents other patients or even nursing staff from over-solicitously helping them in order to get them down to breakfast in time.

Two other major areas of difficulty are cutting up food and bathing. Large-handled cutlery and Nelson knives are loaned or given to patients and a variety of specially adapted cutlery has been made individually

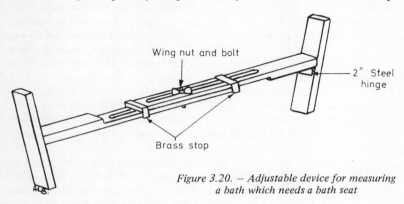

Figure 3.20. — Adjustable device for measuring a bath which needs a bath seat

for those with hand dysfunction. Bath seats are made in the department, often by the patient himself. A very useful aid is a portable bath measure which can be taken on a home visit to simplify taking the measurement of a patient's own bath (*Figure 3.20*).

After injury or prolonged illness, patients often show a marked loss of confidence when faced with traffic or shopping situations, or they may have developed a fear of crowded places, while some may feel conspicuous because of their particular disability. It becomes necessary to reintroduce them slowly into what were formerly everyday activities. Various expeditions are arranged for them to go out accompanied by a therapist who can observe, help and advise on the problems encountered.

DOMESTIC ACTIVITIES OF DAILY LIVING

When a patient works in our ADL kitchen, he or she helps to prepare lunch. As competence increases he does progressively move until the whole meal can be prepared unaided. Cooking lunch has several advantages. It gives the patient a sense of achievement, of having shown realistic ability to do the kind of cooking that will be needed at home; no one can live on cakes and biscuits. Lunch also makes a social occasion when the patient cooks for two, later perhaps for four, and is joined by other patients who stay in the workshops to eat the meal. This gives us an opportunity to help the patient who has difficulty in handling cutlery. No extra cost is involved since the catering officer gives us the ingredients for what the patient would have been eating in the dining room.

Some patients are far more competent functionally in the Centre than they will admit to at home. Two middle-aged women, both with left hemiplegia and histories of cardiac dysfunction, were well able to cook lunch but did almost nothing in their kitchens at home at weekends. (One of them even joined in our weekly social evenings, dancing every dance.) In each case we invited the husband to come and eat the lunch that his wife had cooked in the ADL kitchen, hoping that this would persuade him to be less supportive in future. Unfortunately the habit of many years of indulging a semi-invalid wife prevailed. Both men continued to cook supper after their hard day's work and both women led a boring, relatively useless life, continually bemoaning their hard lot.

Housewives who are going to cook may sometimes be sent out to shop first, to make sure they are fully competent in this area as well. Men too may need help, not only with cooking but also with counselling on how to produce simple meals for one person that are inexpensive, appetizing and nutritious.

When a patient needs to try out housework, the catering officer, who supervises the cleaning of the Centre, allows individual patients to join her workforce for a trial period. Such arrangements need to be carefully planned so that everyone involved knows exactly what he is trying to do. Patients may also be given a specific cleaning or tidying job to do in the workshops, either as a special project or as a regular task.

Occasionally patients want to practise laundering skills. One hemiplegic woman had particularly enjoyed ironing. Since it is always better to encourage disabled people to undertake those jobs that they like doing and to accept help with those that are now even more of a chore than before, we encouraged her. She evolved a complicated system of pinning a garment on to the ironing board to hold it in place. This seemed to us immensely tedious but it gave her great satisfaction.

One patient was offered a job as valet to a retired army officer. This meant that we had to get him to practise brushing clothes, polishing shoes and other valeting activities.

Not all assessment can be carried out in the workshops. Whenever possible and appropriate, a home visit is arranged before a patient is discharged and a follow-up one soon afterwards. Ideally the local authority occupational therapist visits at the same time. In any case, a report of what has been done for the patient and what he requires for the future is routinely sent to the local authority occupational therapist when the patient is discharged.

The relatives are also involved as fully as possible. When it seems appropriate, they are invited to the Centre early on in treatment to give their version of the situation at home. Later on they may be invited specifically to meet the physiotherapist and learn about the exercises the patient should continue at home. At the same time they can discuss with the occupational therapist any outstanding ADL problems.

LIGHT WORKSHOP ACTIVITIES

Some patients who are elderly or who have had a rough passage either before or after operation may be in poor general condition when they first come out of hospital. Even the short walk of 50 yards or so out to the workshops requires some effort. A sedentary activity at a table is about all this type of patient can manage at first. This work may still be therapeutic and develop spinal and abdominal muscles if the position of sitting is arranged with the chair and table at correct working height. As the hands are at bench level the arms will be moved away from the thorax. On occasion, patients who have had thoracotomy operations may be helped by being given an overhead sling to support the arms (*see Figure 7.14,* page 237) away from the thorax. Small accommodating movements of the shoulders and shoulder girdle will call into play the muscles of the torso.

Short walks to the cupboard for tools will entice the patient away from the chair. Tool cupboards set high on the wall will encourage arm abduction and some degree of hyperextension in the dorsal region. If there is an abdominal scar it will be gently stretched by the action involved. As new patients arrive and need more of the therapist's attention the patients who were admitted the week before must become more self-dependent. By suitable devices the patient is led to the expedience of extending activities to suit his own convenience and interests.

Stool-seating

Stool-seating is a simple straightforward activity that produces a good end-product without too much supervision. It is easy to concentrate on the remedial aspects of treatment because comparatively little can go wrong with the craft.

Stool-seating grades itself by becoming increasingly difficult as the seating proceeds. Winding cord round the top of the frame to make a warp is very easy. The cord must be reasonably taut but this does not require very much strength. But when weaving the weft greater concentration and accuracy are necessary, with gradually increasing strength required towards the end of the stool, each thread becoming slightly more difficult than the last.

It also provides a useful bilateral activity. A patient who can only use one hand can have the stool clamped to the table. When there is little use in the hand the stool can still be clamped but the patient can try to hold on to the stool to give himself something to pull against. As the hand improves the clamp can be abandoned so that the patient must use more strength and show greater control with the hand. This activity is useful for patients who have weak grip following a hand injury and also for hemiplegics with only gross grasp, particularly in the non-dominant hand. It is easier to re-educate the affected hand when the other hand is occupied and cannot take over the function of both.

Stool-seating also provides useful work in elevation. Most people prefer to stand for stool-seating. In order to work in elevation they can either be given a taller stool to seat or be asked to work sitting. But it must be possible to see the top of the stool to work out the pattern. When the patient works sitting, the stool can lie on one side with the top facing him.

Patients with back injuries can be given a long shuttle or a long thread according to the stage of the stool. If they work standing they will be exercising their spinal extensors but it is better if they work sitting because then they will also be using spinal rotation.

Stool-seating is useful for assessing semi-fine hand function, concentration, learning ability, ability to count and perception. It is possible to simplify the work by putting web sticks in to mark out the pattern for the patient to follow. Patients can also be asked to compose their own designs. Stool-seating is, however, contraindicated for patients with diplopia.

Some patients, such as hemiplegics, may need help from the woodwork section in assembling their stools; but nearly everyone can manage to sand and polish. A wide choice of stool frames is kept in stock including children's nursery chairs, both with and without rockers, which provide good motivation, especially for grandparents, to work hard. Seating cords of rayon, fibre and plastic are all used. Fibre and plastic are harder on the fingers than the other materials.

Mosaic

This is another simple activity that minimizes the therapist's teaching time, leaving her free to concentrate on treatment and also to treat more patients at one time. A good result is guaranteed and the patients are producing inexpensive, interesting and useful articles. The work can be creative but need not be.

Mosaic work requires continual use of pinch-grip. Most mosaics come already stuck on to net backing so that it can be put straight on to the wall a sheet at a time. The backing must be peeled off, the pieces washed and dried, then glued and placed on the surface to be covered.

Mosaics vary in size from 10 mm ($^3/_8$ in) to 25 mm (1 in) so patients can progress from a coarser to a finer pinch-grip. Italian glass mosaic can be cut up into odd shapes with a glass cutter to make elaborate designs for coffee tables. This requires far more strength and toughness in the hand.

Grouting the spaces between the mosaics requires gentler finger movements and can be used as part of sensory retraining. Mosaic work has been used in the treatment of patients with hand injuries including burns, upper limb injuries, head injuries, hemiplegia, multiple sclerosis and other neurological conditions.

Rug-weaving

Rug-weaving on an upright rug loom will provide exercise for abdominal and spinal muscles at the stage when the patient cannot stand without fatigue. It is also particularly suitable for patients with neck injuries, and for those patients with spinal disabilities who appear to have a functional overlay. It is used in treating patients with shoulder dysfunction and to provide generalized upper limb exercise involving a larger project as a change from remedial games or stool-seating.

Usually flat woven rugs or shoulder bags are made from carpet wool. Occasionally a tufted pattern is incorporated. A fully tufted rug is only woven when the patient requires a specific pinch activity.

A flat woven rug or bag should be completed by one patient. With more than one patient working on the loom, the tension of the weaving will vary and the end-result will be uneven. Tufted rugs can be done by several people and two patients can work side by side at the same time. Even here the standard of work, and the pride in that work, will be higher with not more than two patients involved, especially if one of them intends buying the end-product.

Rug weaving is also discussed on pages 140–142 and 226.

Sewing machining

Sewing machining is used mainly for patients who have an interest in dressmaking or who require practice and assessment for returning to work as machinists. To use it with other patients would take up too much teaching time.

At one time an attempt was made to introduce industrial outwork for the sewing machine. This took the form of webbing arm-slings in four different sizes. Although sewing the webbing together was not difficult it had to be done neatly and it was not always easy to find someone who was both conscientious and interested in this work. We decided that the job was in danger of taking priority over the patients' treatment and now use it more for individual jobs such as special splints.

Printing

Printing is used in various ways as part of a work assessment programme in evaluating the patients' concentration, attention to detail and ability to understand complicated instructions and to carry these out without further briefing. It is also useful for re-educating fine finger movements with or without tweezers for added resistance, and for assessing defects of perception and sight. It is a valuable activity for the more intelligent patient who likes something more challenging to learn as part of his treatment at the Centre.

Because we have two presses, a large foot-treadle press and a small hand-press, we are able to print large hospital forms as well as small letter headings, compliments slips and party invitations. One of our very first jobs was to print large, elaborate certificates for the remedial gymnastic department to hand out to the winning patients at our annual sports day.

Typing

Typing in an occupational therapy department tends to produce problems. Often the typewriter is an old one discarded by the adminis-tration office staff. Even if new it is often poorly maintained, and is very seldom the model that is normally used by the patient who is being assessed for her ability to return to office work. We have been fortunate in obtaining a second typewriter, a reconditioned electric one, which has certainly widened the scope of our clerical section.

Typing is regularly used to provide practice for those returning to this work after a period off sick. It is used to practise fine finger move-ments and manual dexterity and is useful as a non-craft activity for those who dislike craft work. It has been used for patients with severe and permanent hand disabilities who have difficulty in writing; even typing with two fingers will provide them with a better means of communication. Some patients have even begun to learn touch typing in the workshops while others have learned the technique of one-handed typing.

Writing

Writing practice is not only provided for hemiplegic patients but also for patients with other forms of neurological dysfunction and for those with injuries to the upper limb. The occupational therapist's particular function is to analyse the deficits in the patient's movement patterns and to plan treatment accordingly.

There are three basic movement patterns used in writing:

1. The travelling of the hand and forearm over the paper to produce a line of writing. This is usually achieved by slow external rotation of the shoulder.
2. The travelling of the hand to complete each word or group of words. This is normally achieved by extension and ulnar deviation of the wrist.
3. The formation of individual letters by protraction and retraction of the pen which is being held by a pinch action. This is normally achieved by very small extension and flexion movements of the thumb, index and middle fingers. The type of prehension used on the pen will vary with the individual.

When re-educating the patient to write it has been found best to begin with gross movements and progress to fine movements. The first exercise can be to draw long lines across the page to encourage external rotation of the shoulder. Then wrist movement may be practised by drawing short horizontal lines, for example, underlining words on a printed page. This accurately simulates the length of movement that would normally be used. Finally smaller vertical and circular shapes may be practised on wide-lined paper, such as the letters u, o, a, d, g and p. These basic patterns of movement should be well established before attempting to start writing words and sentences.

Sometimes an opponens splint or a narrow strip of Orthoplast moulded round thumb and index finger may be needed to hold a pencil in place. A metal board with a magnetic strip to hold the paper firm is often used, especially with hemiplegics.

Re-educating a hemiplegic patient in the skill of writing is discussed on page 394.

REMEDIAL GAMES

A wide variety of remedial games is used, with different games during one session to provide the maximum amount of movement possible. Virtually any apparatus or commercially available game can be adapted with a little careful planning or used as it is. Notes on the games most often used at Farnham Park for hand injuries, hemiplegics and head injuries, are given below.

Blow football

Equipment and its use   Made in the department, a circular board about 91 cm (3 ft) in diameter with a raised edge and four netted holes for goal mouths spaced at each quarter inside the rim; a table-tennis ball; empty washing-up liquid containers; two sizes of PVC squeeze pump bulbs fitted with rigid plastic tubes.
    Either the containers or the bulbs are used by opposing players to blow the ball into or away from the netted goals.

Therapeutic application   Usually for hand injuries in the middle to later stages of treatment. Can be graded according to strength of blower used: a gross power grip with the container, or a large opposition grip, usually thumb to all fingers, with the PVC bulbs. Blowers can be held differently according to each patient's requirements. Ten to fifteen minutes on this game is usually enough.

Cards

Equipment   Standard pack of playing cards; if necessary, wooden card-holder or upturned brush.

Therapeutic application   Many different card games are played by hemiplegic patients and those with head injuries, from Pelmanism for memory training to more complicated ones, such as whist or cribbage, in the later stages of treatment. Those with hand injuries may also join a group, partly as a social activity if there is some psychological overlay and partly for general dexterity of the injured hand. For any patients who are shy or lacking in confidence, a game like snap or beggar-my-neighbour is an ice-breaker. At times a whole 40 minute session may be spent on this activity.

Chinese puzzle (span game)

Equipment and its use   Made in the department, a board with three pegs; six discs, with central holes to fit over the pegs, graded in size from 20.5 cm (8 in) to 6.5 cm (2½ in) diameter (*Figure 3.21*).

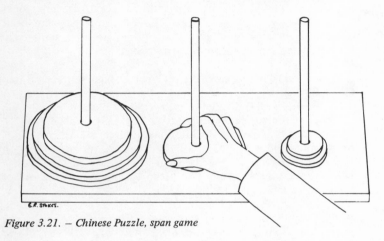

Figure 3.21. – Chinese Puzzle, span game

The game starts with all the discs forming a pyramid on one peg. The object is to rebuild the pyramid on another peg in as few moves as possible, moving only one piece at a time and never placing a larger piece over a smaller one. The minimum number of moves is apparently 63.

Therapeutic application   Particularly useful for hand injuries, to encourage span, extension of proximal interphalangeal joints and flexion of distal interphalangeal joints of fingers. Depending on the size of the disc, metacarpophalangeal joints may be in flexion or extension.

Dominoes

Equipment   Standard set of dominoes; cribbage board and pegs for scoring 'threes and fives'.

Therapeutic application   Used mainly for head injuries and hemiplegics but occasionally for hand injuries, for a short time, for a fairly fine pinch-grip. Involves concentration, number recognition and the use of simple arithmetic, addition and division, for the scoring. The use of the scoring pegs involves fine pinch-grip and good co-ordination. A popular game with most male patients.

Draughts

Equipment   Various types of board and pieces are used, some commercially available, some made in the department:

1. Standard set, with pieces 2.6 cm (1 in) in diameter, each 6 mm (¼ in) high.
2. Large board, with individually turned pieces each at least 3.9 cm (1½ in) in diameter and mostly 2.6–5.2 cm (1–2 in) high.
3. Board covered in black and white Velcro. Pieces are 3.2 cm (1¼ in) blocks of wood with Velcro attached underneath and a loop on top if required for finger extension. 'Kings' are marked with a piece of self-adhesive paper which can be removed at the end of the game (*see Figure 7.14, page 237*).
4. Miniature travelling set.
5. Wall draughts. Board hung vertically, each square having a peg protruding from it to take a draughts piece. These pieces are of different shapes, sizes and weights, the smallest being round, 6.5 cm (2½ in) in diameter and 2.3 cm (⅞ in) thick, the largest 13 cm (5 in) square and 3.9 cm (1½ in) thick.

Therapeutic application   Hand injuries may be graded during treatment from wall draughts, involving a variety of large grips with the hand in elevation, to a much smaller version of the game with resistance if necessary. Mainly opposition grip for most versions of the game but the Velcro draughts may be used for finger extension against resistance by placing the finger through the loop to move the piece on the board. For more disabled patients, such as those with hemiplegia and brachial plexus lesions, the arm may be held in an overhead support such as the OB help arm and the patient may be able to slide the pieces using shoulder movements only. One game at a time is usually sufficient.

Flick ball

Equipment and its use   Made in the department, a board with two end-pieces, one approximately 1.3 cm (½ in) high and the other graded from 3.8 cm (1½ in) to 15.3 cm (6 in) from one side of the board to the other. A wire is suspended between the two ends and may be raised or lowered to increase or decrease resistance by altering the gradient. A table-tennis ball with a hole in it is suspended on the wire. The base board is painted in stripes each approximately 5.1 cm (2 in) wide with scores painted on. Total length of board is approximately 56 cm (22 in) (*Figure 3.22a*).

The aim of the game is to push the ball as far up the wire as possible, by giving it a flick with the finger. If resisted finger extension is required, the thumb pad is gently placed against the finger nail, and the finger must flick against this added pressure (*Figure 3.22b*).

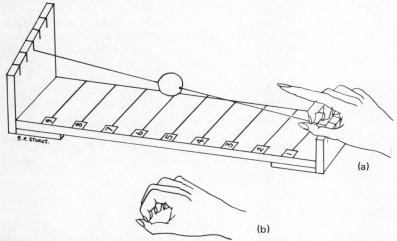

Figure 3.22. – (a) Flick ball game. (b) Resisting finger extension by pressure from the thumb

Therapeutic application   Used for patients requiring active finger extension of proximal and distal interphalangeal joints. Passive extension can be encouraged by using a double or treble finger band (*see* page 344).

Hoop-la

Equipment and its use   Made in the department, a board 46 cm (18 in) square with nine squares painted on it, with a dowel protruding from each; each square has a number. Hoops are cut out of thin plywood or hardboard and painted.

Patient either sits or stands and tosses hoops on to pegs.

Therapeutic application   Rarely used since application is limited. Patient has to hold forearm in supination (not quite full) and forcibly extend wrist when throwing. Elbow is flexed, shoulder in slight ab- duction. Keyhole pinch-grip is required on hoop until it is thrown. Quite good for encouraging wrist extension but other activities, for example woodwork or industrial work, are probably more realistic.

Mastermind

Equipment   Commercially available: plastic board with approxi- mately 0.45 cm ($^3/_{16}$ in) holes in lines of four; small pieces, plastic dome-shaped, and marking pegs, even smaller with holes approximately 0.2 cm ($^1/_{12}$ in) in diameter. Under construction in department: larger wooden board with pegs made from 1.8 cm (¾ in) dowelling, for hand injuries and less co-ordinated patients.

Therapeutic application   Used mainly with head injuries in later stages and with hemiplegics who are alert mentally. Can be used for hand injuries but small pieces are difficult to handle. Has been used successfully with split-hook prosthesis by upper limb amputee. Very interesting and challenging game requiring a great deal of logical thinking, concentration and patience. Progresses quite quickly, so larger version would be suitable for hand injuries.

Nine men's morris

Equipment and its use   Made in department but also commercially available: board approximately 2.6 cm (1 in) thick and 23 cm (9 in) square with pattern marked on and holes drilled to take pegs 0.9 cm ($^3/_8$ in) diameter (*Figure 3.23*). Each player has nine pegs and has to try to form a line of three. Once this is formed he may remove any peg of his opponent from the board. For each turn a player may place one peg on the board or move a peg one space along a line. When reduced to three pegs, these may be moved anywhere on the board. When down to two pegs, the game is lost.

Therapeutic application   Used mainly for hand injuries, either with spring-loaded tongs for opposition against resistance or a power grip (depending on how the tongs are held), or using a fairly fine opposition grip to manipulate the pieces. Some shoulder flexion and extension of the elbow is also involved. Spring-loaded tongs are something like sugar tongs but are graded with different strengths of spring (Epprecht, 1962).

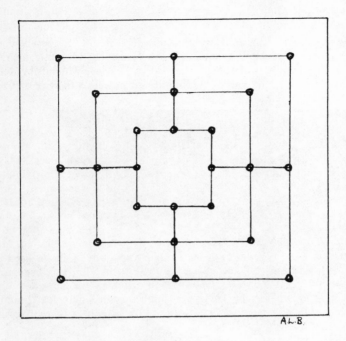

A.L.B.

*Figure 3.23. – Diagram of nine men's morris board showing painted
lines on a square of wood and drilled holes to take pegs*

Noughts and crosses

Equipment   (1) Pencils or felt pens and paper or (2) a board, made in
the department, of hardboard 31 cm (12 in) square with lines painted
on; O's and X's cut out of plywood and painted black or white for
clarity. Players take it in turns to place a piece on the board to form a
line of three O's or three X's.

Therapeutic application   Very rarely used, though (1) may be useful
as light relief for patients doing writing practice, and (2) for hand
injuries or patients with head injuries if they are rather vague mentally.
In any case, used only for very short periods as the game is not very
stimulating mentally. Requires a fairly large opposition grip with
minimal shoulder and elbow movements.

Ring and wire game

Equipment and its use   Made in the department: a loosely coiled copper wire attached to a wooden board 46.8 cm (18 in) long; a copper ring with a handle is attached by a lead to a battery which is housed in a wooden box at the end of the board and powers a light or a buzzer.

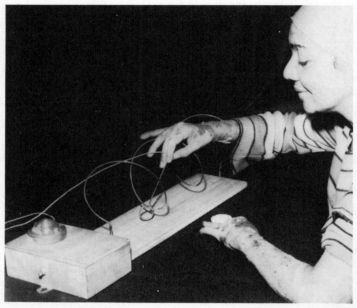

Figure 3.24. − Ring and wire game played by a patient with badly burned hands and arms

The object is to run the ring along the wire without touching it; a touch completes the circuit and activates the light or buzzer. (Our patients complained of the buzz, so this was replaced by a light) (*Figure 3.24*).

Therapeutic application   Suitable for patient with head injuries, disseminated sclerosis and other neurological conditions where co-ordination is a problem, though not when there is an intention tremor. Suitable also for increasing the range of movement at the wrist. This game should be played sitting, and three or four attempts in one session are enough. It can be timed and used as a weekly assessment of speed and accuracy.

Three-dimensional noughts and crosses

Equipment and its use Made in the department, and also commercially available. Four pieces 0.3 cm (¹⁄₈ in) Perspex mounted one above the other, with a 15 cm (6 in) gap between each. Each piece of Perspex is approximately 15 cm (6 in) square. There are 16 holes drilled in each layer, to take pegs of 0.9 cm (³⁄₈ in) diameter. (Pegs are the same as those used for nine men's morris.) The object is to get a line of four pegs either on one plane or going upwards using all four planes.

Therapeutic application Used with or without tongs for hand injuries. Provides opposition grip on the pegs and requires use of elbow and shoulder to reach up to the top level. Also requires good co-ordination and eyesight, and the patient needs to be alert and have good concentration.

Solitaire

Equipment Various types made in the department (but standard types also commercially available). (1) Cotton reels on a peg board; (2) board with holes in to take pegs used with or without clothespegs or tongs (*Figure 3.25* and *see Figure 7.14,* page 237); (3) small board with marbles.

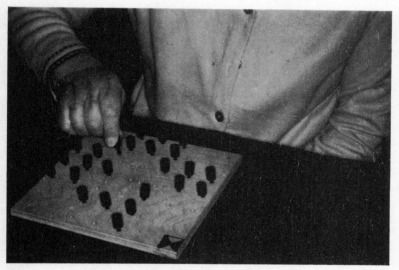

Figure 3.25. – Solitaire board, made in the workshops, with pegs to exercise pinch-grip

Therapeutic application   A useful game for a short time, as the patient can play alone. Becomes monotonous after a while. A good means of quick assessment of hand function. The game may be graded from the cotton reel one, for large pinch-grip, to the clothespeg one, for tough resisted pinch-grip. The version with marbles uses tripod pinch.

DANCING

A dancing class is held every day in the Games Room in the main house. There are six to ten patients in the class which is run by two occupational therapy students, each helping to take the class for two weeks at a time. One student changes each week so that there is always a more experienced student helping the newcomer.

The class originally started as an exercise group for patients with lower limb injuries. The physiotherapy and remedial gymnastic departments were fully stretched and there were no free lathes in the workshops. The patients were already going on daily walks when the weather was suitable but something had to be done to provide further activity. The class proved so successful, particularly in treating those with injuries below the knee, that it was decided to include also patients with head injuries and hemiplegia. This has produced an interesting class where there is not only straightforward exercise but also retraining in balance and encouragement to join in a socializing activity.

There is usually an imbalance between the sexes, and most patients would not know the steps, so waltzes, quicksteps and foxtrots are not really suitable. Country dancing and Scottish dancing are both popular — the current vogue depends on what the student in charge is able to teach. Modern dances like the twist and others that came later are good because there is no need to hang on to a partner, and the patients can just jig around the room. Music is provided by a record-player and records are either bought from general funds or, very often, donated by patients.

SOCIAL ACTIVITIES

Farnham Park is situated about three miles from the nearest town. A proportion of the patients usually visit a local public house near the Centre after supper but occasionally some form of evening entertainment is arranged for them by the head remedial gymnast. The occupational therapy students often stay to help with this. We always have far more men than women patients and many of the men, conscious of their disabilities, often need much encouragement and even persuasion to join in social activities.

It has always been the responsibility of the workshops to make the decorations for the Christmas party with the keen interest and help of the patients, and the department has also helped with other patients' parties. Now it has become the custom that each successive group of students should themselves, during their three months' hospital practice, organize a party for the patients with only a modicum of advice and assistance from the staff. They are expected to plan a theme with appropriate decorations at a minimum cost, and to encourage the patients to co-operate in making and hanging these, in preparing extra delicacies for supper and in running the party itself. The evening's programme must include activities that will involve participation by the more disabled patients as well as those who are relatively fit. It is often very revealing to observe how patients function on such an occasion. The whole affair usually takes some four weeks' preparation and gives the students practice in affording some extra stimulus to the patients' interest.

REFERENCE

Epprecht, E. (1962). *Gadgets and Aids for the Treatment of the Upper Extremity.* 'Milchsuppe', Basel. Sozialmedizinische Abteilung des Bürgerspitals Basel

FURTHER READING

Goldsmith, S. (1976). *Designing for the Disabled.* London; RIBA Technical Information Service
Jay, P. E. (1976). *Coping with Disablement.* 2nd Edition. Consumers' Association

4

Muscle Movement and Posture

The study of human movement is essential for occupational therapists. Fortunately this study is fascinating, will last a lifetime and still holds riddles over which even experts may argue. Fortunately also, at every stage in learning, by observation and application some knowledge will be achieved. This knowledge can be used to help those who need education in muscular control to win the fullest possible degree of function.

The basic principles of anatomy may be learnt from books, a skeleton, and demonstrations or dissections of the subject in an anatomy laboratory. Elementary physics may be called in to help. A bone may be considered as a lever, a joint as an axis, a pressure point as a fulcrum and the slant of the muscle pull as the direction of power. The squares which in the usual diagrams denote the position of weight may be taken to represent another part of a limb or the body, or a tool used on some resistant material in productive work. Analysis of muscle contractions required for holding a position may be made by observation, or special measuring instruments, on one's own body or those of fellow students. All these methods will help to make one familiar with the normal range of movement and extent of contraction available in healthy muscle fibres.

It takes time to appreciate the interplay and balance of muscles working in co-ordination. There is tedium in preparing or reading lists of muscles stimulated into contraction when a series of movements follow each other. This tedium is understandable when it is appreciated that though there is regional representation of body movements in the cerebral cortex, neither individual nor team contractions of muscles are pictured in thought in the untrained brain. The processes by which stimuli initiate contraction and relaxation in muscle fibres have taken scientists as long to unravel as stories recorded in the ancient text of a forgotten language. There are said to be about two hundred

110

pairs of muscles which may be susceptible to voluntary control. It is known that the stimuli which initiate contraction come from motor cells in the spinal cord. These cells receive impulses indirectly from the cells in the cerebral cortex, together with impulses from afferent nerves of sensation. The stimuli are co-ordinated and shared out to muscle fibres in varying degrees of intensity to bring muscles into play. Anatomy and kinesiology must be studied by the therapist and then translated into pictures of action for the patient. Action is a concept that is acceptable to the conscious mind. Even after much time in study, analysis of muscle work takes shape in the imagination more happily as a form of ballet than as lists of muscles tabulated under the roles of prime movers and synergists, primary or secondary fixators. Pictured as a ballet one can appreciate that no principal can play an effective part without supports in the background as well as the fore-ground. What appears as a contraindication is seen as control of opposition. Varying tempos of contraction and relaxation act as foils to each other. The conscious mind acts as a stage director insisting on innumerable rehearsals until balance and economy of movement are achieved.

When performance of a series of actions is satisfactory, action itself fades out of the conscious picture, and the results or associated con-sequences of action occupy the attention. The ordinary adult is forgetful of the practice and concentration that must be devoted to obtain integrated action. The pattern of movement is established and then passes into the limbo of the conditioned reflex. Such automatism may take long to perfect. For example, the baby lying in its cot learns a relationship in distance and direction between the hand and the mouth. Later a spoon may be put into the baby's hand with something nice in it, like jam. The hand still goes to the mouth and the jam is applied to the cheek. Correction and over-correction, growing experience in the amount of muscle power needed to guide the right end of the spoon to the mouth results in the characteristic picture of a baby's face smeared with jam in an arc from ear to ear. At first occasionally, and then habitually, the jam is deposited in the mouth. As the baby grows into the adult, feeding becomes a more complicated ritual. The muscular control needed for coping with various sizes of spoons, forks and knives becomes automatic. The conscious mind is more interested in appreciation of flavours, colour, and all the decorations associated with food, or, untrammelled by mundane considerations, the mind is free to enjoy conversation, creative thought, and plans for the future which have nothing whatsoever to do with the job of eating.

Patterns of movement which become reflex are still dependent on practice for continued perfection. Regularity of practice is dependent on outside conditions associated with the accepted pattern of movement. People who were years in prisoner-of-war camps have told as a joke that for months after their return to good food they had to restrain an impulse to lick the plate, which had become part of the ritual of table manners in prison life.

Habits of self-feeding are a simple instance of conditioned reflexes which are dependent on practice and association repeated on several occasions every day. Many patterns of movement are practised so continually during the waking hours that their stimulation passes almost entirely through the conditioned reflex. The muscles which control general posture when lying, sitting, standing or walking are constantly receiving nervous stimulation. They may contract to reinforce the ligaments around joints, act as stanchions of the skeletal framework, form one part of the body into a stable but elastic platform. They are called upon to redress balance and the effect of gravity. These muscles appear to be in a state of constant tone varying only in degree when there is a change in the external support available such as a chair, a couch, crutches or sticks. It is usually more difficult to learn voluntary control of contractions or of relaxation in these muscles than in those which are called into play to perform productive action for a specific purpose. The mental picture of their function is so much accepted that it has retreated far into the limbo of the conditioned reflex, and it is difficult to recall.

In postural control the head—neck relationship is of extreme importance. The pose of the head is the keynote of the posture of the trunk, it has great influence in the shaping of adult spinal curves, and so in the distribution of the bodyweight. When the head is carried high, with the chin up and slightly tucked in, the whole body looks well balanced, at rest, and yet prepared for action.

The muscles concerned with respiration form a group which respond to stimulation from a mental picture of movement, and can be developed under voluntary control. They also respond to reflex stimulation to act as fixators of the trunk when the movement of the limbs occupies the conscious attention. These muscles also act in response to the chemical processes of living. The intercostal muscles and the diaphragm continue their rhythmic contraction and relaxation during sleep or under anaesthesia, and the stimulus created by a demand for more oxygen will call into play muscles of the shoulder girdle and the abdomen to assist thoracic expansion.

There are said to be about 75 pairs of muscles whose contractions affect movement or position of the skeletal framework. All the muscles of the trunk seem to share in a particularly intimate relationship in the co-ordination of movement in normal life. It would be difficult to differentiate posture and some patterns of movement which seem instinctive, from those which we have been taught in early life, and from others which we have observed in people whom we admire and try to imitate. Throughout our lives we spend a lot of time learning new patterns of movement or in speeding up and adapting old ones to suit a change of purpose. There is pleasure in learning new patterns only when there is an underlying expectation that these will soon retire into the limbo controlled by the conditioned reflex, leaving the conscious mind free to enjoy the results of expertise.

It must be appreciated that the development of such expertise differs enormously with the individual. The student of human movement must watch the passer-by in the street, the fellow-passenger in the railway carriage, people at work and at play, and so learn to observe and appreciate the multitude of postures and patterns of movement that are composed by the permutations and combinations of muscle pulls conditioned by various habits of life. Only by such study can one learn of the possibilities of muscular balance and imbalance, and begin to appreciate the disabilities which may be avoided or cured by re-education of the postural reflexes in all types of activity.

Many phrases are used to describe both physical posture and mental attributes. Stability and balance are qualities valuable both mentally and physically. Grip and grasp and balance are used as descriptions of mental attributes as well as physical descriptions of movement. Perhaps we may again learn from Shakespeare's power of observation when we remember that he made Touchstone start on his chosen task of livening up a drab uncouth girl when he adjured her 'Bear thy body more seemly, Audrey'.

SOME EFFECTS OF BED-REST ON POSTURE

The modern trend in medicine is to cut down both the period of bed-rest and the amount of restriction imposed on movement to the minimum needed to ensure the efficiency of specific treatment. It is appreciated that inactivity has a bad effect on the general condition, and prophylactic measures are taken under medical ordinance by nurses, physiotherapists and occupational therapists so that patients maintain some of their capacities for mental and physical activity. At the same time it is obvious that rest almost always accompanies early treatment, even when not forming a specific part of it, and patients differing in age and habits of life will differ widely in their rate of deterioration in power and control of movement. With no intention to paint too black a picture of the side-effects of bed-rest, it may be of interest to note some of the resulting disabilities that require treatment by rehabilitation, and discuss the proximal cause of discontent between the corporate consciousness and the body after a period of rest.

The effects of illness or injury will interfere with more than the intimate function of an organ or a limb. The postural muscles of the trunk seem to be peculiarly vulnerable on all counts. The muscles and skeletal frame of the trunk are susceptible to disease or injury equally with the limbs. Muscles of the spine, thorax or abdomen must be divided when organs or structures inside them require surgical intervention to improve their function. Scar tissue in these muscles has the same tendency to contraction as scar tissue elsewhere. The patient is just as disinclined to initiate movement which causes discomfort or pain when the scar is in a trunk muscle as in a limb. As well as being directly affected by injury or disease, movements of the trunk must often be restricted during treatment primarily directed to restoration of function in a limb.

Restriction of movement is known to result in bulk wastage of muscles. This occurs more quickly in muscles such as the glutei, which are habitually in a state of action or preparedness to preserve the erect position of man. The glutei are superficial and their bulk wastage is easily observed. It may be assumed that deep-lying muscles principally used to maintain posture will deteriorate with disuse as quickly as those whose wastage and flaccidity can be seen and felt. It may not always be easy to assess muscle wastage by diminution in bulk. Often with idleness there is an increase in interstitial fatty tissue, or oedema due to a slowing down of the lymphatic circulation which depends so much on localized muscle contractions. This latter type of muscle deterioration, when there is an increase in bulk, is more difficult to treat than the former, as the bodyweight is the same or greater than before illness whilst the power available to move it is less.

The uneven wastage of various muscle groups accounts for some of the inco-ordination of movement that may be observed. Another cause is the interruption of the practice of muscle control. Patterns of movement become misty and forgotten with disuse, just as the muscles themselves are weak, slow and uneven in their response to the stimulation of a dimmed mental picture of action and its results.

Bed-rest is inevitably a most disrupting factor to the conditioned reflexes of postural control. During normal life the human frame is accustomed to some hours of relaxation in a comfortable chair or bed, and the conscious mind will relax too, receptive when listening or reading, passive when thoughts or dreams pass in and out, or unresponsive in deep sleep. But when the human frame is kept lying down through long waking hours, the conscious mind expects to be kept occupied with impressions from the outside world. It is natural to want to read or to watch what is going on around. To keep the eyes in the viewing position the head must be raised, supported by pillows pushed up from behind, or poked forward by an unaccustomed and tiring activity of the muscles at the front of the neck, shoulder girdle and abdomen. The normal head—neck relationship is put out of gear. The spinal curves revert to the long C shape of the baby, the dorsal curve increased and the lumbar curve flattened out. In this position the spinal muscles have little reason for activity. Their disuse occurs mostly in the stretched position which encourages a rapid deterioration of muscle fibre. The diaphragm, thoracic and abdominal muscles are cramped in the concavity of the C shape. There is reduced expansion or contraction of the thorax as inactivity lessens the demand for oxygenation of the blood. Even small demands for air entry into the lungs are made difficult to meet by the resistance both of atmospheric pressure and of gravity. These are increased with the greater area exposed to their influence when the body is extended than when it is erect. The muscles of the abdomen as well as the thorax are at a disadvantage. Everyone who has been nursed in bed will remember the difficulties of defaecation when using a bed-pan lying down. The whole metabolism of the body depends on some habits of life which involve changes of position, opportunities of movement which involve contraction and relaxation of muscles stimulated by conditioned reflexes. The general tone of trunk muscles plays an important part in the satisfactory performance of vital organs in the thorax and abdomen.

Spinal and thoracic joints may have only a small range of individual movement, but they are accustomed to frequent use. Like other joints, when immobilized or used in less than their habitual range, they become stiff, the capsules and surrounding soft tissues losing their elasticity. The vicious cycle of disuse will have altogether a more widespread and, therefore, a more harmful effect on the general condition when inactivity includes the trunk than when only a limb is immobilized.

The degree of disorganization of habitual posture which results from bed-rest will, of course, be relative to the amount of restriction of movement and to the duration of time for which restriction has been imposed, as well as to the individual reactions to restriction. Prophylactic measures by nursing, physiotherapy and occupational therapy may do much to lessen residual disabilities. The muscles of the spine, thorax and abdomen are supplied by nerves which are susceptible to voluntary control. Control may be learnt and some muscle power retained by exercises and the practice of work carefully taught and supervised. Special bed-tables, arm supports, and back supports may be designed to enable the bed-fast patient to carry out activities in positions which are as little cramping as possible. But these measures must all be secondary to the specific aims of treatment which have included a necessity for rest, and must take their place as an episode in the day's programme which must already appear a busy one to the patient in bed. And although all imaginable treatments may be prescribed to maintain some elasticity and power of movement, these will all take place in bed, and not in the erect positions, sitting or standing, which are customarily held by the reflex contraction of postural muscles during the waking hours of normal life.

There are other factors which will disorganize normal habits of posture and movement. For example immobilization of a limb or the spine and inhibition of muscle contraction have their after-effects as well as the paresis or paralysis discussed in the chapter on hemiplegia. Immobilization of limbs or spine includes splintage applied externally or internally. External splintage requires further subdivision into rigid splintage such as is provided by plaster-of-Paris casts, semi-rigid splintage such as jointed calipers or polythene moulds and lively splintage, giving spring support to some joints. These limit the range of movement to within that which could be harmful to paretic or painful muscles and the joints which they control and prevents the overstretching of tendons and capsular ligaments around these joints. Internal splintage necessitates a surgical operation, and may involve such things as the insertion of a pin down the length of a fractured bone, plating with screw fixation and bone grafting of bones affected by disease or trauma. Such surgical treatment will involve some bed-rest but is often carried out to avoid prolonged bed-rest. The application of rigid or semi-rigid splintage is usual before weight-bearing activities are permitted, though weight-bearing is used later to encourage the formation and consolidation of callus. External splintage may be continued for months or years and during this time activities must to some extent be limited. It is obvious that, without support, for some patients many activities would be impossible or fraught with insecurity and pain or discomfort, with their deleterious effects.

With removable splintage patients may be treated with physiotherapy and remedial exercises to a gradually increasing range of movement without resistance except that of gravity or the weight of the limb. A smooth supporting surface, or better still a therapeutic pool will do much to help eliminate gravity or weight when such exercises are performed. In occupational therapy there must always be some resistance in carrying out work, however light this may be and whatever external supports may be provided. Occupational therapists must learn to increase such resistance and decrease assistive supports with discretion as well as with medical guidance.

Inhibition of muscular contraction will somewhat surprisingly often be observed. This may occur after operation or trauma involving bone or only soft tissue. Inhibition is especially easy to observe in the quadriceps, and will benefit very obviously from re-education which is sometimes started by a physiotherapist using faradic stimulation. This produces a muscular contraction both seen and felt by an observant patient. Until this inhibition is overcome to some degree, specific exercise of individual muscle groups will be without value. Wide group muscle activities carried out with remedial exercises and occupational therapy will assist recovery. Muscle contractions are so interdependent that wide activities involve an overflow of stimulation spreading even to inhibited and paretic muscles. This stimulation does not produce contractions easy or possible to observe in the early stages of treatment. But the writer is convinced that such overflow of stimulation to contraction and relaxation occurs and will speed recovery. Occupational therapy must always involve the activities of many if not all muscle groups of limb or trunk. The attempted segregation of activity is useless and fatuous, and may even have the effect of increasing inhibition, just as when a patient himself tries too hard to achieve a muscular contraction by voluntary effort. In occupational therapy the patient's attention is largely attracted by the productive results of his work and little attention is paid to muscular contractions. The latter is the duty of the occupational therapist devising the treatment. The division of the patient's attention is not wholly a disadvantage as reflex and overflow stimulation of the affected group may occur when the attention is focused on a broad group activity. The writer has observed contractions in a paretic tibialis anterior after anterior poliomyelitis. Faint contractions are difficult to observe in a large group of muscles such as the quadriceps. It is reasonable to suppose, however, that as the quadriceps are habitually used in conjunction with the glutei as well as all other leg muscles in walking, apparently inhibited quadriceps will react to reflex and overflow stimulation when the glutei are actively used. Such active use occurs on a foot-power lathe when the patient sits on a bicycle stool and the affected leg is lightly slung under the lathe.

It should be stressed that such treatment should be carried out in close co-operation with physiotherapists and remedial gymnasts, and timed to follow these. After treatment by exercise under dry heat or in a therapeutic pool the limb will be warmer and more supple than before. The patient's attention will have been focused for a short time on specific contractions. When his attention is distracted the reflex and overflow stimulation will be the more easily spread to include apparently inhibited muscles. Co-operation and co-ordination of various treatments are essential to obtain good and rapid results. Emphasis on one or other treatment is the duty of the prescribing medical officer, the appreciation and carrying out of the prescription the duty of the members of professions supplementary to medicine.

In every programme of treatment where progression is planned, after rest or limitations of mobility have played their part, there comes a time for the increased resumption of activity. For most people the idea of activity includes an intention to move from place to place without help from others and maintaining something approaching the erect position with balance and control. The use of the hands may be the goal of achievement, but the torso and legs provide the base, pivot and positioning for their use. After enforced rest, inco-ordination of posture and movement becomes apparent in any activity, and though some generalized weakness may have been expected by the patient, the loss of the sense of balance comes as a surprise. For some patients balance in the prone position has become habitual, for others sitting up in bed has progressed to sitting in a wheel chair. Ambulant patients' balance has been adapted to include carrying the weight of a plaster. Even the change from plaster to walking caliper needs readjustment of balance. As all forms of support such as crutches, sticks, belts or collars are gradually discarded, further readjustment of balance is necessary.

Such readjustments are more obviously difficult for patients suffering from disabilities of the lower limbs or spine, but lack of good balance may also be noticed amongst patients with disabilities of the upper limb. An arm paralysed from anterior poliomyelitis or peripheral nerve lesion is a dead weight on one side; trauma may require splintage which is an added weight. Many disabilities involve the application of a sling which transfers some of the weight to the opposite shoulder or to the wrist. Imbalance of the shoulder girdle becomes apparent when necessary splintage and slinging are discarded, even if this be gradual.

The necessity to relearn both postural control and patterns of movement arouses some resentment in the corporate consciousness. When muscle control was first learnt in early life it was an adventure. The world was small in those early days, as a baby cannot see far. The control of the small muscles which focus the eyes was learnt as slowly as other patterns of movement. Then there were few distractions from the job of learning how to move, and if such distractions were unpleasant, such as an unfastened pin in a nappy, it must have been some relief to voice that displeasure. It is not so easy for the adult. The world is large for him to see, and there are many distractions that are difficult or painful, as well as some that are perhaps too pleasant. Adult pride will prevent appealing against difficulties with a furious howl. The adult will prefer to emphasize the importance of distractions which provide an escape from the tedium of incessant practice necessary to recondition the postural reflexes. Yet this alone permits regainment of the fullest possible functional activity and permits freedom of the mind to enjoy its results.

It has been noted that when lying down in bed the spinal curves conform to the large C shape of the baby. When sitting up with a back support, the head-forward position will persist to balance the legs, whether outstretched or supported by a knee pillow. Starting to get up, a patient will often begin to walk in much the same way as in early childhood. The toes are put down before the heels instead of using the adult heel—toe rocking action. The body, accustomed to the angle of hip flexion in bed, leans forward. The head is poked forward and the eyes look anxiously down to the feet. All the old patterns of movement seem to be forgotten and the impression is given that this is as much due to the poor distribution of bodyweight as to general flabbiness of musculature.

In teaching any pattern of movement as a part of rehabilitation the importance of the head-neck relationship must be stressed as the basis of good posture. As the poise of the head is relearnt, the other spinal curves will fall into place and balance will improve. Exercises carried out in front of a mirror will do much to help the development of good posture. Many persons have an accepted picture of themselves in activity which is quite unrelated to their state when the practice of movement has been interrupted. Exercises carried out with the bodyweight supported by water in a therapeutic pool will help to develop the sense of position and enable the patient to put joints through a full and increasing range of movement. Free exercises will progress to those against resistance and the bulk and power of muscles will improve. But it is almost impossible for a patient inexperienced in pure movement to keep the attention fixed on contracting or relaxing groups of muscles for any length of time. Even when considerable emphasis is laid on the necessity to practise exercises, this can only be carried out periodically and may easily become just an incident in the day's programme. There still remains the problem of relearning postural control, and this must be done whilst carrying out many jobs in life which entirely engross the conscious attention.

The significance of therapeutic occupation is not always appreciated when considering the treatment of patients whose primary disability is situated in the trunk, or who have developed the secondary disability of deterioration of postural muscles. It is easy to see the value of occupational therapy for disabilities affecting the upper or the lower limb. It is obvious to the patient as well as to the doctor. The limb on the affected side can easily be compared with its partner, and there is some standard of mobility and power available as an incentive for effort.

In a simple analysis of function of different parts of the body the legs act to transport or to support the trunk, which in its turn supports the head. The trunk also provides the pivots from which the hands are brought into position to perform those actions which transform into reality the ideas formulated in the brain. It is in their capacity as stabilizers of the limbs that the muscles of the trunk can be brought into play and their power developed. The practice of work entailing the use of arms and legs will restore old patterns of movement. But if the postural reflexes are to be reconditioned to their best advantage, it is essential that such work should be specifically planned and supervised so that it is carried out in a good position.

Some occupational therapists complain that they are directed to work with patients in a way that is classified as 'diversional'. Further study of the problems of posture would suggest directions to include aims which are 'prophylactic'. By appreciating the dangers to reflex tone of postural muscles that must accompany bed-rest, it may be possible to prevent some of the secondary disabilities that occur whilst primary disabilities are being treated. Other occupational therapists say that the prescribed aims of treatment are indicated as being 'general tonic'. Such a prescription is not to be despised. It does imply recognition that all the muscles as well as the personality of a patient need toning up during or after a period of inactivity. Here again the study of posture may lead to wider and more interesting developments of the therapeutic use of occupations.

It must be recognized that all patients do not need prophylactic or general tonic occupational therapy. Perhaps the period of their incarceration in bed can be foreseen as short, and their personality or musculature judged to be of the type which is not disposed to rapid deterioration. Some people are the better for a period of comparative idleness when they can study, repose, and have time to think and get their ideas into perspective. Others again may benefit more by short periods of breathing exercises in bed, and for the rest of the time not filled by medical treatment or investigation, may be safely left with a large pile of detective stories or crossword puzzles which will amuse and occupy the superficial mind and its demand for a logical conclusion.

Occupation in itself is not the aim of an occupational therapist. The stress must be laid on the idea of therapy — a treatment of some condition. The necessity and probable or possible value of any treatment for any condition must be assessed by the medical officer who undertakes the responsibility of treatment. This assessment must take place before the aims of treatment can be seriously or honestly considered and indicated.

Diversional, prophylactic, general tonic are all terms that have their uses but may also be employed to cover a lot of vague and muddled thinking. It must be stressed that occupations must be specifically planned to encourage the maintenance or the development of good postural control whilst diverting the patient's attention from the boredom that attends the path of continued practice. Economy and co-ordination of movement of a limb can only be achieved when the trunk muscles stabilize the platform on which the limb pivots. Success may only be claimed when general balance and reflex control of the postural muscles are maintained whilst the conscious mind is engaged and free to enjoy the results of movement.

The physiotherapist and the gymnast have certain advantages in working with the patient in gym shorts or bathing dress in a pool. The doctor in his clinic may see the patient undressed. These people can measure the range of joint movement or the circumference of a limb more accurately than the occupational therapist who works with the fully-clothed patient. Naturally measurements taken in a therapeutic pool will show better results than elsewhere, because of the warmth and support of the water. Individual exercises with spring or weight resistance or assistance may show different measurements. The doctor's clinic has an unfortunate effect on some patients. A limp, stiff back or stiff finger may be exaggerated either through an exhibitionist desire for sympathy or increased palliative treatment, or through a nervous anxiety to show off which brings on increased spasm in muscles and so spoils the effect. Too frequent measurements in various departments may well make a patient over-anxious, so that a disability looms unreasonably large. It has been considered therefore that actual measuring should be reduced to a minimum in occupational therapy workshops. Notes are made at staff conferences of when and where measurements have been made, and these are checked up with observations of patients' movements at work. Such observations made in workshop or garden have some advantages as the patients are in something approaching their natural surroundings. On occasion a much freer range of movement can be seen from a distance than is available when the patients feel 'on parade'. By receiving reports from different departments at staff conferences a medical officer can check up on his own findings at a clinic. Some patients look upon a doctor as one to whom people must make complaints and report symptoms. Sometimes the complaints and symptoms are not borne out by general behaviour and habits of movement carried out in everyday conditions. That team work in rehabilitation includes the combination of all observation and knowledge of the various specialized departments, can never be too often repeated.

RE-EDUCATION OF THE POSTURAL REFLEX

The process of re-education of the postural reflexes always seems to begin with the head—neck relationship. The use of head balance to lead off a push or pull with the help of bodyweight may be observed in many activities. In twisting round the die holder in cutting a screw thread on a bar of metal the operator will push his head forward to counter-balance the weight of the body thrown back to reinforce the pull of the arms. Some pianists on a concert platform are interesting to watch. The hands are the principal tools of his art, but emphasis on loud sudden chords will be accompanied by a head thrust forward, the shoulders braced, and the bodyweight thrown into the scale for good measure. Long slow notes seem to be drawn out of the piano with the pull back of bodyweight, led by a backward head movement. It would be impossible not to include every muscle in the body if one were attempting to analyse the movements involved in playing a piano.

It is fascinating to observe the head—neck relationship and see how much this is used to balance and lead the flow of movement. So when observing a new patient starting on work, one may first consider that general posture and co-ordination of movement are poor. Then one notices that the head dips forward to increase power and backwards to regain balance in a jerky, useless manner. The hand will follow, jabbing at the work. It is easy for the patient to see that uncontrolled movement has resulted in a scratch on a piece of metal, an ill-beaten thread of weft on a loom, or a crooked saw-cut. It is essential for the therapist to demonstrate smooth rhythmic movement, and a capacity to handle tools with efficiency and control. To make tools do their work neatly, co-ordination of movement, poise and control are more necessary than power, and more easy to imitate. The patient will begin to want to make friends with the tools, and to feel that they must be controlled as a specialized part of himself if they are to do their job properly. The disposal of bodyweight increases the effect of muscle power, and stabi-lization of the head—neck relationship makes possible the use of bodyweight to its best effect.

It is obvious that for the production of work that will stir a patient's ambition to succeed, good tools and materials are necessary. Workshops with good lighting are one of the first essentials for encouraging a satisfactory head—neck relationship. The patient must be able to see what he is doing without poking the head forward, as would be natural for anyone working in inadequate light. Chairs and benches must be adaptable to people of various heights and stable enough to give con-fidence. But it is not sufficient for the occupational therapist to design or choose workshops and equipment. It is necessary to learn to observe the patient's posture, sitting, standing, walking and working, and to be able to demonstrate and teach smooth and economic movement as being dependent on good posture, and applicable to each individual patient.

This teaching must be carried out with clear and simple explanations and tact, so that the patient does not feel 'nagged at'. It must be stressed that reconditioning the reflex is sometimes a slow job. The co-operation of the patient is needed, and to get this the therapist must win confidence. Learning to appreciate the difficulties of this is an early step in training the therapist. The value of gaiety and laughter in a therapeutic workshop is difficult to exaggerate. The tense, edgy patient must sometimes be wheedled, bullied or teased into laughter that will assist relaxation. Inco-ordination of movement is often due to spasm in muscles, which may be the result of anxiety, lack of confidence and insecurity. These may be eased when there is some confidence in the hope of enjoyment. Laughter may be one way to achieve that relaxation which is the beginning of co-ordination in movement. But the technique needed to produce an atmosphere in which postural control may be developed, and smooth reflex conditions, is as indefinable as the colours of a sunset.

FURTHER READING

Brunnstrom, S. (1972). *Clinical Kinesiology*. Philadelphia; F. A. Davis Co.

5

Disabilities Affecting the Spine

Patients suffering from disabilities affecting the spine are usually in need of reassurance. All too often they have not had the opportunity to discuss their problems with anyone who can really help. Doctors do not usually have time to listen and the only people who have the time are frequently uninformed about spinal conditions. It is worthwhile for the occupational therapist to take time at the initial interview both to listen to what the patient has to say and to stress that he may come back for further discussion.

Before planning treatment it is relevant to ask the patient where he experiences pain, how often and what activities trigger it off. Some problems may appear more important than others and these may usefully be tackled first. Someone who has difficulty in sleeping or wakes up in pain during the night may find that a mattress on the floor provides a better night's sleep. Fracture boards to go on the bed under the mattress, from at least the back of the neck to the sacrum, can be made in the workshops. Boards that cover the whole bed are better because they cannot slip out of place, while a sheet of 12 mm (½ in) plywood cut to the size of the bed is best. Any support must be the full width of the bed so that it lies firmly on the sides of the frame. If the frame is wooden the support may be fixed with a few screws. Some patients with spinal disabilities have sexual problems and if the therapist can provide an opening will be relieved to discuss them, though this will only be helpful if the therapist can suggest a solution. For example, the position recommended for intercourse with a pregnant woman may be equally suitable for both men and women with spinal disabilities.

Patients who have suffered pain over a long period of time tend to lack confidence in treatment techniques. We have found that confidence can be improved if the therapist can make the patient understand her belief in the treatment offered at Farnham Park. She explains that what a patient does in the workshops is all part of a concerted effort by all the staff to improve the condition of his back during a full day's programme of exercises and activity, carefully graded to his individual needs.

Keeping in touch with other members of the treatment team is always important but particularly so when treating patients with back injuries. Treatment in physiotherapy aimed at correcting postural defects must be reinforced in occupational therapy; work in the remedial gymnasium is carefully graded so that the patient is not too exhausted to work in another department for the next session. If the patient forgets his back and shows more functional competence in the workshops than in the doctor's clinic, other departments will need to know this in order to grade their treatment accordingly.

Doctors differ in their approach to the treatment of back injuries, some putting emphasis on spinal rotation at an early stage, others on extension followed by flexion. These preferences must be respected, particularly when patients are referred for treatment prior to possible surgery. Sometimes this conservative treatment will prove so successful that the need for surgery is eliminated. At other times treatment is used diagnostically to highlight the patient's problems. The way he reacts in the workshops and in other parts of the Centre will give a much more objective assessment than when he is seen only in a consultant's clinic. When surgery is inevitable, conservative treatment will help to build up the back muscles pre-operatively and so produce better post-operative results.

Normal function of spinal muscles requires movement of the trunk in order to place the shoulder girdle and upper limbs into a position where they may be used with the greatest mechanical efficiency, and be maintained in this position for as long as is needed to perform a particular task. When standing or sitting with the arms hanging loosely at the side of the body, gravity is pulling down through the trunk; in order to maintain normal erect posture, the spinal muscles are doing minimal work. When the arms are brought forward and upward into a functional position, the muscles of the spine come into action more strongly to maintain the required position. This working position is used in the early stages of treatment. As strength and mobility improve, bending forward to work at a lower level increases the pull of gravity and hence the work of the spinal extensors. This working position is therefore adopted in the later stages of treatment.

It is always essential that muscle power should be developed one step ahead of joint mobilization as an unstable joint is a serious liability and, without the balanced contractions of the stabilizing muscles, tendons and ligaments around joints would soon suffer from stress.

The stability and alignment of the vertebral joints have a special importance. The spinal cord is held in place, supported and protected in the neural arch of each vertebra. The nerve roots pass through the foramina between the pedicles. Any injury, instability or deformity of the vertebral joints which causes malalignment may lead to pressure on the spinal cord or the nerve roots. Such pressure can cause paralysis of the muscles, the nerve supply of which is damaged, or intense and exhausting pain from nerve root irritation. Numbness and loss of joint sense may also be a symptom. This pain and paresis is experienced in a limb, and it is not always easy to convince the patient that the damage is in the alignment and stability of the spine and not in the limb of which he complains so bitterly. In all stages of treatment it is essential to watch the patient's posture, and to re-educate the postural reflexes by seeing that chairs, benches and other equipment are suitably adjusted. It will take some time for the patient to connect cause and effect, and to understand and then put into practice therapeutic movements relieving pressure and irritation of the nerve roots.

A large proportion of spinal disabilities are treated by fusion or bone graft between the vertebrae, an internal fixation intended to maintain the spinal column in such a position that pressure on the spinal cord or the nerve roots is avoided or relieved. In certain diseases, such as ankylosing spondylitis or spinal caries (a tubercular condition) ossification of the vertebrae will produce rigidity of the spinal column. In the past the patient was kept for a long time in the optimum position whilst this ossification was developing. When treating patients with long-standing disabilities of these types extreme forms of rigidity of the spine will be encountered. In other cases removable collars or corsets are supplied to limit the range of movement of the spinal column. Such supports may be necessary for only a few weeks or months; sometimes they may be worn more or less permanently when work requiring any strain is being carried out. It is usually the policy of the Centre to wean the patient off such external support. Often he has become so habituated to its comfort that the aims of rehabilitation are directed towards developing a musculature that will be adequate for the maintenance of correct posture without external support.

In occupational therapy, when a patient is of necessity working against a certain amount of resistance, it is essential that little effort should be made to increase the range of movement of the spine before there is full assurance that the muscles will be capable of controlling that range. Free exercise under the eye of the physiotherapist is less fraught with danger and may be carried out without the resistance of gravity or with the assistance and support provided by warm water when the exercises are carried out in a therapeutic pool. This will be enough to keep free or gradually increase the range of movement with safety. The occupational therapist will be fully occupied in developing sustained and controlled power in the postural muscles as well as developing the patient's capacity to adapt his mode of life to the range of movement which is safely inside his measure.

There are various curves of alignment and ranges of movement in the cervical, dorsal, lumbar and lumbosacral regions of the spine. Range of movement in each joint is small; the gross range of movement of the vertebral column of the normal person is extensive. This gross range appears to be more limited by a disability affecting one or two vertebrae in the living body than would appear likely when studying the vertebral column of a skeleton. This is explained by the muscular attachments, which, by overlapping each other, govern the movements of the whole region of the spine wherein the affected vertebrae may be situated, and beyond into the neighbouring regions.

When considering the treatment of patients with spinal disabilities it has been found convenient to divide the patients into groups according to the region of the spine principally affected. The occupational activities have been chosen and adapted to develop the postural muscles within such limitations as have been imposed by the regional disability.

LUMBAR SPINE

In the lumbar region the vertebrae are much larger than elsewhere. These vertebrae carry not only the weight of the torso, arms and head, but also the pull of the powerful muscles which control the wide range of movement available in this region. By reason of the shape of these vertebrae, their spinous and transverse processes, there is a much wider range of movement in all directions in the lumbar region than in the dorsal. In comparison with the cervical region, extension may be about the same but forwards and sideways flexion, and rotation to either side, are much more free.

Trauma in the lumbar region is less likely to have fatal results than higher up in the vertebral column, as spinal nerve roots and connecting links with the sympathetic nervous system, controlling the reactions of the vital organs, mostly leave the spinal cord in the cervical and dorsal region. The bulk of each lumbar vertebra provides considerable protection to the spinal cord in its own area. It is perhaps the free range of movement available between the lumbar vertebrae which makes the effects of trauma in this region not fatal but crippling. Long-standing pain, spasm of muscles and limitation of movement are the symptoms commonly met amongst patients who are sent for rehabilitation. These symptoms make the patient anxious, lacking in confidence to return to work and a normal life. They are apprehensive of making a movement which may start the pain again or intensify it. This apprehension is in itself enough to cause inco-ordination of movement and muscle spasm. It is often easy to say that a symptom is functional or that someone is lacking in moral stamina and desire for independence. But it must be remembered that to the patient the pain is very real and may have been real for a long time and that this pain is often eased by prolonged rest, and renewed or intensified by activity. Patients will also have heard many an 'old wives' tale' about spinal disabilities and injuries which form the opening chapter to the story of a bedridden life.

The number of patients sent for rehabilitation with disabilities primarily affecting the lumbar region is large in comparison with other spinal disabilities. This group is not only important numerically, showing the comparative frequency of disability in this region, but important in that members of it have been difficult to treat, apprehensive in their approach to occupation and demanding much attention and encouragement from the therapist. Successes there have been, but many have only been partial: an alleviation of symptoms, some restoration of confidence, an acceptance of disability and acquiescence in return to a life which may be rather different from the previous one of activity.

In the lumbar spine the muscles must be in a condition of constant tone acting as fixators when any movements of hand or foot alter the position of bodyweight. This condition of tone easily passes into spasm. Something can be done to ease this spasm by learning smooth co-ordination of movement, neither easy to teach nor to learn. The first step is restoration of confidence. It is essential, therefore, that the early stages of treatment by occupation should not make too heavy demands on power and range of muscle movement, but should rather develop their co-ordination. The bodyweight must not be shifted jerkily, but in a smooth rhythmical manner, otherwise pain or spasm will result, thus causing the patient to regret his initial confidence in the value of rehabilitation.

Back pain is usually part of a vicious circle. Pain is caused by inflammation or overstrain or damage, such as from a prolapsed intervertebral disc or pressure on the sciatic nerve. The reaction to this pain is loss of alignment of the spine in order to remove the pressure and so reduce the pain. But the loss of alignment will itself provoke overstrain, swelling and more pain. The first aim, therefore, is to correct the alignment of the vertebrae and simultaneously strengthen the muscles to retain this realignment. Symmetrical muscle power is important. If there is weakness in the muscle to one side of the spine, the stronger muscles will pull the spine the opposite way. Similarly, if there is spasm in one group of muscles, the spine will be pulled in that direction. Postural training must therefore be combined with an increase in muscle power.

In the early stages of treatment it is important to build up the erector spinae. The patient should work with the spine in a stable position and with the vertebrae well balanced, not using either forward or lateral flexion at this stage. But the intervertebral joints must be mobilized to improve the circulation and reduce the spasm in any affected muscles. When using the spinal extensors to keep the spine erect and therefore stable, it is possible to promote, at the same time, smooth voluntary rotational movements which will use the spastic muscle in a rhythmic pattern. Using rotational movements in this way achieves partial mobilization of the joints without affecting the stability of the spine. This mechanical stability must be maintained in order to improve posture and so reduce pain. If the spinal nerves are no longer being impinged on by slipping movements due to mechanical derangement, there will be a reduction in the swelling which accompanies inflammation. Building up the spinal muscles and improving the patient's general condition will help him to improve his posture and maintain a mechanically correct upright position.

At Farnham Park the medium of treatment for back conditions is usually woodwork (*Figure 5.1*). This activity can be very easily graded and gives both a physical and psychological boost to the patients. Men feel that they are doing something reasonably tough. Women are not only amazed that with a spinal condition they can attempt woodwork but also enjoy the attention they inevitably get from the other patients in the woodwork section who are mostly men.

The patient should stand at a high bench with his work no lower than elbow level. If necessary the wood can be raised in a vice for sawing. The height of the working bench is of the greatest importance and the varying height of patients has led to the development of various methods of heightening not only work benches but also looms and other equipment in the occupational therapy workshops. *Figure 5.2* shows one simple method of putting an adjustable raise on a bench. Another method is to use a system similar to bed blocks but with the hollowed-out space in the block deeper than usual, to give extra stability. Two blocks joined together by a plank of wood the width of the bench will be more stable (*Figure 5.3*). Yet another excellent method is to use a dentist's hydraulic chair. The base of such a chair, with a bench top fixed on it, may be easily raised and lowered; it is particularly suitable for a printing table since some patients will work sitting and others standing. One of the woodwork benches at Farnham Park is kept permanently raised for the convenience of early-stage patients but even

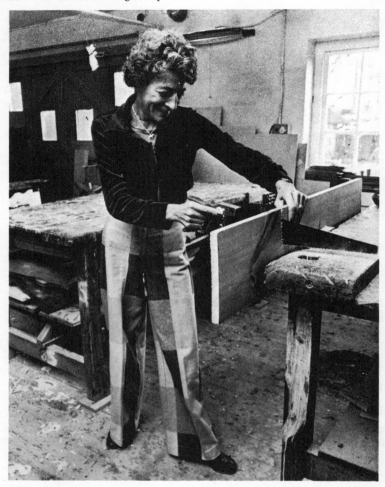

Figure 5.1 – Patient with low back pain and general debility in the earlier stages of a programme to build up working tolerance and spinal musculature

this needs to be adjustable. One patient with a lumbar disc lesion was 2 m (6 ft 7 in) tall. His bench had to be raised to nearly 122 cm (4 ft) to enable him to do woodwork, and the bicycle stool, on which he sat occasionally when working, was stretched to its limit.

Some patients may need to adapt permanently to a higher working surface. One patient was a highly skilled engraver and designer for a

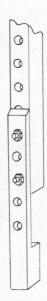

Figure 5.2. – Detail of extension leg for a woodwork bench or upright rug loom. This is not stable enough for a large bench

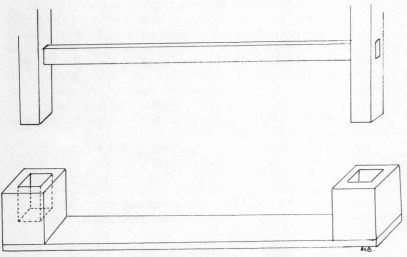

Figure 5.3. – Method of raising a bench to a fixed height

famous firm of goldsmiths and silversmiths. He was not at all confident that he could carry on with his work, as he could neither sit nor stand for any length of time with comfort. The writer visited him in his workshop about a year after he had completed his course of rehabilitation, and saw that he was carrying on quite well. He had adjusted his workbench so that he could sit on a high stool or stand to work, and had become accustomed to working either way.

When choosing an article for the patient to make in woodwork, something large and simple will be most suitable. Small pieces of wood and intricate jobs will only provide static work. Long working movements are necessary to give active extension and rotation of the spine; sawing, planing and sanding are all appropriate. Complicated joints should be avoided, half-lap joints or gluing and pinning being much better. Articles of sufficient size to demand the correct movements will include coffee tables, step ladders, cupboards, large toolboxes, bookcases, clotheshorses and trolleys. The patient should stand with his feet apart, facing the bench. His spine will rotate gently as his arms move but, because he needs to watch his work, his head will remain in the same position. The movement in the lumbar and dorsal regions will also provide rotation and extension exercise for the neck. It is good practice to provide work which demands that the spine exercises as a whole unit. This technique can also be adapted in treating injuries of the cervical spine.

Patients with back conditions must be given adequate rest while in the workshops, especially in the early stages. Rest periods should not last for more than five minutes but they must provide proper rest and be supervised by the therapist until the patient learns the art of relaxing. Effective positions will vary and may be sitting, standing and leaning against a wall, or lying down, if necessary on the bed in the ADL unit. Patients are often reluctant to rest on a bed, feeling that they are giving in to their condition, but must be reassured and persuaded to accept this as part of their treatment if they cannot rest properly in another position. Suitable resting positions are shown in *Figure 5.4a, b* and *c*. To begin with, patients may work for spells of, say, ten minutes interspersed with five minute rest periods. Activity is upgraded by lengthening the work spells. Providing rest periods for patients with back trouble is much more difficult than for those with limb injuries. For the former, leaning against a bench is contraindicated and is not a therapeutic way of resting, although putting one foot on a stool when standing, to flex the hip and knee, thus flattening the back, gives temporary rest and increased comfort.

Patients with spinal disabilities need to keep reasonably warm. Feeling cold will not only be uncomfortable but will make the back tense and exacerbate muscle spasm. (Some patients have found warm body-belts of more value than supportive corsets.) In the workshops it will be necessary to choose a place to work well away from draughts, especially after a session in hydrotherapy.

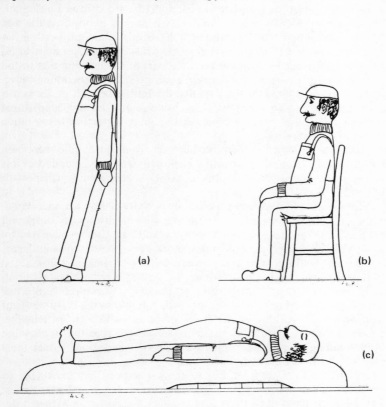

Figure 5.4. – (a) Resting in the standing position. (b) Resting in the sitting position. (c) Resting in the lying position

Although most patients with spinal disabilities go straight on to woodwork, this is not always possible and the more nervous patients with long-standing histories of symptoms may be best started on light sedentary work. Particular care must be paid to the height of the chair on which they sit. This must be set low so that the knees and hips are at right angles and the feet firmly planted on the ground with the weight carried on the heels. The sacrum should be against the back of the chair and the lumbar spine supported; the shoulders should be back and the shoulder blades pulled down. It may be useful to have one or two chairs with back-rests that are adjustable in height and angle, for those who do not get adequate back support from a conventional chair. The provision of foam-rubber cushions which may be used on the seat of the chair, or occasionally at the back, has been found useful. Attention paid to comfort in seating is well worthwhile in the treatment of all patients and is particularly important as part of the introduction to the workshops of patients with spinal disabilities. The therapist's sympathetic attitude towards the patients' disabilities will do much to win their confidence. This makes it much easier to suggest occupational activities which can be graduated fairly quickly up to those demanding an increase of exertion.

Industrial outwork, using the bilateral overhead handle, has been found useful for patients with low back pain who need a period of less active work during their treatment. This is described in Chapter 3, page 62.

Stool-seating is sometimes used as an activity before starting woodwork, and may be carried out either standing or sitting. The work will get harder as the stool nears completion, and can also be increased by using a closely woven pattern so that more work is involved in each row of weaving. Wall draughts and warping up on a warping board attached to the wall are other useful activities.

In good weather a proportion of patients much prefer to work out-of-doors. Hoeing and raking are both suitable in the early stages of treatment and working in the fresh air often makes the patient feel generally more fit. However, patients are always told that if they get tired standing they should come back to the workshops, either for a supervised rest or a change of activity.

Patients with disabilities in the lumbar region may have loss of sensation or paraesthesia in the lower limbs, or they may have sciatica. The origin of these conditions should be explained to the patient. Any sensory defect should be carefully assessed and reassessed to monitor improvement or deterioration. If there is sciatic involvement there is likely to be residual weakness in the leg muscles following a period of time with a painful leg and possibly a limp. All the lower limb machines can be of value in providing bilateral exercise. Since the referral of these patients usually includes a warning to avoid forward flexion of the spine, sitting at the lathe on a bicycle stool, leaning forward at the hips towards the lathe, enables this precaution to be observed. At the same time there is good demand for active contraction of the glutei and hamstrings. These muscles are very commonly wasted after a spinal lesion which has caused pressure on the nerve roots in the lumbar region. A few patients have shown considerable wasting of the dorsiflexors of the ankles. One such, a man aged 23 years who had just

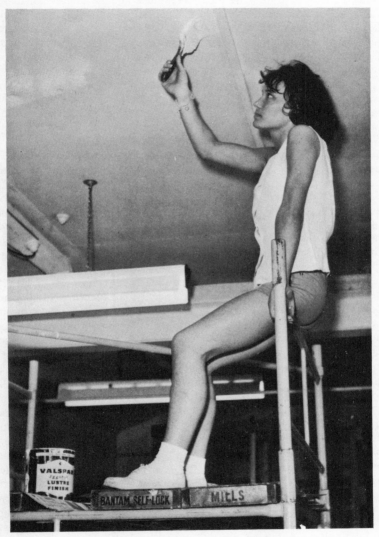

Figure 5.5. — Patient who had a laminectomy of the 5th lumbar vertebrae following prolonged back pain, painting the ceiling in the woodwork section

completed his training as a master plasterer, wanted to make himself an elaborate signboard. He cut the letters of his name and qualifications out of sheet brass. Working on the ankle-rotator saw with a metal fretsaw blade gave him the required exercise for the dorsiflexors, and filing the letters on the bicycle filing machine exercised the glutei, hamstrings and quadriceps. He sawed, planed and polished the oak board on which he screwed the letters. It was a fine job when it was finished. He averred that it only cost him a fraction of what a commercial firm would have charged for such a high class board.

While patients are still working in extension in the workshop, they will be going through their maximum voluntary range of spinal movement in the gymnasium and in physiotherapy. They will not necessarily be flexing in the standing position but may be when lying down. They will almost certainly be while exercising in the heated pool.

Patients may arrive for treatment wearing lumbosacral supports. It is usually the policy of the Centre to help patients to give up wearing corsets by developing their spinal muscles to do the work instead. Sometimes this takes time because the spinal muscles have already atrophied through prolonged lack of exercise. The corset is first taken off in the gymnasium where the patient is doing pure exercise, and retained in the workshops. Gradually it is worn for only half a day, then perhaps for one session, then just in the evening and finally discarded.

Patients need to be constantly reminded about good posture until it becomes a habit even when they are concentrating on other things. The patient should be told to draw himself upwards from the crown of his head, with his neck neither in flexion nor extension. The therapist can help by putting one hand on the centre of the patient's back and the other about 4 cm (1½ in) above his head, and then asking him to push up to reach the upper hand. His shoulder blades should be drawn back and down. His feet should be slightly apart and close to the bench when working. It sometimes helps to chalk a toeline on the floor.

Upgrading the patient's treatment may be done by increasing the time spent on any activity, and in wood-turning by increasing the thickness and/or the hardness of the wood to be worked. When the erector spinae are stronger and posture is improving, it will be time to begin mobilizing the back by working at a lower bench (*Figure 5.6*). If the patient is very tall this may mean progressing from an extra-high bench to a standard one. As the back continues to improve, increased mobility can be demanded by getting the patient to cut out wood on the sawing stools. Kneeling on a large sheet of plywood between two sawing stools, to saw it through, is a good working position but scares some patients. An alternative is to place the plywood so that it overlaps the edge of a low working bench, and then kneel on the top of both the plywood and the bench. In this position the spine is 'slung' between the shoulders and the hips, and gravity pulls the spine towards hyperextension. The

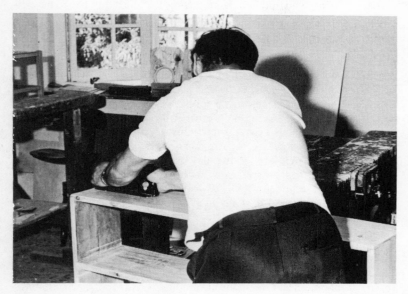

Figure 5.6. – Patient upgraded to work at a lower level to increase mobility of the spine, and using large sweeping movements as he planes a bookcase

spinal extensors are working as fixators but not as strongly as in other working positions. Some patients find this a very comfortable position for work but it is contraindicated for anyone with sciatic stretch pain.

Sometimes it is possible to provide work at floor level, either kneeling, semi-kneeling or bending right over. One patient who had been able to achieve only minimal spinal flexion in the doctor's clinic, was seen in the workshops the same afternoon bending right down to floor level to mark the correct length to be cut off the legs of his coffee table to make it stand even.

Cross-cut sawing on a sawing horse is good heavy work for the later stages of treatment. Many patients with spinal disabilities never really trust the man at the other end of a double-handed cross-cut saw. These patients prefer to saw logs on their own, being nervous of the other man pulling too quickly, before they have finished their own pull, and so jarring the spine. It has been found that a single-handed cross-cut saw cutting on the push out is more satisfactory for this type of patient, as it requires spinal rotation without much flexion. The latter movement may be taught to take place in the hip joints.

One patient who did cross-cut sawing had hurt his back, he said, while working as a 'sewer man' and had not worked officially for two years. After four weeks of exercise, bench work and cross-cut sawing he decided he would accept suitable work if offered by the 'town services' — it was surmised that this meant road sweeping. This man was not an easy proposition. He had seven children and his weekly packet of 'benefits' came to about 25p less than he had been in the habit of earning. His general reaction to work was not unwilling nor did he appear fatigued by working on a cross-cut saw, at least not as fatigued as one might reasonably expect from his history of official unemployment.

It is to be expected, of course, that some patients will be sent for rehabilitation rather late in the day when their own hospitals have whistled all the tunes they know, without the successful result of the dance leading the patient back to work. A change of surroundings will often speed rehabilitation. One such case was a railway fireman, aged 26 years, who had minor wedging of the first lumbar vertebra as a result of a fall from the tender of a railway engine. Two months' immobilization was followed by outpatient treatment at his local hospital. Eleven months later he was sent for rehabilitation apprehensive to a degree. As frequently happens, such apprehension caused widespread spasm in his muscles. Gradually in the therapeutic pool, and with work that interested him, he started moving more easily. He did woodwork and wood-turning. Eventually he was sent for short periods to our local Skill Centre, where he was employed in helping to repair the roof of a lorry with the aim of regaining his confidence in working above ground level. After a total of 13 weeks' rehabilitation he went to work in the railway stores, but said he intended to return to work in his own job.

Patients with lumbar spine fusion have had to learn to adapt their co-ordination of movement to the limitations of spinal rotation and flexion enforced by the fusion. It sometimes surprises even an experienced occupational therapist how smoothly these patients with permanent limitations of movement in the lumbar region can learn to move so that their disability becomes unnoticeable. It has been found that this improvement in postural movement is much more easily achieved when there are several patients with the same disability at different stages of recovery being treated at the same time. The competitive spirit is easy to arouse, but there is also the unconscious instinct of imitation. Good carriage and posture are essential in therapists themselves if they expect patients to learn to walk, stand and sit correctly.

A contrast has been observed between those patients whose pain has been relieved by laminectomy and those who have felt no benefit. The latter have no confidence in treatment. 'Lack of moral fibre' may be attributed to some, but persistent and unrelievable pain may wear thin the fibres of courage in many of us. The threshold of pain wears low in the passage of time as do the marble steps of an old cathedral. The relief, mental as well as physical, is startling amongst those in whom surgery has found a further organic lesion. These patients have suffered from the fear that the 'evil lay in themselves', in their thoughts and not in their backs. This fear has only found expression when it has proved groundless.

Patients have often been referred for treatment for low back pain. When the first edition of this book was published, the writer was criticized by an eminent consultant because low back pain is not a diagnosis. Nevertheless it is now accepted as a syndrome which may be either physical or psychological in origin, or a mixture of the two. Treatment will be similar to that outlined for other disabilities of the lumbar spine but particular emphasis will be placed on getting the patient interested and involved in his work, to get him to relax, to rebuild his confidence and to give the therapist the opportunity to observe his functional level.

Until pain can be accurately measured and evaluated, there will always be some doubt about the condition of patients when no formal diagnosis of specific spinal disorder has been made. These doubts also apply to patients who have an outstanding case for compensation. At the same time it must be realized that spinal disorders are not easy to diagnose, and that because no cause has been found for pain this does not mean that pain does not exist. When a patient has a claim pending, this may prove a relevant factor in his recovery. The workshops and the large gymnasium are where the staff are most likely to discover if he is pretending to greater disabilities than actually exist.

DORSAL SPINE

The natural curve of the dorsal spine is concave forwards, balanced between the cervical and lumbar curves which are convex forwards. The ribs spring forward from their articulations with the dorsal vertebrae to form the staves of the barrel of the thorax.

What is described as hyperextension in the dorsal region is a muscular effort to straighten out the normal dorsal curve. The effect of a straight back is increased by pulling the scapulae together and flattening them against the posterior wall of the thorax. When one looks at an articulated skeleton, it is not easy to appreciate how little space there is available between the dorsal vertebrae and the ribs, and how easily nerve roots may be compressed.

With any damage to bone tissue that can be demonstrated by radiographs there must be some damage to neighbouring soft tissue, which together will cause local effusion and oedema. When these occur in the neighbourhood of an already narrow foramen there will be nerve-root pressure, resultant pain and spasm in the area applied by sensory or motor nerves through the affected nerve root. The movement that is most likely to cause narrowing of the foramina is forward flexion. Hyperextension will expand the foramen. The difference in the range of movement from forward flexion to hyperextension between vertebrae in the dorsal region is very small, but it is enough to be of first importance in the planning of an occupational therapy programme for patients who have any lesion in the dorsal region. Rotation of the spine does not cause acute narrowing of the foramina, and it can be combined with hyperextension in much productive work. Forward flexion must be avoided until it is specifically in the medical directions for progressive treatment.

Some patients with fractures of the dorsal spine may go back to their own jobs after a week's rest and treatment for shock because their jobs are well within their scope of muscle power and range of movement. The patients who have continued to suffer pain may be sent for rehabilitation. Some are nervous of movement because they have not understood the mechanism that is causing pain and are afraid of aggravating their symptoms. This fear is in itself enough to cause spasm and disability. Others again have muscles that have wasted from weeks of disuse, except for short bouts of exercise that they have not continued to practise when away from supervision. These are the symptoms which must be treated by rehabilitation. In nearly every case it has been found that the patient was as much lacking in confidence as in muscle power or range of movement and that general improvement in all these conditions occurred together and not independently. The aims of treatment were directed to co-ordination of movement with a view to the patient regaining confidence as much as to the development of firm muscle.

Activities described as appropriate for treating disabilities of the lumbar spine can equally be used in treating disorders of the dorsal spine. In addition weaving on an upright rug loom has been found therapeutic. These looms also require some foot-power work on the pedals to change the sheds, and so give practice in general co-ordination. Their main value has been found in the development of hyperextension in the upper dorsal spine, as well as giving some opportunity for spinal rotation. The position of work is good and the general movements of arm extension and flexion all have their values in shifting the body-weight, which does so much to improve the tone of the postural muscles.

Upright looms as normally made should have extension legs added to them to ensure that patients stretch up to reach the beaters; the normal height of these looms requires little stretch and so provides less exercise. The patient must be taught to pull down the beater with the hands as far apart as possible, the elbows bent and in line with the

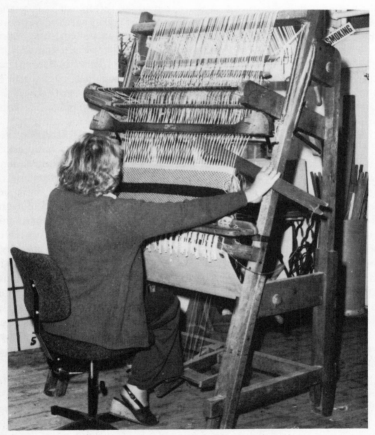

Figure 5.7. — Weaving on an upright loom, sitting on a low chair to encourage extension of the whole spine, especially the cervical and dorsal regions. The large shuttle necessitates wide movements of the arms, and shoulder girdle activity

shoulders. Then the long back muscles will get their exercise in the most beneficial position of hyperextension in the upper dorsal region, and the rhomboids will pull the scapulae together. The rhomboids are particularly useful to the occupational therapist as they are superficial and their action can easily be felt through the clothes. In teaching weaving on an upright rug loom the demonstrator can ask the patient to lay a hand on the spine between her shoulder blades before the demonstrator checks up in the same way on the patient when pulling down the beater. The rhomboids, in some books on kinesiology, are classed as having leverage of the third class on the scapulae. They are not very large or powerful muscles but they act in such close co-ordination with others, such as the middle and lower parts of trapezius and latissimus dorsi, that one may well assume (except, of course, in a patient who has had poliomyelitis) that these other muscles are getting their share of exercise when one can feel the rhomboids harden and pull the scapulae together. When the scapulae are held back there is much more opportunity for expansion at the sides of the thorax. The intercostal muscles come into play and the thorax expands as the ribs lift upwards and outwards to balance the movement of the arms.

One patient, a girl aged 26 years, with compression fractures of the eleventh and twelfth dorsal vertebrae came for rehabilitation 12 weeks after her accident. She tried rug-weaving on the upright loom but it was found that this increased the pain in her back and had to be discontinued. This happened before the writer had had enough experience with injured spines to observe that there is a considerable difference in the effect of pulling down the beater in several sharp bumps, and pulling it down slowly and gently to press the wool into place. The latter method has proved to be more effective in developing the back muscles, and safer in that it avoids any tendency to jolt the spine. It makes just as firmly woven and beaten a rug as when using the customary method of bumping down the wool into place. In this case the girl had to change to sedentary occupational therapy. After four weeks she returned to her work as a Post Office telephonist which she did sitting. It was considered that the reaching up for the telephone plugs would be work suitable as a continued form of exercise for her postural back muscles.

Another patient was a housewife aged 57 years. She came for rehabilitation 12 months after a road accident when she sustained a compression fracture of the twelfth dorsal vertebra. She did rug-weaving very successfully, using the gentle pull-down method. After six weeks' treatment she returned to her home duties.

We have also treated a number of patients with multiple injuries which have included fractures of the dorsal spine. It is perhaps invidious to select just one of these for comment; the injury and disability was however, very dramatic and the recovery so satisfactory that it is hoped that the choice will be of interest.

A young man aged 26 years, a university graduate in mining and geology, fell 21 m (70 ft) down a mine-shaft. He sustained a compound fracture-dislocation of the left ankle which could be set and put up in plaster, but there was also a fracture-dislocation of the twelfth dorsal vertebra. It was found necessary to carry out an open operation to unlock the articular processes of the twelfth dorsal and first lumbar vertebrae. He was about six months in a plaster-of-Paris jacket. He had a considerable degree of paraplegia which gradually cleared up, and when he came for rehabilitation 13 weeks after the accident, he could walk on elbow crutches. He still had marked weakness of both ankles, the left, naturally enough, being the worse. He could just move round the foot-piece of the ankle-rotator saw with his right foot and was entirely unable to do so with his left. He could work on the bicycle saw. He was very keen to progress and was apt to over-exert himself, and after the first week he had to be put on to rest in the afternoon for about three weeks. This was gradually diminished and he returned to a full programme. The bouts of exercise on the bicycle saw had to be kept short, and in between times he learnt typewriting as a sedentary job. About six weeks after admission he started wood-turning, sitting on a bicycle stool, keeping to short periods of 20 minutes to half an hour at first. In another six weeks he could work on the lathe for one hour without fatigue. He was, rather sporadically, practising on the ankle-rotator saw, but being of an impatient nature, he needed some firm handling to persuade him to work steadily in a good position, as he could see more results from his efforts if he waggled his leg from toe to hip rather than rotating the foot on the ankle with a minimum of knee and hip movement. (The original ankle-rotator made at Farnham Park did not have any attachments to stabilize the knee.) However he steadily improved and was walking reasonably well when he was discharged after 25 weeks of treatment, though there was still some weakness in the glutei and quadriceps which gave him a rather undulating gait. He returned to study medicine at his university and the following year bicycled down 25 miles each way, just to show off his complete recovery, to our great satisfaction.

CERVICAL SPINE

The range of movement between the cervical vertebrae is almost as free as that between the lumbar vertebrae. The vertebrae are specialized, the first and second being singled out by special names. It is between these two vertebrae and the occipital bone that most of the rotary movement of the head takes place. Fractures and displacement of the cervical vertebrae are not commonly met in an active rehabilitation centre for the reason that they are often so serious as either to cause immediate death or a paraplegia so complete that ambulant rehabilitation is out of the question.

When sitting or standing in the best position to anticipate controlled movement, the head is carried on the neck with the chin held slightly up and tucked in. The articular surfaces of the occipital bone rest plumb on the atlas, the first cervical vertebra, but allowing for the curve, concave posteriorly, the neck would appear to form an angle of about 45 degrees with a line drawn from the external occipital protuberance to the point of the chin. When a plastic collar is employed it does not hold the head firmly enough to prevent some rotation, but the flexion will be very much limited both forwards and sideways.

The occupational therapy arranged for patients who are in an external support must take into consideration the limited area of vision that is possible in the prescribed position. The article which is being constructed must be fairly small and of a type that can be kept fixed on a bench at eye level when the patient is sitting and later on when he is standing at work. It is very fatiguing to hold work up as high as this even with the arms supported. It is essential that a vice be available. This further limits the choice of the article that can be made. Leatherwork by saddle-stitching or thonging may be held in saddlers' clamps which are themselves held high in a vice. A small easel with an adjustable slanting frame such as that used for a deck-chair will be found useful. Paper may be fixed on it for the patient to practise writing or drawing. A small warping board can be adapted in the same way and later on a table loom tilted up at the back will allow the patient to see the weaving comfortably. Plywood, or pieces of sheet metal, may be held high in a vice and cut out with a fretsaw to make toys or brooches.

Netting also requires the use of both hands freely and equally even if one or both require support. This can be carried out sitting or standing, without encouraging neck flexion. Industrial outwork using the bilateral overhead handle (*see* page 62) has been found useful for patients with stiffness in the neck, for example, following cervical spondylosis.

When a patient starts to discard the external support, it has been found wiser to carry on at first with the same type of work. It demands enough effort to continue the same movements without support. Rotation of the head will develop naturally in the desire for a wider field of vision. Sideways flexion, which cannot be carried out without some degree of rotation, will develop next. Forward flexion is the last movement to be encouraged, and will take the longest time to regain as it is very much inclined to cause pain and aching. As a patient becomes accustomed to doing without support, he will find it natural to work at a more normal level in woodwork or in the garden. Picking up a fallen tool may be done at first with a sweeping stoop, bending mostly at the knees. Economy in the use of movement is an incentive to more natural movements.

Nearly all patients with disabilities affecting the cervical spine have shown some degree of paresis in the arms. For these patients sling arm-supports are essential for any productive work to be possible whilst the patient maintains reasonably good posture. The buoyancy that is obtained for exercises by carrying them out in a therapeutic pool should be imitated as much as possible. There may be some advantage even over pool exercise in the spring and sling arm-support, as the assistance given can gradually decrease with any sign of returning power in the muscles that need development.

We used to make our own spring and sling arm-supports. These had a freely swinging metal overhead section attached either to the back of a chair or to a woodwork bench. Guthrie-Smith springs between the overhead support and the arm-sling provided buoyancy and the following case histories illustrate this system. We now use the OB Help Arm, which works on a different system (Ellison, 1971). This can also be used for a similar programme of treatment with diminishing arm support.

A man aged 43 years had a sudden onset of pain and paresis of the arms which responded to bed-rest. When the symptoms returned 18 months later a laminectomy was performed and the disc between the sixth and seventh cervical vertebrae removed. He started rehabilitation one month later, free of external support for his neck, but needing a spring-loaded sling to support his right arm. This spring assistance started at 15 lb, and was gradually reduced to 5 lb, before being discarded. He had had a varied industrial history from lorry-driving to roof-tiling. It was decided that it was inadvisable for him to return to such heavy work, so the therapist was directed to develop fine hand movement and to assess his adaptability to factory work. He worked on a small electrical screw-cutting centre lathe and learnt to use small taps and dies in making up screws to hold together a loose-leaf photograph album. After eight weeks he returned to work as a maintenance fitter in a factory. Fifteen months later he reported he was in the same job. He still complained of numbness of his right index finger.

Another patient, a man aged 27 years, had been a physical training instructor. He had injured his neck, and three years later a diagnosis of prolapsed intervertebral disc between the fifth and sixth cervical vertebrae was made. There was no obvious wasting of the muscles but he complained of inability to use his right arm. No operation was advised and five months later he came for active rehabilitation. He did rug-weaving on an upright rug loom, at first with a spring-loaded sling for his right arm. The spring tension was 25 lb and was gradually reduced to 5 lb before being discarded. He progressed to woodwork. He was also tried out at the local Skill Centre where he was considered suitable for training in centre-lathe turning. After seven weeks' rehabilitation he left to start this course which he reported three months later as satisfactory. Fifteen months later he was playing badminton.

ANKYLOSING SPONDYLITIS

This is a rheumatic condition, affecting more men than women. Patients are given considerable anti-inflammatory medication and are usually sent for rehabilitation before the spine has become stiffened and deformed. Treatment is aimed at building up maximal power in the spinal extensors in order to prevent flexion deformity. Treatment also aims to build up general fitness and muscle strength but to do this without causing undue fatigue. Patients follow a similar routine to those with other spinal disabilities but need to work more gently and with particular emphasis on rhythmic movements. Hip joints are usually affected as well and tend to go into flexion. Patients need advice on posture and appropriate working positions.

When patients are admitted after a degree of stiffness is already established in the spine and hip joints, treatment must be aimed at helping the rest of the body to adjust so that maximum function is possible. This may include work in physiotherapy to improve chest expansion. The extent of the stiffness and the position in which the patient is fixed vary widely; for example, some have stiffened in the sitting position, others in standing.

Patients who cannot sit comfortably on a chair may prefer a bicycle stool. One with a motor cycle saddle is ideal because it is well sprung and therefore comfortable; also, being very narrow at the front it is suitable when hip abduction is limited. A padded back-rest to lean against will add comfort and make the patient feel more secure.

Very often patients need advice about suitable employment, particularly because of the prognosis of the disease. Wear and tear of the inflamed joints should be avoided and heavy work is therefore contraindicated. Outdoor work is also unsuitable because these patients should avoid both cold and damp. Consequently, since many of them have spent their early lives doing heavy unskilled work, in or out of doors, they frequently require retraining or resettlement in a walk of life which is less demanding on physical power or capacity to stand up to all weathers. The bicycle fretsaw and filing machines have been found useful in helping the therapist to assess the patient's capacity for accuracy in fine work, as well as for improving mobility of hips and knees without much strain. The electric screw-cutting lathe and the use of hand hacksaws will provide other opportunities for judging if the patient is interested in and really enjoys fine work. Some people have the advantage of a straight eye and light touch without knowing it, as they never needed to use them. They may regret giving up work out-of-doors, but they will find some compensation in opportunities to develop their talents. One patient who had been a driver of heavy lorries and excavating machines, had a mitral stenosis as well as anky-losing spondylitis. He came for rehabilitation in fine summer weather and at first he could not bear the idea of working indoors. Gradually, as his confidence in our advice grew, he agreed to try indoor work. He found he had a pretty touch on the electric lathe and that life still held some pleasure with a growing interest in indoor work. On discharge he was soon resettled in an assembly job in a factory near his home and he has adjusted himself very well.

It may be pure chance, but it has been observed that patients who have ankylosing spondylitis have been very much easier in their adjustment to their disabilities than those suffering from other spinal disabilities, such as prolapsed disc. It is difficult to understand why this should be, as they have often gone through long periods of backache. They know that the disease may not be arrested though it may be relieved by treatment, and quite often they have seen other members of their families severely crippled. But these patients seem to be blessed with courage and good temper, qualities which stand them in good stead in the effort to surmount their disabilities.

LIFTING

Any patient with a disability of the spine should be taught how to bend, lift and carry, Indeed, those without such a disability could also benefit. It is especially important for housewives and nurses to learn the correct movements for bedmaking, cleaning the bath and moving furniture or lifting heavy objects. Many jobs entail heavy lifting and some employees, such as firemen and factory workers, are usually taught, in the course of their work, how to lift but a great number of others, such as labourers and drivers, are not.

The use of correct lifting methods will enable people, both at home and at work, to lift loads that they would not otherwise be able to manage. As well as avoiding backstrain and preventing accidents, people who lift correctly will be able to continue lifting heavy loads when they get older and their muscles lose strength.

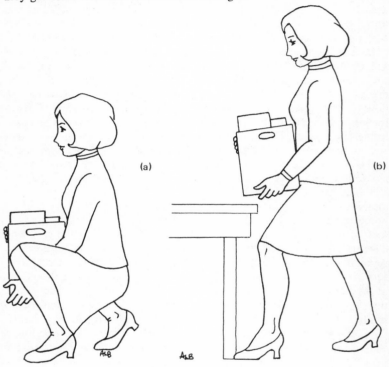

Figure 5.8. — Lifting correctly. (a) Head up, eyes forward, chin in, back straight, elbows held in to body, good grip using palms of hands, load close to body, hips and knees bent, one foot in front of the other. (b) Legs straightened, rear foot pushes off, front foot points in direction of lift, bodyweight used to lift load forward on to table

With careful planning it is possible to eliminate some lifting jobs and to make others much easier. Most furniture can be fitted with castors; some items like wardrobes can be permanently fitted in the room and will never need moving. Choosing a car with a rear door and a high platform inside will make loading and unloading the shopping much easier than bending over the back seat, or into a low boot. If the article to be moved is too heavy or too bulky, it should be left until someone else is available to help with the lift. Unessential heavy lifting or moving should be avoided altogether by those with spinal disabilities. Putting anything heavy on the floor if it will need lifting later should also be avoided. For example, when there is no room on the draining board, a bowl of wet clothes may be put on a stool or the kitchen table, instead of on the floor.

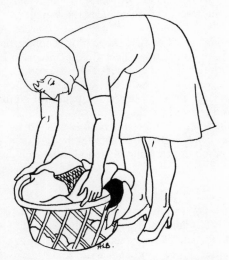

Figure 5.9. – Lifting incorrectly. Back bent, legs straight, feet together, arms away from body, gripping load with fingers

When lifting is necessary, certain basic rules should be followed (*Figure 5.8*):

1. Position the feet slightly apart with one foot a little ahead of the other. The leading foot should be pointed in the direction of travel so that once the weight is lifted it can immediately be carried to its destination.
2. Straighten the back, raise the head and keep the chin tucked in.
3. Take a deep breath before the lift and hold it while lifting. This utilizes the diaphragm and lungs to provide muscular and pneumatic support for the spine by filling the thoracic cavity with a cushion of air.

4. Reach down to the load by bending the knees and keeping the back straight. This is not always possible because the quadriceps muscles may not be strong enough to lift both the body and the load. Exercises and work to strengthen the quadriceps may be a necessary precursor to lifting.
5. Take a proper hold of the load. Grip it with the palms in close contact, not with just the fingers. Hold the load close to the body with the elbows tucked well into the sides. This reduces the length of the levers and so reduces the weight of the load on the hands.
6. Use the bodyweight to help when this is appropriate. Sometimes it is necessary to tilt the object first, in order to get a good grip on it. Use the body as a counterweight to do this.
7. Lift by stages if this makes the job easier. For example, lift the object from the floor on to a stool, pause for a moment and then lift it from the stool to wherever it is going.
8. When something must be put on a high shelf, do not try to lift above the head with arms outstretched. Use a stable pair of steps and climb up, carrying the load in the usual way.

WORK ASSESSMENT

Building up work tolerance and assessing the patient's ability to return to work is an important part of occupational therapy. This is discussed in detail in Chapter 13 but patients with spinal disabilities have particular problems which are considered here.

What does the patient's job entail? Many work situations produce problems for these patients and so the requirements of the job must be carefully analysed. How many hours can he work? How heavy work can he do? Can he bend, lift and carry loads similar to those at work? Can he manage ladders? Can he work for a prolonged time in awkward positions as dictated by his job, for example, as a plumber, electrician or aeroplane body worker? Can he work in high stretched-up and low bent-down positions, as a painter and decorator? Can he sit for a long time at an office desk? Does he have the right kind of postural chair? Can he sit in a car, or lorry, for long periods? Does he have the best type of driving seat? Should he return to a driving job?

Various ways can be found of simulating work situations in the workshops. Sheet metal workers can practise lifting and stacking sheets of plywood. These are just as unwieldy as sheet metal, although not as heavy, and the therapist can use the exercise to correct lifting techniques. It is essential to have a set of stackable metal boxes containing heavy components, for lifting practice. These should be in a selection of weights ranging from 9 to 45 kg (20–100 lb). Further lifting practice will be given in the gymnasium, for instance, learning to lift sacks and to give a fireman's lift.

Other activities which have been used in work assessment include painting and decorating, window cleaning, car cleaning, tidying out the stores, general maintenance work of varying kinds, tree felling, cross-cut sawing, chopping up wood and gardening.

Sometimes returning a patient to work is mainly a question of building up confidence together with general fitness. One patient had fallen off a step-ladder at work while mending a fuse and had not worked for several years since then. Nothing appeared wrong with his back although he was out of condition and said he could not bend down. He was a co-operative and obliging man and was admitted at the time we were building our ADL section. After some time on woodwork, which he did well, he was asked to go and help another patient, a carpenter by trade, who was making our new kitchen cupboards. He acted as a carpenter's mate, passing tools and materials, but never getting down to floor level. Then came disaster, the carpenter was discharged fit for work before the kitchen cupboards were completed. His mate spent the next two days doing minor jobs that were within his reach. The next thing we saw was that he was on his hands and knees working on the sliding doors of the cupboards. He could not bear that our cupboards should not be finished, and not even his back was going to stop him. Some weeks later our ADL section was completed and he was discharged to suitable work.

REFERENCE

Ellison, P. L. (1971). *The O.B. Help Arm*. Nottingham; Nottingham Handcraft Company

FURTHER READING

Advice on Housework for Patients with Low Back Pain. Noel Wilson Ltd, Graphic House, Craghead, Stanley, Co. Durham

Cailliet, R. (1968). *Low Back Pain Syndrome*. 2nd Edition. Philadelphia; F. A. Davis Co.

Health and Safety Booklets. Lifting and Carrying (1958) (11, 360840 3). London; HMSO

Chartered Society of Physiotherapy. *Lifting in Industry*

Health and Safety Executive (1970). *Seats for Workers in Factories, Offices and Shops* (11, 360830 6). London; HMSO

6

Disabilities of the Lower Limb

The lower limbs have never been honoured with the title of 'organs' as have the hands in medical and legal language. Their function is, crudely considered, to support or balance the rest of the body when it is stationary or sedentary, or to transport it hither and thither as required. The movements and control of the lower limbs absorb much attention in early youth, and later may be elaborated in other activities such as athletics when close co-ordination is developed between hand, foot and distribution of bodyweight. Muscular contractions required to perform in such co-ordination soon become almost automatic. It is only when age, illness or trauma interfere with the function of the lower limbs that they again become important in conscious thought. When freedom and independence are hampered the activities of the lower limbs are the centre of attention.

Even the fascination of agility and control in the hands takes second place, as they are only needed to grip sticks to aid in walking, or to hold on to a stable object to help standing. Unfortunately the desire for mobility is easily satisfied. The patient is anxious to gain independence in the choice of his immediate locality and seldom gives much attention as to how this is attained. Immediate freedom may be won without troubling to relearn the tricks of movement and balance which once held interest.

Learning to walk in childhood has certain advantages beyond the question of absorbing interest. A child is short in height and light in weight. A tumble to the floor is a slight matter and easily forgotten. For the adult the distance is greater and bodyweight is not only greater but otherwise disposed. Previous childish experience in learning how to walk therefore would be of little value even if it were easy to recall. The adult must learn to walk again as an adult and not as a child. The importance and difficulties of learning the technique of movement are relative to the period during which its practice has had to be abandoned owing to bed-rest.

Often the patient's first slither or hop to the lavatory is achieved with no instruction. Physiotherapists teach walking first as an exercise between parallel bars, which help with support and balance, long before the patient's embarkation on crutches or sticks is allowed. Occupational therapists can do much in workshops by giving opportunity to practise muscle movements of the lower limbs whilst the patient is sitting. In this position bodyweight is near floor level and there is little fear of falling, so that relaxed and smooth movement may be expected. It is necessary to provide machines which are worked by specific movements used in walking whilst the patient's attention is to some degree attracted towards the work done by his hands in guiding tools or material. Such machines are not like factory machines, designed to economize on human endeavour, but rather to encourage and exploit the efforts required to put thought into action. At the same time it must be stressed that an even and steady movement of the legs must be enlisted to work the machine efficiently.

The occupational therapist cannot only be concerned with patients working on machines for re-education of movements in the lower limbs. The teaching of walking is the province of the physiotherapist, but the supervision of all activities in the workshops is the responsibility of the occupational therapist. The patient's mode of walking needs constant supervision. The therapist gives thought to finding work that is therapeutic as well as of interest to the patient. The patient appreciates the opportunity to make something he wants and will hurry to do so. Occasionally the appearance of haste may be assumed to impress the therapist or to disguise a time-lag that has intervened whilst he has loitered with a cigarette between the gymnasium and the workshops. Whatever the cause may be, the effect of hurrying is the same. The patient lurches carelessly into the workshops with little thought of the exercises he has just been practising before a mirror. This limp, swing and lurch is frequently seen when he goes to fetch a tool, or leaves a lathe when he has had his turn. With or without crutches and sticks this method of progression is little regarded by the patient whose work is in his thoughts. The writer has found it necessary to insist that good walking should be practised at every opportunity even if the distance is but a few steps, and insistence has been carried to the point of asking the patient to return to his starting point and repeat the excursion with balance and control.

The practice of walking by the patient with a paretic leg, who can only hold one stick, is discussed in Chapter 10. For patients suffering from disabilities of the lower limb only, the writer has always had a personal preference for the programme which replaces two crutches with two sticks and insists that two sticks should be used until both can be abandoned. This makes it easier for the patient to learn the habit of walking with an even distribution of bodyweight. Many authorities prefer that the patient should use one stick for an interim period before embarking on complete independence from external support. There are also patients with residual disabilities for whom one stick may be a more or less permanent necessity, especially when walking out-of-doors on rough ground. The stick then serves not only to give the patient support and confidence, but to warn passers-by that special consideration must be given to one whose security of balance would be easily upset by the careless pushing past of those who are accustomed to move quickly in the hurly-burly of pedestrian traffic.

The same principles may be used in supervising the walking of patients on two crutches, two sticks or one stick. The bodyweight is evenly distributed between the disabled leg and the stick held in the good hand, whilst the 'best foot is put forward'. Because the leg is weak, the first step may be short. The patient must be taught that the following step, with the good leg as the pedestal, should be of the same length. This helps to ensure the patient's appreciation of an even pace. There are many theories and methods of teaching walking. The writer has only described the one she has found preferable.

Early treatment to prevent ill-effects of bed-rest

When a patient has had an amputation of the lower limb, say at mid-thigh level, it is taught in most schools of nursing or physiotherapy that there is a part of the procedure as important as bandaging the stump to shape it. This consists of turning the patient over or teaching him to turn himself over so that he lies in the prone position for regular periods during the day. During these periods he is taught to practise contractions of the glutei and the adductors of the thighs, whilst the position of prone lying helps to stretch the hip flexors. He is taught also to exercise the erector spinae. Some help may be given by the addition of pillows under the chest, and another under the elbows which are treated with surgical spirit and talcum powder to harden the skin. This is done to ensure that when the patient starts standing between crutches he can control the position of the stump. Later on when learning to walk between crutches he is taught to pull all these muscles into contraction in the natural pattern of walking. Then he will more easily learn the control of a prosthesis.

An amputee gets a good deal of attention as playing lead in a dramatic and tragic incident. He is usually a short two or three weeks in bed unless there are other complications. Some other patients with injuries to the lower limb stay in bed far longer. It is understandable that people with bad hearts which may accompany a rheumatic condition cannot be turned over to the prone position. But there are many others for whom this position would not be detrimental. Patients on traction for above-knee or below-knee fractures must lie with a C-shaped spine, and hips flexed for a long period. But then comes the time when traction is removed and the patient is free in bed. This period could be put to good use, and the patient encouraged to turn over to the prone position. At first, perhaps, it might be necessary to allow a pillow or rubber cushion to ease the stretching of contracted hip flexors. This is a period when the hip flexors should be gradually stretched, the glutei exercised, and contraction of the spinal extensors taught. A couple of pillows under the chest and one under the elbows should ease the discomfort of the prone position. With such preparation for standing and walking it might not be so easy to pick out the newcomer for rehabilitation. Usually such a patient is seen pointing his nose as far forward as the toe of the leg he is carrying, his weight so far forward on his crutches that one sees nose and toes coming round the corner before the rest of him. He has the C-shaped spine, and both hips seem permanently flexed. Muscular imbalance and postural re-education must first be taught before the true aims of rehabilitation are attempted. These may be indicated as mobilization of hip, knee and ankle of one or both legs. The rehabilitation period might well be cut in half if it were started, as we are all taught that it should, in the ambulance going to hospital. All members of the rehabilitation team should appreciate that in the later stages those who have put over the idea correctly in the earlier stages are the real instigators of good posture. Regular evidence of their work would make short the invalidism and crippling incompetence often observed in patients who come for rehabilitation.

ARTHRODESES OF HIP OR KNEE

Arthrodeses are rarely performed now, for two very good reasons. Antibiotics are available to control infections and therefore patients no longer sustain severe damage to their joints, caused by tuberculosis or osteomyelitis. Technical development of inert materials has so improved methods of arthroplasty that this operation has a high success rate and is the preferred operation for patients with joint damage due to osteoarthrosis or rheumatoid arthritis. The few patients who come for treatment with an arthrodesis either have had an arthroplasty which failed or an arthrodesis several years prior to admission.

The patient who has had an arthrodesis of the hip can lie on his face in the gymnasium and work the muscles below hip level against spring resistance. The patient with an arthrodesed knee can lie on his back and exercise the hip muscles. In occupational therapy neither type of patient can be given work on any of the machines so far designed for developing muscles in the lower limbs, without risking a strain on the arthrodesed joint.

Some help may be provided for the patient with a stiff hip by a bicycle stool and table adjustable in height. These must both be very stable and heavy as they cannot be bolted into position. If the patient finds difficulty in getting on or off the bicycle stool further assistance may be given by a substitute for the arms of a chair. This is constructed as an open square which surrounds the chair or the bicycle stool (*see Figure 2.1*, page 21). It is made of electric conduit piping an inch in diameter. When suitably braced a few inches from floor level it is stable. The patient can then hoist himself by holding on to the arms of the chair to gain the completely upright position.

The hip is usually arthrodesed in a slightly forward position, to allow the patient to sit. It has been noticed that many patients with an arthrodesed hip complain of backache in the lumbar region. Sitting in an ordinary chair or lying in bed they are apt to go into a position of lordosis which may affect both sides, though usually the pain is more marked on the side of the arthrodesed hip. With medical permission, the writer has found it helpful not only to use bicycle stools in the workshops, but to advise the patient to put a small pillow under the knee in bed to relax back strain. He may have to continue to do this after rehabilitation as nothing can be done to remedy this lordosis when lying on the back. Several specialized bicycle stools have been made for patients with stiff hips. These they have taken with them on discharge for use at home or at work.

Another aid to those with the hip fixed in flexion, however slight it may be, is the raised shoe. Such flexion shortens the affected leg in comparison with the other and spoils the level of the pelvis. Scar contraction of muscles and capsules severed or separated at operation may continue for some time, though malalignment of the pelvis may be slight in the beginning and as the patient feels it so little he is unwilling to wear a raised shoe. It has been noticed that this malalignment has increased in many patients who return to pay a social call long after they have ceased to attend the surgeon's clinics. Scoliosis too may have become marked and probably fixed. There have been complaints of pain in the back which the writer feels might have been prevented by suitable adjustments to shoes. In recent years the smallest malalignment of the pelvis observed in a patient when walking or at work has been reported immediately to the medical director.

The patient with a stiffened knee can sit on an ordinary chair when he still has hip flexion. In the early stages such patients often have considerable oedema of the leg and have always been given foot-stools of various heights within reach. They have been taught to keep the leg raised high, and then lower it themselves. In this way postural drainage will help the circulation. The patient can learn to feel when the leg feels 'full' and then to keep it high. The periods between high and low foot-stools and leaving the foot at ground level will gradually even out until the foot can stay at ground level without swelling and discomfort.

Therapeutic occupations for patients with arthrodesis of these joints have been indirect in application. The scope of occupations includes bench woodwork and wrought ironwork. Wood-turning on the foot-power lathes has been found not only possible but beneficial. The patient is taught to stand on the stiffened leg and treadle with the other. Every muscle on the affected side will be exercised in keeping the stance regulated to maintain the balance of the torso and the handling of tools on the revolving wood. This work has been found especially useful for the patients who complain of ache in the lumbar muscles after a hip arthrodesis. If the hip cannot bend then the lumbar curve is straightened out and the back extensors in the lumbar region work strongly in the outer range. These muscle contractions are not static though the rhythmic activities occur in a small range of movement. Such exercise will help to correct the lordosis to which these patients are inclined, and the spasm which results in the lumbar muscles. This spasm is stronger on the side of the arthrodesed hip and, if it remains uncorrected, will result in scoliosis with all its subsequent disabilities. It is maintained that occupational therapy should be used as a preventive as well as a remedial treatment. Methods of treatment should include indirect activities of muscles used correctly to maintain good posture and balance, before bad habits of movement can become established.

THE HIP TREATED BY ARTHROPLASTY

A number of patients have come for rehabilitation after operations designed to make mobility of the hip joint mechanically possible. Such mobility will be of little practical use to the patient until he learns to control it by muscular activity, since stability of all joints in the lower limbs is essential for the enjoyment of mobility. All these patients have had long histories of pain and stiffness in the joint before operation. With modern techniques of arthroplasty patients are fully weight-bearing as soon as they are allowed out of bed. They may however need crutches or a walking frame for balance until they have relearned a good pattern of walking. One can observe the patterns of movement long established by pain and limitation of movement. Much may be done to disrupt the incorrect patterns of movement accepted by the patient as inevitable before operation, and to lay down a basic pattern of movement which is nearer to the normal movements used by the patient before the onset of disability. Typically there is the rolling, swaying movement used in walking. The patient will swing the hip and leg forwards using muscles and joints in the lumbar region to avoid the pain brought on by attempted hip movement. The glutei on the affected side have become markedly wasted, and the adductors may have become shortened by constant contraction in the effort to maintain the balance of the torso, the weight of which is principally carried on the unaffected side.

The aims of treatment in occupational therapy are therefore to encourage development of muscles in the region of the hip wasted by disuse, and to encourage relaxation and restoration of elasticity in the adductors of the affected side by encouraging abduction. Care must be taken to avoid any possible forced movements and some surgeons stress that sitting cross-legged is contraindicated too soon after the operation. A patient should work within his own limits of voluntary activity and should not force his hip joint movement. The therapist may need to restrain the over-enthusiastic patient.

Besides training in walking, patients will need help with climbing stairs. They may also need assistance in getting in and out of the bath, and with dressing the lower part of the body.

In the early stages of treatment work on the bicycle machines with suitably adjusted pedal cranks will provide gentle mobilization. As power and mobility increase the patient will follow the usual programme of those with disabilities of the lower limbs working on foot-power lathes. The programme must be graduated to the general condition of the patient. Patients with hip arthroplasties are usually in the older age-groups, and not capable of heavy types of work. There was one memorable patient, a girl still under 30 years, whose hip arthroplasties, originally of the Judet pattern, were bilateral and both required revision. She had several spells of rehabilitation after different operations and returned to work in a clerical capacity after each incident. It was natural that she was depressed and apprehensive when she came for rehabilitation after the first revision operation. It is not easy to encourage activities when a patient keeps a worn and discarded prosthetic head of her femur in her handbag and constantly reminds the therapist that its mate is still in her other hip.

All that has been written about balance and control of movement before pushing on with increased range must be reiterated when the treatment of these patients is considered.

THE KNEE TREATED BY MENISCECTOMY

Patients who have had meniscectomy for injuries of one or both semi-lunar cartilages form the largest group of patients with the same disability sent for rehabilitation. They have usually been young men who lead a reasonably active life during the week but are extremely active at the weekend. An accident when playing football is most commonly blamed for the injury. The knee joint, by its structure, is particularly vulnerable to a sudden wrench or twist, unless the quadriceps are well developed and can save the knee from unguarded movement. The internal part of the quadriceps, vastus medialis, is a muscle in constant tone to main-tain the extension of the knee required by the erect posture, though it cannot easily be felt in strong contraction except when the knee is slowly extended against resistance. A quick, jerking extension does not seem to call for its contraction. Vastus medialis wastes quickly with disuse, the result of injury and the fear of pain previously experienced in full extension. The patient who has injured a cartilage may complain of incidents of pain and locking in the knee on several occasions before submitting to operation.

When walking or running both legs work together in sequence, but when one leg is used for a specific purpose the other is not inactive, and its muscles are in contraction to secure support and stability of the torso. The muscles of the supported hip and leg are necessarily in play to stabilize the pelvis and so give a firm basis for action to the one leg capable of productive work. Therefore any work that is carried out with one leg supported and in elevation does not imply that the leg will be at rest and the muscles relaxed. Small or static contractions of muscles round the hips will call on similar though less strong con-tractions farther down the leg. The quality of contraction depends to some degree on previously formed capacities for control of balance, but these are often disrupted by disuse consequent on disability. The accepted patterns of activity stimulate contractions in the muscles of both legs which are fundamentally reciprocal in character.

As so many patients have been sent for rehabilitation after meni-scectomy and, like all other patients, come for occupational therapy several hours a day, it is possible to give a detailed history of the treatment of a typical patient. The aims of treatment are directed to the restoration of power in the quadriceps, and particularly in vastus medialis, to give stability to the knee. In the early days of treatment the muscles can only be developed by static contractions which do not necessitate knee flexion and extension. There may be stitches *in situ* which could be torn by flexion; there may be effusion in the knee which is being treated by a tubular elastic bandage and kept in ele-vation; or the patient may have an extension lag.

An extension lag occurs when, despite a full passive range of extension, the patient is unable to lock his knee in extension because vastus medialis cannot contract sufficiently strongly to hold the knee in the locked position. This lag is tested by asking the patient to sit on the floor with knees outstretched, contract the quadriceps of the affected knee and lift the leg off the ground. If the leg lifts quite straight in the locked position, there is no lag. If the knee flexes slightly, the locking mechanism is not working and there is an extension lag. Allowing a knee to work in flexion before an extension lag has been overcome makes re-education of vastus medialis much more difficult. It is therefore contraindicated.

An extension lag should not be confused with an extension block. With a block there is not a full range of passive extension. The defect is mechanical rather than muscular. It may be due to gross swelling, intra-articular fractures, fractures near to the knee, loose bodies or osteophytes. Treatment of an extension block will include measures to reduce any swelling and, when appropriate, manipulation.

In occupational therapy static contraction of the knee can only be achieved by work which requires balance from the affected leg which must be treated in elevation. Then small or static contractions of all the leg and hip muscles are called into play to stabilize the pelvis on the side of the affected leg, and so create a sound foundation for the unaffected leg to work in independent movement. It has been observed that someone with experience in the economical use of muscle power and balance can work with one leg and make little demand on the other in elevation, but this phenomenon has not been encountered amongst patients. When the patient is allowed to bear weight on the affected leg and begin to mobilize the knee, productive activities are used to stimulate the muscles to increasing contraction. Mobilization always follows in the steps of development of power and control of muscles in an affected region. This is constantly reiterated as being an important feature in our treatment of patients.

The patient may come for rehabilitation with the stitches still in, and with a tubular elastic bandage round the knee. He is warned not to bend his leg, and if he cannot contract his quadriceps voluntarily, he will be taught this by faradic stimulation. On the next day he comes to the workshops on crutches and is shown the foot-power lathes and some of the processes of wood-turning. Then he sits at a table with the affected leg raised and supported on a foot stool. This stool is about the same level as the chair on which he sits. The stool does not support the heel itself but is arranged just behind it (*Figure 6.1*). This prevents hyperextension at the knee joint which might cause pain and result in spasm of the muscles lying in relation to the knee. When sitting he is shown drawings as well as finished table lamps. He can choose the colour and grain of the wood he prefers, medium hard wood which is easy to turn. At various times these have included sycamore, beech, lime, plane, mahogany and walnut. Oak is not recommended for

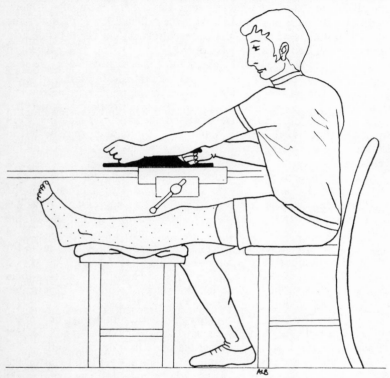

Figure 6.1. – Patient working with oedematous leg supported on a cushion on a stool which is the same height as chair so that his leg is horizontal. Patient is wearing a Tubigrip stocking

turning by the inexperienced as it has a hard tough grain which is easily torn. The patient is encouraged to draw the outline of a table-lamp on graph paper to give himself an idea of the contours he would like to follow when turning.

Then taking the drawing and perhaps clutching a folding foot-stool with his crutches he goes to the wood workshop and saws out the block of wood for the stem of the lamp, about 50 mm (2 in) square and up to 41 cm (16 in) long according to his design. This he does sitting with the leg raised, and continuing in this position he planes the block of wood in a vice on a low bench. The wood must be shaped to a rounded bar.

By the sixth or seventh day after operation these preparations are completed and the patient may start turning the stem of his table-lamp. He sits on a bicycle stool with the affected leg slung under the lathe. The sling is of rather stiff canvas about 38 cm (15 in) wide held up by a hook bolted to the back of the lathe bed. The sling is arranged to support the leg from just behind the knee to just above the heel (*see Figure 2.9*, page 39). He is taught to treadle the lathe with the good leg at the pace of 80 or 85 strokes to the minute. A metronome is used at first to ensure the appreciation of this timing, which has been found to produce active contractions in vastus medialis. Even when the affected leg is slung, some static contractions may be felt in all the muscles of the leg in the efforts required for balance of the pelvis. He may require some help in treadling at first.

The patient continues to work with the leg slung until the stitches are removed or have dissolved, any effusion is so minimal that the tubular elastic bandage has been discarded and any extension lag has been overcome. The patient is then allowed to put the foot of the affected leg on the back of the treadle and use the extensors of both legs to work the lathe. He will still only be working on the lathe for about half an hour at a time, and when not so occupied he saws a square block for the base of the lamp, and planes it on one side to an even surface. When he has finished this stage of work he will probably be allowed to use the scroll saw (*see Figure 2.13*, page 47) to cut it to a round, about 150 mm (6 in) in diameter. The scroll saw may be worked sitting with both feet at first in a small range of extension and flexion. As the range of movement increases the saw cuts more efficiently.

When the patient is fully weight-bearing a week or so after the stitches are out, he can work on both lathe and scroll saw standing. He stands alternately on the affected and the unaffected leg, using the other for treadling. Both when sitting and standing he is advised to keep his feet parallel to each other so that he keeps the knee joints in alignment with the femur and the tibia. This is an essential point, because if the foot is turned out the knee is inclined to sideways flexion on the inner side which might strain the internal lateral ligament.

As the patient gets stronger he can work longer on the lathe, and he then works the extra time helping a patient weaker than himself to treadle. Turning the 150 mm (6 in) base of a table-lamp is much heavier work than doing a stem 50 mm (2 in) in diameter. The table-lamp is therefore found to be an ideal piece of work for a meniscectomy patient. He can then progress to making a larger bowl which he should easily complete within the average five to six week period of treatment. The patient will also normally spend at least 10 minutes every day on the bicycle fretsaw with the pedals suitably adjusted, to help to improve his range of movement and muscle power. Making small toys, jigsaws, group projects or projects for other patients prove suitable for such short periods of treatment, allowing each patient in the group of leg injuries to have a turn.

If a patient has chondromalacia of the patella his leg should not be worked against resistance when the knee is flexed at over 90 degrees. Great strain is put on the underside of the patella when the knee is in acute flexion. Wood-turning, with the patient correctly positioned, is a safe activity but bicycling should be avoided unless against minimal resistance.

It must be pointed out that it has not been possible to work out the average period of each stage in treatment, nor for completion of rehabilitation. There have been patients whose rehabilitation has been delayed by gross effusion or haemarthrosis in the knee after operation. There have also been some elderly patients whose rate of recovery does not approach that of the typical young man. Football is not the only cause of injuries encountered. Falling off a chair when putting up curtains, or even slipping on the edge of a mat, as well as other quite simple activities may be blamed. Any untoward strain will affect the knee joint when the tone and condition of muscles are inadequate for a sudden demand for movement.

Occupational therapy for elderly or weak patients has included work on the bicycle machines with the cranks of the pedals suitably adapted, if work on the foot-treadle lathes proves too heavy. Often, however, such a patient will be allowed to help treadling on a lathe. The young patients have always been found considerate and co-operative in the treatment of the elderly.

FRACTURES AND OTHER INJURIES ALSO AFFECTING THE KNEE

The patients who have had fractures and other injuries of the lower limbs, including patellectomies, have followed much the same programme as those who have had meniscectomies. The rate of progression is naturally slower. The leg in plaster, or non-weight-bearing, must remain slung under the lathe and the patient must be seated; the exception to this is the fractured femur which must never be slung since this puts undue pressure on the healing fracture site and may cause a refracture. The unaffected leg does the active work of treadling, but the muscles round the hip on the affected side can be observed to work on the other side to keep the torso upright and balanced. A bicycle stool (*see Figure 2.2,* page 22) makes the strongest demand for balance, and allows freer movement of the working leg; it is therefore preferable to a chair but sometimes a high plaster may cut or pinch the leg when the patient uses a bicycle stool, and then a high chair with a foam-rubber cushion has been found more satisfactory. It has been found that such patients, for whom a long period of rehabilitation is foreseen, can turn the legs of a stool or coffee table, and carry on with the bench wood-work necessary when they have done their daily stint on the lathe. By the time they are out of plaster and fully weight-bearing they have learnt the art of turning well enough to turn a bowl, which demands more skill as well as power. The general physique of the patient as well as the specific requirements for muscular development and range of movement have always been taken into consideration. A salad bowl of 31–36 cm (12–14 in) in diameter requires considerable exertion as well as craftsmanship in turning.

The scroll saw will cut through wood up to 75 mm (3 in) thick. It is particularly useful for cutting out the round before turning a bowl (*see Figure 2.13,* page 47). Its use requires much more power than the bicycle saw and its full thrust gives opportunity for a wide range of knee movement including full extension.

One patient must be mentioned who was unwise enough to voice the opinion that there was not work available which was heavy enough to cause him exertion of his quadriceps. He found himself cutting out the saddle clamps for the V-blocks using a junior hacksaw blade in the scroll saw. These were made from ½ inch (12 mm) mild steel, and he made no demands for heavier work. Other patients have cut out the angle brackets for ironing boards. This is much lighter work as the mild iron plate is not more than $\frac{1}{10}$ inch (2.5 mm) thick.

The period that treatment lasts has varied widely. Some patients come in newly fitted plasters, just out of bed, others in walking plasters, others in a caliper, others again free of all outside support to regain a range of movement lost during earlier periods of treatment by immobi-lization and rest. The patient with a long leg plaster shown in *Figure 3.15* (*see* page 84) came to us in a very early stage when non-weight-bearing, with toes that quickly turned purple and blue unless the leg was raised high. A sling had to be attached to a copper-beating block and his foot raised to about 122 cm (4 ft) to counteract the effects of the poor circulation which produced these colourful symptoms. His progress was satisfactory but it took several months for him to walk without any support.

Another patient was sent in without support but with a knee bend of only about 40 degrees after a compound crush fracture of the femur. He was discharged after 6—7 weeks' treatment with a knee bend of 70 degrees. He was a ship's carpenter and said he would get all the knee-bending exercise he wanted on his own job. Two years later he paid us a social call and demanded that the range of knee bend should be measured. It had improved about another 50 degrees.

Patients who have had a patellectomy tend to take longer to get a fully mobilized knee than those who have had a meniscectomy. Often the patient will be discharged with limited knee flexion but follow-up reports have indicated that this continues to improve. One patient, who had had a patellectomy after a motor cycle accident, returned 10 years later to pay a social call. By then he had a knee bend which allowed him 'to kick his own bottom'.

It would be uneconomic from either the point of view of the patients or the Health Service to continue treatment to these standards of recovery. The really important thing is for the patient to learn how to continue his own treatment using to the full the activities available in his own job and his own recreations.

DISABILITIES OF THE LEG BELOW THE KNEE

The conditions most commonly treated at Farnham Park include fractures of the lower third of the tibia and fibula, Potts fractures, fractures of the os calcis (usually bilateral), lesions in the Achilles tendon or pain in this tendon treated by decompression (a sports injury), and sprained ankles.

The aims of treatment are to reduce oedema if this is present, to increase the range of movement of the joints of the ankle and foot, to strengthen the affected muscles and to improve the pattern of walking.

Most patients who have been immobilized in plaster are put into Tubigrip as soon as the plaster is removed; this prevents oedema. When this procedure has not been followed the patient may come to the Centre with oedema in the calf, ankle and/or foot. His leg will then be encased in Tubigrip from the toes to the knee and the foot of his bed will be put on blocks. In the physiotherapy department he will be given gentle mobilization in elevation and in the workshop he may be given work to do with his foot elevated on a foot-stool. This foot-stool should be the same height as his chair so that the hip is at a right angle. The seat of the stool should support the leg from above the knee to above the ankle. It should not support the heel because this would force the knee into hyperextension. A folding stool with a canvas sling top or a wooden stool with a cushion will be suitable (*see Figure 6.1*, page 161).

A selection of such stools of varying heights to fit different chairs should be kept.

In the early stages of treatment patients usually come for rehabilitation when partially weight-bearing and with any plaster removed. Provided there is no oedema they will start wood-turning on a treadle lathe, sitting on a bicycle seat, and with both legs together on the front of the treadle so that the affected leg is assisted by the unaffected one. Patients also work on a suitably adjusted bicycle fretsaw against minimal resistance.

In the intermediate stage of treatment the patients become fully weight-bearing. They will continue with wood-turning, standing at the lathe and using alternate legs to treadle. They will be encouraged to treadle with just the toes on the foot-plate, rather than the whole foot, because this position ensures optimum work for the leg muscles. The bicycle fretsaw will be adjusted to require a greater range of movement of the ankle, and the cutting resistance increased to build up muscle power in the lower leg.

In the later stage the patients will be working for increased plantar flexion and dorsiflexion and for stronger muscles in the lower leg. They will now stand at the back of the lathe and treadle with the heel on the axle, pushing down in plantar flexion on the foot-plate. This method of treadling is harder work because of the loss of mechanical advantages in having a shorter lever arm. (This is also a third class lever; treadling from the front was a second class lever.) Work in this position is limited to sanding or polishing. At this stage in addition to the treadle lathe and bicycle fretsaw, patients can work on the ankle rotator for strong circumductory movements and also on the plantar-flexion adaptation in the industrial outwork section.

When the lower limb is injured below the knee the patient tends to stand and walk with that foot turned outwards for greater stability. As a result the arches of the foot in eversion become flattened. Tibialis anterior and the peronei are of the greatest importance in supporting the medial and lateral arches, and the intrinsic muscles support the arch of the metatarsal heads. These muscles can all be well developed by practice on the ankle-rotator saw (*see* pages 35—37 and *Figure 2.8*).

Observation of the patients walking about in the occupational therapy department will be necessary as well. The therapist can do much to help by instruction and advice on the problems of walking correctly and by ensuring that the patient stands with his feet parallel to each other when he is working on the foot-power lathes. The same precautions are taken when the patient is working on the bicycle saw or treadle sewing machine.

When it is considered particularly important to mobilize the small joints of the foot, the patient may work in plimsolls which allow the foot to move more freely, or even without shoes. On the lathe, plimsolls would give some protection from a falling chisel. Working a bicycle fretsaw without shoes will provide gentle, rhythmic movement of the metatarsophalangeal joints. Similarly, using a treadle sewing machine will provide static work for the lumbricals which should help to strengthen the transverse and longitudinal arches of the foot. Working an ankle rotator without shoes requires a 'pawing' action which gives good exercise for the forefoot.

Although patients with painful feet are frequently told to buy stout, supportive shoes, we have found that some types of sandal can provide good exercise which strengthens the small muscles and reduces pain. 'Flip-flop' sandals, which only attach to the front of the foot, either at the great toe or across the toes, and leave the ankle free, are kept on the foot by contracting the lumbricals at each step. This lifts the sole of the sandal to meet the sole of the foot with a 'flip-flop' sound. Patients need to be taught to walk in this way; a shuffling gait, as if wearing sloppy slippers, has no therapeutic value. This method is not suitable for a patient with claw toes since, instead of pressing the toes against the sandal he will flex them into an even more clawed position.

FOOT-PADS WORN INSIDE THE SHOE

Padding inside the shoe may often help a patient to walk better. Various types of patients suffer from feet which are tender or painful when weight-bearing. There are those patients with traumatic foot conditions, such as fractures of the os calcis, other tarsal or metatarsal bones; others with rheumatoid arthritis which has resulted in deformity from the growth of exostoses. Patients who have had anterior poliomyelitis may suffer from weakness of the intrinsic foot muscles with the result that the bones which support the weight-bearing scaffolding of the foot are not in alignment. Others again have long-standing deformities from various causes such as hallux valgus. These patients may suffer from tender or painful feet for a time, even after the original cause has been corrected by surgical treatment or whilst other physical treatment is being given.

It has often been possible to ease the pain, and so inculcate the principles of correct weight transference in walking, by the provision of foot-pads to protect the tender points of bony formation. A variety of foot-pads is available commercially and these should be tried first. When they do not provide relief the occupational therapist should be able to make pads or insoles to fit the individual patient's needs. They can be made from standard or high-density Plastazote 12 mm (½ in) thick which will compress slightly on weight-bearing. Biscuit-coloured or black Plastazote is particularly suitable for insoles. They can also be made from closed-cell high-density rubber sheeting, supplied in 10 mm (³⁄₈ in) and 4.5 mm (³⁄₁₆ in) thicknesses. The thicker sheeting may be sufficient but if the patient has loose enough fitting shoes and generally painful feet, he may benefit from a further insole made from thinner sheeting to cover the whole sole and fit over the special os calcis insole.

In the case of a patient with tenderness on the tuberosity of the os calcis, the sheeting should fit inside the shoe, under the heel and extending well forward. A paper pattern is made by drawing around the patient's foot. The point below the centre of the longitudinal arch, usually in line with the front of the tibia, is marked with an arrow. If just a heel-pad is required, this point will indicate the anterior border of the pad. If a whole insole is needed, the whole pattern is used.

A heel-pad is cut out in 12 mm (½ in) Plastazote, and the anterior border is chamfered or bevelled to eliminate the 'ridge' (*Figure 6.2a*). An insole is cut out in 6 mm (¼ in) Plastazote and placed over the heel-pad. The pad or pads are put in an oven at 140°C (284°F) for five

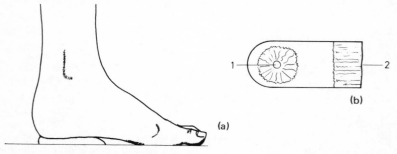

Figure 6.2. – (a) Medial aspect of left foot showing 12 mm Plastazote heel-pad. (b) Upper aspect of heel-pad made from rubber sheeting showing (1) funnel-shaped hole for tuberosity of os calcis; (2) bevelling on distal border of pad

minutes, slipped into the shoes and the patient is then asked to stand on them to mould the pads to his feet. When the pads are cool they are trimmed as necessary.

When the insole is made from rubber sheeting this must be cut to shape instead of moulded. A heel-pad is cut out following the pattern described above. The under-edge, lying on the sole of the shoe, is bevelled round with a pair of scissors so as to fit into the sides of the uppers. The distal edge is bevelled on the upper side so that it fits smoothly under the foot. A small hole about 6 mm (¼ in) in diameter is then cut out of the upper surface just under the point of the tuberosity of the os calcis. This hole is bevelled out all round to make it funnel-shaped (*Figure 6.2b*). This funnel-shaped hole should fit round the pressure point and so take a lot of the weight off it. A full insole should remain in place but a heel-pad will need sticking into the shoe with either an adhesive, such as Evo-Stik, or with double-sided adhesive tape. The latter has the advantage that the pads can be removed for washing, provided that the patient is given spare strips of tape. It may be necessary to make several insoles for different pairs of shoes.

When the pain is situated in the fore part of the foot, a metatarsal bar may assist in taking the pressure from the front arch. This can be made from Plastazote moulded by the method previously described for

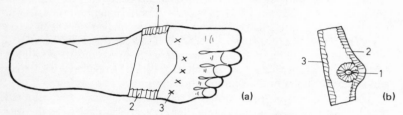

Figure 6.3. – (a) Plantar aspect of metatarsal pad in place on left foot showing (1) and (2) bevelling of medial and lateral borders of pad; (3) position of heads of metatarsal bones. (b) Upper aspect of metatarsal pad showing (1) extra raise stuck in position; (2) and (3) bevelling on proximal and distal borders of pad

heel-pads, or from rubber sheeting as detailed here. The metatarsal bar is usually made in the shape shown in *Figure 6.3a* and *b*. An extra pad or raise (1 in *Figure 6.3b*) may be added to the bar, just lateral to the ball of the big toe, if extra support is needed in this position. The bar should be made to fit slanting to match the slant of the front arch of the heads of the metatarsals. The lateral and medial edges of the pads should be bevelled on the under (sole) aspect to fit the sides of the uppers. The distal and proximal edges are bevelled on the upper side so that there are no sharp edges to give untoward pressure. If the extra pad (1 in *Figure 6.3b*) is found necessary this also should be bevelled all round so that the extra raise is evenly distributed. This extra pad should be stuck on to the metatarsal bar, usually on the upper side.

On occasion it has been found necessary to make a ring-pad to protect the metatarsal joint of the big toe when this is grossly deformed by arthritis producing an extreme form of hallus valgus. This is made on the same principle.

A commercially produced metatarsal pad may have an elastic loop which fits over the foot, or one which loops over the second toe, either of which helps to hold the pad in place. A 'home-made' pad is also usually best worn inside the sock or stocking, since this keeps it in place whilst the foot is being inserted into the shoe.

The plans given are mere indications of the shapes needed to fit the disabilities mentioned. The idea is to protect a painful pressure point by spreading the area on which the pressure is taken. Patients with painful feet usually wear rather loose-fitting shoes but some care must be taken to ensure that the pads do not make them too tight.

If these pads are made of rubber they may cause the foot to become hot and sweaty. This is particularly noticeable when the patient has rheumatoid arthritis and is taking large doses of aspirin or its compounds. It has been found helpful to puncture the rubber pads all over with holes about 13–25 mm (½–1 in) apart. A wad punch is found useful for this and 6 mm (¼ in) holes are necessary as smaller ones tend to be occluded when the foot is weight-bearing. The sweatiness can be helped by teaching the patient to rub the foot with spirit and to powder it with talc at least twice a day as well as washing it regularly with soap and water. In this way the skin may be kept in good condition.

The description of these foot-pads has been added as it is considered that the work of making and fitting them is very appropriate to the role of the occupational therapist or physiotherapist who sees the patient frequently. The pads require individual fitting and may require daily adjustment at first to make the patient really comfortable. Sometimes a patient finds it difficult to describe the exact locality of painful pressure because he has become used to generalized discomfort. His posture and movements may be so much improved by this local attention that the time spent in fitting and adjusting is well rewarded by the result. It is however, necessary to remember that if a patient is made comfortable by supports, he may be disinclined to make the effort to practise assiduously those exercises which might make the intrinsic muscles of the foot adequate in weight-bearing without assistance. In such cases, particular attention must be paid to the supervision of exercises.

THE TEMPORARY SHOE RAISE

Many patients after fractures of the femur or tibia and fibula have some shortening of the affected leg. Fixed flexion at the hip or knee will have the same effect. When this lack of extension is expected to be temporary and can be remedied by suitable exercise and work, no extraneous adaptations should be suggested. But when the shortening of one leg for any reason is considered unalterable and permanent, a shoe raise will do much to restore correct alignment of the pelvis and to prevent resultant scoliosis of the spine. The latter may develop gradually in the patient's attempt to keep the head straight and the eyes level so that the world at large is observed with comfort.

The permanent shoe raise is manufactured by the orthopaedic shoe expert. Before the exact height and shape are decided by the doctor or surgeon, he may request that the shoe raise be tried out temporarily under observation. This experimental work has frequently been carried out in the occupational therapy workshops, and methods used have been modified with experience. The medical director or orthopaedic surgeon has indicated the additional thickness required when the patient stands on blocks of various thicknesses. The walking sandal with varied thicknesses of sole has not been found practical in a quickly moving clinic.

A shoe raise is usually only requested when there is more than 13 mm (½ in) shortening, since with less than that the patient can adapt to the deficit without detriment to the spine. A raise should be as light as possible so as not to add unnecessary weight. A shoe that is very much heavier than its pair, worn on a foot supporting a leg that is weaker as well as shorter than the other, will do more harm than good and will prevent rather than encourage good balance in walking. Cork is the best material for a shoe raise because it is light in weight and yet durable. If composition cork is used it must be flexible, of high resilience and waterproof. Cork can be attached to the shoe with a suitable adhesive, such as Evo-Stik, and coloured to match with shoe dye. Composition rubber sheeting as used by shoe repairers is glued under all shoe raises to protect the cork and to provide a hardwearing, non-slip walking surface.

When a raise of 13–19 mm (½–¾ in) is requested, this can be made by raising the heel without a corresponding sole raise, provided the raise is tapered towards the front so that the shoe stands flat (*Figure 6.4*). This not only looks less obviously raised but leaves a more flexible sole so that the patient can continue to bend his foot naturally when walking. It may be necessary to remove a rubber heel or one layer of a leather heel to provide a flat, firm surface on which to glue the raise. This extra height should be included in the raise.

For a raise of more than 19 mm (¾ in), both the heel and sole must be raised but it will be less obvious and just as effective if the sole raise is tapered towards the front (*Figure 6.5*). Cork will allow some flexibility in the sole.

Often the old and comfortable shoes provided by the patient for such temporary raises are convex on the sole, both crossways and

172

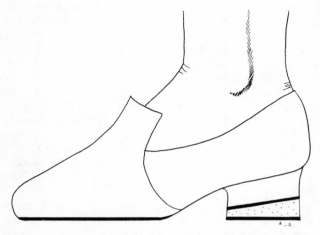

Figure 6.4. – Heel raise 12–19 mm (½–¾ in) can be supplied without a corresponding sole raise, provided the raise is tapered towards the front so that the shoe stands flat

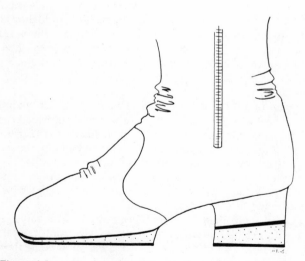

Figure 6.5. – Shoe raise 19–25 mm (¾–1 in). The raises on both heel and sole are tapered towards the front to make the adaptation less obvious

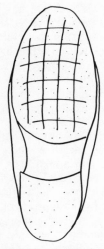

Figure 6.6. – Raise on an older shoe with a worn, curved sole. The cork is scored on the underside, before it is attached to the shoe, to make it more flexible

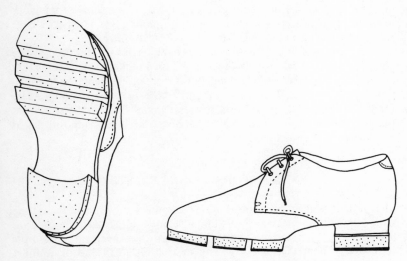

Figure 6.7. – Shoe raise higher than 25 mm (1 in). This shows the positioning of the sections, in line with the metatarsal heads, under a left shoe

lengthwise. It may be enough to shape the cork with a rasp or coarse sandpaper to the necessary concavities. If the curvature is very pronounced the cork can be scored on the underside (*Figure 6.6*). It will then bend to the shape of the sole and stick more effectively in place.

When a raise of more than 25 mm (1 in) is requested, and when it is considered particularly important to allow maximum flexibility in the sole, three sections of cork aligned with the slant of the metatarsophalangeal joints can be glued to the sole (*Figure 6.7*). This enables the patient to bend the foot in walking and to regain mobility and a gait that is not unlike the normal. It is usually easy to find the correct slant by looking at the crease in the shoe when the patient lifts his heel whilst keeping his toes on the ground. The distal section ends nearer the toe than the crease observed. The other two sections are 25–38 mm (1–1½ in) wide. For a high raise to be stable, it is essential that the shoe is of a type that is laced or strapped firmly to the foot.

Though an occupational therapist should know how shoe raises may be quickly and temporarily tried out, the patient can often be taught to do the work for himself, or another patient can help him to do it when neither is actively employed in work that is directly therapeutic. Many patients claim some experience as a 'snob' or amateur cobbler. This work cannot be easily carried out by a patient who must remain sedentary, for the three-footed iron last used by the amateur must be used on a firm bench or block of wood, and some of the work must be carried out with the operator standing. He must also have reasonably strong and mobile hands to do it efficiently.

Some doctors like their patients to have a raise on the shoe of the good leg when a walking plaster is raised on a rocker. This ensures that when the patient is standing the pelvis is level and leg lengths are equal. Other doctors take their view that the plaster is there to compensate for the lack of ankle movement in walking, and that a patient will not rise up on the curve of his rocker as he walks if the opposite leg is lengthened by a shoe raise.

ROCKERS FOR WALKING PLASTERS

The patient with a fracture of the lower limb may spend some time with the leg in plaster. Whilst non-weight-bearing this presents no problem, but when weight-bearing begins there have been many attempts to provide some means of keeping the plaster clean and dry, whilst permitting the patient to walk about freely in and out-of-doors. Sometimes special plaster boots are provided which have the advantage of keeping the toes and the plaster clean, warm and dry. Their expense is,

however, a consideration. All other means of preservation are founded
on the old-fashioned patten which the ladies of Cranford strapped on
their shoes to raise them out of mud when taking a walk out-of-doors.
At Farnham Park the writer has designed a wooden rocker which can
be fixed on the original non-weight-bearing plaster with little trouble
and its shape makes possible a reasonable gait.

The rocker is shown diagrammatically in *Figures 6.8* and *6.9*. The
bottom is shaped to an ellipse with a flat area to come under the
ankle joint so that the patient has a steady base when standing at a

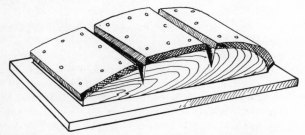

Figure 6.8. – Wooden rocker for application to a walking plaster

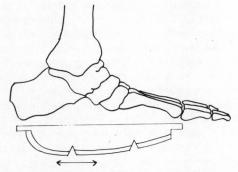

*Figure 6.9. – Rocker showing flat surface to give firm stance with
weight transmitted under the ankle joint*

workbench. The elliptical curve is longer at the front of the foot than
under the heel to ensure that the patient walks with the correct rocking
movement and prevents the development of the 'ball-iron' gait which is
so difficult to eliminate when once acquired. There is a shelf of about
6 mm (¼ in) on the upper surface to allow for fixation with plaster
bandages, and one or two saw cuts through the rocker help to give space

for the plaster bandage passed all round. The walking surface of the rocker must be covered with some non-skid material, such as rubberized canvas used for machine belts in a factory. Sometimes the tread of an old motor-tyre which has worn thin has been used. The rocker itself is of 38 mm (1½ in) thick deal, and is made in three sizes:

	Width	*Length*
Large	100 mm (4 in)	175 mm (7 in)
Medium	87 mm (3½ in)	162 mm (6½ in)
Small	75 mm (3 in)	137 mm (5½ in)

The general posture of the patient must be watched so that balance and co-ordination of movement are quickly regained. If the shoe on the 'good' foot is put up on a temporary raise when a walking rocker is first applied to a plaster splint, the patient should never acquire a limp. As soon as the short plaster allowing knee bend is permitted, he can work standing at a foot-power lathe and develop still further his sense of balance and co-ordination. One patient in a long plaster was able to chop wood. He was also able to swing a 31 kg (14 lb) sledge-hammer on the wedges to split logs (*see Figure 3.15,* page 84). He said that he could dance a slow waltz though he could not manage a quickstep.

Whilst on the subject of shoe raises and the patients who require specialized adaptations of the shoes, it may be convenient to note that many patients walk badly because they wear down the heel on one side of the shoe. While disabled they have some difficulty in getting their shoes repaired. If it is not possible to arrange for shoes to be repaired locally (this could be the excuse for an expedition to the shops for another patient who needs to try public transport) it is usually possible to buy suitably sized do-it-yourself heel sets from Woolworths to be put on in the department. It is also useful to have a supply of soling material so that more major repairs can be carried out. The writer has observed that patients with widely varied disabilities can be taught to walk and stand, maintaining a greatly improved posture when the heels of their shoes are regularly replaced and kept level. This work can be done by the patients themselves.

PLASTAZOTE SANDALS

These sandals are made at Farnham Park for patients who have had decompression of the Achilles tendon. The foot must be held in plantar flexion and no pressure should be taken on the incision site. The sandal must therefore have a raised heel and be open backed.

Although not many occupational therapists treat patients with this particular condition, they do make sandals for those with deformed feet caused by rheumatoid arthritis and for post-operative conditions of the feet. Some of the sandal designs that have been published are very unsightly, although they may be comfortable. A recent survey of patients' attitudes to wearing surgical shoes showed that a high proportion were very concerned about the appearance of their feet and resented wearing ugly shoes which drew attention to their disability.

The Farnham Park sandals are of a simple design and do not make the foot look too conspicuously disabled. They are made in white Plastazote, which has been found more acceptable than pink. Patients who no longer need to wear them have asked if they can keep them for use at home. The details of how to make the sandals are included here because the basic method can easily be adapted for other patients by leaving out the raised heel and the open back.

To take a pattern, sit the patient on a low chair with his knees flexed at right angles and his ankles directly below his knees. He will be balancing on the ball of his injured foot and should hold his ankle

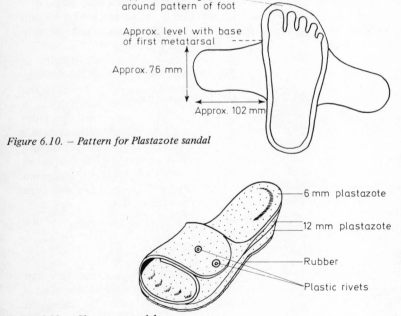

Approx. 12 mm gap around pattern of foot

Approx. level with base of first metatarsal

Approx. 76 mm

Approx. 102 mm

Figure 6.10. – Pattern for Plastazote sandal

6 mm plastazote

12 mm plastazote

Rubber

Plastic rivets

Figure 6.11. – Plastazote sandal

in as much dorsiflexion as possible. Measure the distance from his heel to the floor to work out the raise required. Draw the outline of the foot and mark where the straps will come; this will be approximately 7.5 cm (3 in) towards the heel, varying with the size of the foot. Draw two outriggers approximately 11 cm (4¼ in) on either side to act as wrap-over straps (*Figure 6.10* shows overall shape). Add 1 cm ($^3/_8$ in) all round the foot outline to make a basis for the sandal.

Using 12 mm (½ in) Plastazote cut out the foot pattern twice, and also as many heel pieces as are needed to produce the required raise. Chamfer the front upper edges of the heel pieces on the electric buffer or sander so that they slope gently towards the toes. Using 6 mm (¼ in) Plastazote cut out the foot pattern again and also the outriggers.

Stack all the pieces together with the 6 mm (¼ in) layer on top, the heel raise pieces in the middle and the two thicker base layers underneath. Place them in an oven preheated to 140°C, and leave for 8–10 minutes.

Remove from the oven and, with the patient in the original seated position, place his foot on the sandal and strap the pieces over the front of the foot (*Figure 6.11*). Hold the sandal in position for 2–3 minutes.

Finish off the sandal by securing the strap pieces with plastic rivets, buffing the edges with an electric buffer or sander, and by gluing a piece of ripple rubber under the sole for added strength and safety.

FURTHER READING

England, M. D. (1973). *Footwear for Problem Feet*. London; Disabled Living Foundation

7

Disabilities of the Upper Limb

The number of patients with disabilities of the upper limb has only
been a small proportion of the total treated at Farnham Park. Yet the
discursiveness of this chapter has become inevitable. The hands are the
means through which therapeutic occupations are directed to other
parts of the body. Disabilities of the hands have been observed to
affect not only the general posture but the mental outlook. Observation of the use of the hands has given opportunity for assessment of
capacities of accuracy and adaptability. These may have lain dormant
in a patient whose history gives no indication of a hopeful future.
Study of the uses of the hands has influenced the writer's approach to
many problems in the treatment of patients with various disabilities.

Elasticity of soft tissue in the upper limb

The late Professor Wood Jones in his *Principles of Anatomy as Seen in
the Hand* has devoted a chapter to the study of the fasciae. He writes
of the elastic stocking formed by the deep fasciae of the lower limb
being thick and complete in compartments enclosing the muscles. He
describes this as being of particular value in resisting the pressure of
'passive fluids' which are liable to gravitate downwards in a limb usually
vertical in waking hours. He contrasts the fasciae of the neck, shoulder
girdle and upper limb. This may be fairly thick on the posterior aspect
or the extensor surfaces where less movement of the skin is required.
On the anterior aspect and the flexor surfaces the superficial fascia is
abundant, lacy in structure and lax. The skin is mobile and elastic. The
superficial and deep fasciae constitute gliding planes between the skin,
muscular bundles, joint capsules and ligaments, as well as providing the
scaffolding which carries the nerves, arteries and veins on their several
occasions.

It is suggested that co-ordination of movement in the hand and upper limb is as dependent on the elasticity and mobility of the fascial structures as on the quick intention of thought which instigates muscle contractions. To fulfil the functions of the hand, muscles of the upper limb appear to change their grouping quickly, some acting as prime movers, others as fixators or opponents in a complexity of patterns of movement found nowhere else in the body. The fascial investment of muscles which can perform such intricate activities must play a singularly permissive role, allowing structures to glide over each other in various positions.

Reference has already been made to the effects of rest and immobility on structures of the trunk and lower limb. Rest must be expected to play its part in the early stages of treatment of most disabilities. The ordinary positions of rest for the upper limb have perhaps more noticeable effects on the structure of the fasciae in this region than elsewhere in the body. The patient will not be kept in bed for as long as when the disability occurs in the trunk or lower limb. When an arm is injured and there is danger of oedema the arm will be slung high in elevation whilst bed-rest is indicated.

Dr Boyes (1970) commented that 'the deep fascia enclosing the long flexors in the forearm is tough and unyielding, so that pressure developing within its enclosure from trauma or obstructive engorgement squeezes out the blood supply and Volkmann's ischaemia results.' In the acute condition which might result without surgical intervention in ischaemic paralysis, the occupational therapist can play no part, except through the provision of a soft woolly ball suspended within reach. This may make it easier for a patient to carry out instructions to keep the fingers moving in catching and clutching it.

Later on, if there is still residual oedema though a patient may be allowed up and be sent for rehabilitation, elevation at night may be directed by the medical authorities. The swing arm supports described later (pages 236—237) can be used for this purpose. The hand and arm may be supported in the prescribed elevation whilst permitting some freedom of movement to the patient without the discomfort which would disturb sleep.

When the patient is allowed up, the hand itself may be kept high in a sling (*see Figure 7.15*, page 238). The general position of rest for injuries of the upper limb includes the upper arm hanging by the side with the forearm supported only just above a right angle. Examples may be quoted. Gravity can count as a help to pull into alignment the lower end of a fractured humerus. The capsule of a dislocated shoulder must be allowed to heal in a position shortening the fibres of the lower aspect which have generally been torn by the incident of dislocation. Fractures of the radius and ulna must be immobilized in a position which will help to prevent cross union. Hand injuries may require fixation to the abdominal wall to obtain good skin coverage in preparation for further stages in plastic surgery. The positions of immobility or comparative fixation as well as the occurrence of damage will have their effect on fasciae, superficial and deep. Without the continual small stretchings of normal movement, fascial structures will lose their elasticity. The lubricating exudates, which should be minimal in quantity and fluid in quality, lose these characteristics. Tissues which should slide smoothly over each other become adherent or move sluggishly and stickily.

The restoration of mobility and elasticity to all fascial investments are aims which must never be forgotten in occupational therapy. These are of primary importance in treating disabilities of the upper limb. To achieve these aims sudden and strenuous movements are not found to be successful. They may even be deleterious in tearing apart structures that have become adherent or inadequately lubricated through disuse. Such tears can only be repaired by scar tissue, and this will spoil the structure of fascial investment. Manipulation of stiff joints under anaesthetic may be the last resort of the surgeon. Manipulation without anaesthetic by encouraging sudden or over-forceful movements is no part of occupational therapy.

Occupational therapy for disabilities of the upper limb

Occupational therapy programmes have been planned to use the whole of the upper limb as fully as possible. The disability may have affected principally one region, but the whole arm has been affected by the rest or immobility needed to treat that region.

To some extent this is true even when the disability only affects one finger. It has, however, been appreciated that a disability affecting the hand requires a rather different approach from that directed to the upper limb above wrist level. There may be some annoyance at an inability to manoeuvre the hand into its customary positions of usefulness when the arm is disabled, but this cannot be compared with the affront of a disfigured hand, and the distaste for having it in full view added to the annoyance of poor function. It has therefore been found reasonable to divide disabilities of the upper limb into broadly two groups, one of disabilities above the wrist and including the shoulder girdle, and the other of the hand. Amputation of the thumb or of individual fingers will be discussed after hand injuries.

Postural defects which develop as a result of injuries to the upper limb

The occupational therapist in practice soon learns to appreciate that almost all 'purposive activities' of the body are geared towards giving the hands opportunity to carry out their manifold functions to the best advantage. It is by the results of their actions that conscious thought achieves reality. This eager insatiable desire to make full use of the hands has, on occasion, attendant dangers. Postural defects of the shoulder girdle may easily be developed, followed by unbalanced activities of the spine. It has been observed that many disabilities become exaggerated and permanent as a result of efforts to discount malalignment of bones, or weakness or spasm in muscles, which hamper the hands as servants of conscious thought. Only by considering the individual as a whole is it possible to foresee and to prevent structural changes which may be irreversible or postural habits which will require much time and attention to correct. The maximum efficiency of the body as a whole will eventually give full opportunity to the functions of the hands. But this picture of balance and control is difficult for the patient to appreciate. It is a necessity that the occupational therapist study the functions of the hands and observe their influence, so that 'purposive activities' can be of truly therapeutic value.

THE SHOULDER GIRDLE AND ARM ABOVE WRIST LEVEL

Anatomists and surgeons interested in phylogenetics give the opinion that the arm above the wrist and the shoulder girdle have developed in more recent specialization than has the hand. It is suggested that this has occurred as a result of the growing desire to improve the functional capacities of the hands by increasing the area of the environment in which the hands find scope to fulfil their services to conscious thought.

The observation of two patients with congenital defects of the forearm has made the writer appreciate how much the hands are dependent on the reach and mobility of the upper limb. One patient had bilateral absence of the radius and ulna. Her beautifully shaped hands were attached to the elbows. She was an expert seamstress and did exquisite embroidery whilst in hospital for operations on her legs to enable her to walk. But she could hold no article much larger than a handkerchief as there was so little space between her body and her hands in which to turn her work. She could not reach out to use a sewing machine or a loom. The second patient was a young man with complete fusion of the radius and ulna on the left and partial on the right. His elbow extension on both sides was limited, and pronation and supination non-existent. Surgical intervention attempted to improve forearm rotation on the right side by excision of the head of the radius. But little improvement was noted. He was a gardener and returned to this work, but the limitations of forearm movement threw considerable strain on his wrists and shoulders. It was felt that the outlook when he grew older was not encouraging in view of the abnormal wear and tear to which these joints were subjected.

The aims of treatment in occupational therapy always direct the therapist to regain mobility and controlled power. Mobility would seem to be the most important aim for treatment of the upper limb, as distribution of bodyweight can do much to assist in the achievement of forceful activity. This may be contrasted with the aims of treatment for disabilities of the lower limb and the spine where stability is the first necessity, and bodyweight cannot be used so effectively to reinforce the power of muscle contractions.

It is of interest to consider some of the movements which will habitually be called into play to compensate for reach and mobility in the upper limb. Such compensatory movement may have to be encouraged and developed if a shoulder or elbow joint has been arthrodesed. In other cases it must be guarded against. The movement of the scapula sliding forward on the wall of the thorax, pivoting on the sternoclavicular joint, is usually employed to assist abduction and forward flexion when the scapulohumeral or elbow joint are at all stiff. Side flexion of the spine in the lumbar region will lift a hand about seven to nine inches without moving the elbow joint from a right-angle. Sometimes backward swing from the hips or increase of the normal lumbar curve will add to the lift.

If the shoulder has been arthrodesed the scapular movement must be encouraged, and the lumbar movement discouraged. It is wiser not to develop spinal imbalance which would lead to scoliosis or lordosis and to learn to make the best use of the upper limb in the limited range made available by scapular movement. A large group of powerful muscles controls scapular movement. The deltoid is accustomed to contract as part of this group, and it has been observed that after arthrodesis of the scapulohumeral joint, the deltoid will continue to maintain its bulk and tone to some degree, whereas if the circumflex nerve has been affected in a brachial plexus lesion, rapid wasting of the deltoid will occur. The bulk and tone so maintained in the deltoid may be of considerable value in cushioning the point of the shoulder girdle.

One patient, a man aged 46 years, had a fracture-dislocation of his left shoulder which could not be satisfactorily reduced. Four weeks later his surgeon performed an arthrodesis with the humerus in slight abduction and forward flexion. After a further eight weeks the patient was sent for rehabilitation with a note that this position had been chosen to enable him to return to his work as a bricklayer. He started by knocking down an old brick wall, which was not very heavy work as the cement had become very friable. His left arm was, of course, weak after three months of immobilization, and when it became tired he sat down and did some basketry with the arm in a spring-loaded sling to give buoyancy with support. In gradually lengthening periods of work at his own job he cleaned off the bricks and built a wall to make an open shed into a woodstore for the occupational therapy workshops. In the beginning it was interesting to note that his elbow and forearm movements were as weak and uncertain as the movement of the shoulder girdle fused with the humerus. He handled the bricks clumsily and used a lot of lumbar movement not only to lift his arm but to make up for the lack of rotation in the shoulder joint which he was accustomed to use to increase the range of pronation and supination. Before he was discharged after nine weeks of rehabilitation he could toss a brick over and round with all the style of the expert. His lumbar movement decreased with supervision and explanation of its dangers, as his forearm and shoulder power improved. He returned to his own job straight away. He still felt that he had lost some of his pace at work, but in his follow-up reports he wrote that he was employed on work that needed skill and finish rather than rapidity.

The late Dr C. J. S. O'Malley when director of the Medical Rehabilitation Centre, Camden Road described the plight of another bricklayer, who had a fracture of the lower third of his right humerus. The surgeon, in early days of treatment, told the patient he would not be able to return to his trade. Immediately after discharge from hospital he was sent to an Employment Rehabilitation Centre. There he was found unco-operative and it was decided that he was not suitable for retraining in other work. He went home and apparently was not employed for a period of two years dating from the accident. He was then sent to a Medical Rehabilitation Centre, and after some weeks started bricklaying of his own free will. He returned to this trade with success.

O'Malley's case A.B. was told he could not return to his trade whilst our patient was assured, in the early days of treatment, that he could do so. Our patient was sent for rehabilitation under medical supervision four months after the original incident, whereas A.B. remained without treatment for two years and was judged untrainable in the meanwhile. It would appear that the comparison of these cases would make a strong plea for reassurance by the surgeon from the beginning of treatment and early rehabilitation under medical guidance and the supervision of personnel trained to work with patients.

Compensatory movements of the scapula must be discouraged when there is no 'bony' reason for it. To illustrate this point, and also the previous remarks about the importance of fascial elasticity, one example of patients who suffer from 'frozen shoulder' may be cited. A woman aged 53 years had had a bad attack of shingles. After this had passed she had acutely tender areas round her neck and shoulders. She had heavy domestic responsibilities and learnt willy-nilly to use her right hand and arm, this being the master side. But she must have managed without her left arm, as in spite of various episodes of physiotherapy for eight months she had to be sent for a full programme of rehabilitation. This of course included hydrotherapy and exercises. In occupational therapy she started with the arm slung with a 25 pound tension spring to give her support and buoyancy. At first only a small range of movements was attempted and she wound rug wool around rings of cardboard to make the woolly balls useful in the treatment of patients with badly damaged hands. Then she progressed to weaving on a horizontal loom, making a rug on a 76 cm (30 in) wide warp. The length of shuttles she used was gradually increased until she had reached about 80 degrees of abduction with spring assistance. Then the springing was gradually decreased. After 11 weeks of treatment she could achieve about 80 degrees of active abduction with spring assistance. Then the springing was gradually increased. After 11 weeks of treatment she could achieve about 80 degrees of active abduction without much scapula movement. She was an out-patient, and regular inquiries were made about the housework, high dusting, cooking and washing she did in the evenings and at weekends. In her follow-up reports at three, six and 15 months after discharge, she still complained of pain in her left shoulder, but this was not preventing reasonable activities. She had gone back to the office-cleaning job which she had done before she got the shingles, as well as doing her housework.

always been taught that the biceps is peculiarly liable to become contracted if the elbow is kept long in flexion, and that such contractions must never be pulled out forcibly or with jerky movements.

These may even irritate the fibres of this muscle enough to give rise to the condition of myositis ossificans when spicules of bone are formed in the muscle fibres, tendons or fasciae. It has therefore been found necessary to encourage extension by light work which requires the use of the triceps. Sawing and planing are both useful, but the therapist must be careful in the choice of wood used. Oak or beech are often too hard and even deal must be carefully chosen to avoid hard knots in the grain which might cause a sudden jar to a joint or jerky movement in a muscle. Often plywood may be found the most suitable as its consistency is even.

The second precaution that must be remembered in treating the arm even above wrist level is the condition of the skin of the hands. The 'son of toil' will not be 'horny handed' after a period of rest or fixation of the upper limb. The thickened layers of skin peel off, and the skin is left as soft and easily blistered as that animal which must be almost as extinct as the dodo — the lady of leisure.

It has been found also that certain hand disabilities which have required lengthy plastic surgery suffer from noticeable wasting of the forearm and upper arm. It is impossible to provide occupational therapy sufficiently demanding to redevelop these wasted muscles without running the risk of damaging a recently grafted area. Suitable exercises to develop the muscles of the forearm and upper arm can however be carried out against spring resistance in the gymnasium; and only light work, with smooth materials such as mosaic, or handling a paintbrush or weaving, used in the workshops. It may take some weeks to harden up the skin of the hand sufficiently for work with heavy or rough materials.

THE HAND

The *Oxford English Dictionary* defines 'the hand' as 'the terminal part of the arm beyond the wrist, consisting of the palm and five digits, and forming the organ of prehension characteristic to man'. This definition satisfied the Lord Chief Justice in giving judgment (1957) to allow for the appeal of an injured person, when there was some question as to the hand being an organ or a limb. The definition would not satisfy an anatomist, a physiologist, a neurologist, or an occupational therapist.

Wood Jones (1920) says: 'We shall look in vain if we seek for movements of the hand which a man can do, and a monkey cannot. But we shall find much if we look for purposive actions which a man does do, and a monkey does not.' It is the scope of the hands, their relationship to the brain, and the effect of 'purposive actions' on the balance and activities of the body as a whole that are of particular interest to the occupational therapist.

Wood Jones, elsewhere in the same work, makes it clear that the hand of man has changed less anatomically in evolution from its primitive state than would appear possible 'when we study its wonders as a functional organ'. He also discusses the implications of evolutionary changes in the foot and other structures leading to the erect posture adopted by man. It would appear that other parts of the body have been gradually adjusted or differentiated to allow for full development of capacities in the hand, and that a relationship has been established between the hand and the brain which has been of 'great importance in developing the destinies of man as a species'.

It is a necessity that the occupational therapist study the functions of the hands. These may be considered in their main categories as organs of appreciation, expression and commission.

Sensory appreciation in the hands

The term 'sensory appreciation' includes a variety of impressions related to objects in the environment outside the body, and to conditions existing in the body itself. The former class of impressions is received by specialized cells, conveyed by nerve paths, and delivered to cells in the cortical area of the brain where conscious thought may accept the impression and incorporate it in the picture of the environment which absorbs the attention. The impression may be rejected when it does not fit into a desirable picture, and then the individual may be described as 'not to have noticed feeling' some particular quality of an object in the environment. The presence or absence of notice and awareness may fluctuate in the same individual. This fluctuation will depend on the interest and attention focused by conscious thought. 'Awareness' is a capacity which can be trained and developed into specialization of some or many aspects of sensory appreciation.

The second class of sensory appreciation concerns the conditions, positions and relationship of various parts and tissues of the body. These sensations are conveyed to various parts of the brain through devious routes with close interchanges. Conscious thought may be trained to pick up information if it so desires. For example one can think of the position of a hand in the dark, or the tension exercised by muscle contraction. But one is not ordinarily aware of the many details of sensory appreciation which have gone to build up this picture in thought. The skilled person such as the dancer, the musician or the engineer who gives the impression of exercising highly co-ordinated movement must have been able to train his talent for sensory appreciation of position without knowing the hows or whys. His awareness of the results has enabled him to develop a relationship between sensation and activity. Various tissues in the body will develop in their capacities as a result of demands made by conscious thought. It is not too fanciful to imagine that nerve paths constantly carrying impressions of environmental or deep sensation may react more quickly, and become more alert in their constitution with practice, and that this may occur to a greater degree in some people than it does in others.

Wood Jones (1920) quotes other authorities as well as his own observations to demonstrate 'how dominant in the cortical area is the representation of the hand as an appreciative organ'. In this capacity the baby starts using its hands. The first movements are practised in relation to the earliest area of sensitivity — the snout. Fingers, then toys and toes are clutched and crammed against or into the mouth. Eye muscles are not yet under control and one watches the baby squinting in efforts to get into focus objects that can be touched, held and felt. The eyes soon take over from the mouth in a partnership with the hands. Together the eyes and the hands develop power and capacity. Conscious thought is modelled through their associated activities. We memorize experiences and learn to guess and to judge position, relationship, contours and textures of objects in our neighbourhood. The descriptive words we learn to convey to others our impressions of our environment have their significance based on the appreciation of touch as well as of sight. It is difficult to imagine what words we would use to describe a velvet dress worn by a woman seen at a distance except by using the word 'velvety', which has significance gained by touch and then referred to sight.

Boyes (1970) has described the nerve cells which have the specialized function of stereognosis, the perception and recognition of objects by touch. These nerve cells are distributed in profusion over the area of the finger-tips, especially of the thumb and index fingers. This faculty with other sensations will be intercepted by a peripheral nerve lesion in that area. It is interesting that occasionally a lesion in the receptive area of the brain, caused by embolism or thrombosis with accompanying hemiplegia, may affect the function of stereognosis alone when other senses, such as appreciation of heat and cold, are intact. This situation was observed in a patient who had bilateral parietal abscesses. After these had been aspirated he could feel objects in his pocket, but found it impossible to distinguish between coins with a milled edge and those which were smooth. He could with difficulty distinguish between a Yale key and a coin. He also complained that he was unable to control the amount of power of grip he exerted. If he held his little daughter's hand when taking her for a walk, he found that he might hold her hand so tightly that she cried out with pain. He could distinguish between a soft finger and a hard metal cylinder of the same size, both by temperature and by consistency.

The loss of the various senses of appreciation is a most interesting study for the occupational therapist. It will be encountered as a by-product of so many various disabilities. The peripheral nerve lesion and the lesion in the conscious area of appreciation in the brain are but two causes. The replacement by plastic operations of part or whole digits will produce a tool which may be trained comparatively quickly as an organ of expression or commission, but very slowly as an organ of appreciation. Crush injuries to the fingers are another problem. Perhaps the oedema which is so markedly characteristic of this type of injury has an ischaemic effect on sensory nerves.

Sensory nerves lying in the epidermis are less cushioned than motor nerves lying in the muscles and interstitial tissues. Co-ordination of movement can be re-educated by imitation and practice to some extent, but complete co-ordination of movement can only be achieved by re-education of all forms of sensory appreciation.

To achieve this, the occupational therapist must first learn to observe in herself the feeling and appreciation of texture, the feeling of position and the feeling of tensions caused by movement. Then she must be able to translate these appreciations to her patient. The obvious necessity to avoid risk of further injury to tissues which are just recovering is the first appeal to reason. The importance of observation and the trans-position of vision in its relationship to sensation by touch is the next step. The sense of touch educated the appreciation of vision in early days of life. Now the occupational therapist must use the patient's appreciation of vision to re-educate the dimmed sensations of touch.

The hands as organs of expression and commission

These faculties of expression and commission appear to merge into each other. The development of the use of the hands in expression is very active in some people. The musician or conductor of an orchestra expresses with his hands thoughts that beggar anyone's vocabulary, whilst he might appear hopelessly inefficient if he were asked to hammer a nail into the wall to hang a picture. The writer may find it difficult to dictate coherently though words flow from his pen in embarrassing abundance. By racial habit some people accompany their speech with expressive gesticulations. In some inarticulate individuals the material and solid result of the work of their hands expresses more personality and imagination than would be credited to them if judged by their speech or writing. 'By their works ye shall know them.' The activities of the hands in expression and commission are as varied as people's interests and occupations.

The linking together of the functions of the hand

Conscious thought links together the functions of the hands. The *Oxford English Dictionary* is not as limited in its definition of the hand as first appears. 'Prehension' is defined as 'grasping, seizing or mental apprehension'. Words are not always easy to use in clarifying the meaning of other words. The hands as organs of appreciation present information about their environment to the brain. This then instructs them in their capacities as organs of expression and commission to create something which will satisfy a desire for reality pictured in conscious thought. When appreciation, expression or commission fall short of desire the hands are set to practise their functions. The satisfaction can seldom be found as the pictured result is always a step in advance of skill. The hand as an organ of appreciation might be labelled as INTAKE; when occupied in expression or commission as OUTPUT. Yet all these functions are used together and at the same time. These are the 'purposive activities' described by Wood Jones as being important in developing the destiny of man as a species.

The hands in normal life

Some organs of the body such as the heart, liver, spleen and stomach exist singly. Others are duplicated, one on each side, such as the lungs or kidneys, but we are not conscious of this in normal health without special study. We may not be conscious of one-sided dominance of eye, ear or foot without considering the matter, but such dominance exists on test. By nature or by habit people will claim to be dominantly right-handed or left-handed. It has been found tiresomely pedantic to repeat in writing right or left dominant hand, and the phrase master or slave hand has been adopted for brevity. The terms are being used as a relative indication of what the individual patient counts as being of importance and not in a derogatory sense when referring to the slave hand. The position of the hands as master and slave is only in doubt to those few who are ambidextrous and can lead with either hand at will. Amongst a sample of healthy schoolchildren 49.3 per cent were found to have completely right-sided dominance of eye, ear, hand and foot, 4 per cent were wholly left-sided and amongst 46.7 per cent one or more organs were varyingly dominant. Yet in many activities it is difficult to distinguish between master and slave hands in either power or agility. Who would say that in playing the violin the left hand that holds down the strings, sometimes with powerful and controlled vibrations, is in a slave relationship to the right hand that holds the bow to stroke out the music from the strings?

In past years left-handed dominance was frowned upon and children were forced to learn to write with the right hand. Nowadays one notices an increasing number of young people who have been allowed to retain left-handed dominance in writing and many other activities. It is usual to hear parents say that the only activities they insist that a left-handed child should carry out in the more common right-handed manner are in handling a knife and fork at table because this looks more comely, and batting when playing cricket, because it wastes time to change over the fielders. It should be observed that the handling of knife and fork differs from country to country. In Britain the knife is held in the right hand and the fork in the left hand when eating meat in its solid form. When the meat is cut up, such as in mince or stew, the knife is seldom used, and the fork is held in the right hand. In other countries the solid meat may be cut up as in Britain, but then the knife is discarded and the fork transferred to the right hand for the purpose of conveying the morsels to the mouth. That these activities should be so carried out appears acceptable and reasonable to the young, possibly because both require an equal use of both hands. Writing is really one of the few activities that require full dominance of one hand. Type-writing is taught using both hands and all the fingers, though one often notices the self-taught typist using only the index fingers and thumbs. Most tools require the use of both hands, though one remains the master and the other the slave. The ordinary potato-peeler is one of the few tools mass-produced for the left-handed person, but the demand is said to be less than 1 per cent of the total, so apparently few left-handed people bother to avail themselves of this convenience. It would appear as easy to revolve the potato on the peeler as the peeler on the potato.

Carpenters with good training insist that a woodworking gauge should be used with the left hand, the wood being steadied against the bench block with the right hand.

All factory machines are designed for the use of the right-handed. A wood machinist uses his left hand to hold the wood against the guard which all but covers the rotating blades, whilst the right hand is at the back pushing forward the wood. The press operator uses the right hand to press down the switch or pull down the lever to put the machine in motion whilst the left hand places the material in position. In these cases the left hand will be in the position of danger at work. An electrically operated circular or band saw makes equal demands on both hands pushing forward the material and both come into the danger zone. The engineer, fitter or machine setter uses both hands together in most operations. One engineer and toolmaker has mentioned that though usually right-handed, he finds himself using only the left hand to work a small tap or die as he appears to find the left hand more sensitive.

Under these circumstances it is easy to appreciate that either hand, master or slave, may be involved in an accident. In a sample of 398 patients with various injuries directly involving the upper limbs, only 6 were strongly left-handed, and out of this small number only 3 were affected on the left side. For the rest of the picture, there were 193 patients with injuries of the right hand or upper arm, and 176 with similar injuries of the left. Such differences are statistically insignificant except that they go to show that the occupational therapist must be prepared to rehabilitate the slave hand as well as the master.

Disfigurement of the hands as a personal affront

When studying the close relationship between the hands and conscious thought it is easy to appreciate how disfigurement of either or both hands will shock the personality. The shock is only comparable to that endured from facial disfigurement. In fact to many it may be worse.

> 'My face is ugly, let others mind it.
> I can't see it, I'm behind it.'

But the hand is continually in front when it is being used. Its uselessness and disfigurement are ever present. The affronted patient hides the offence to save his own feelings as well as those of his neighbours. This gesture of concealment is a natural reaction of something like disgust, a disinheritance, a severance of the close relationship which has taken all the previous years of life to establish. If a hand is disfigured by trauma, the early stages of treatment, dressings and bandages, will have acted as a screen. The interest and preoccupation of the doctor and nurse have given them an authority over the injured hand far greater than the patient's ownership. These are the factors which produce that disassociation one observes when a patient comes for rehabilitation after a hand injury. He regards the hand as a 'sort of a something' for which he has neither liking nor responsibility. Professor Lane's warning that a scar on the mind may be more crippling than a scar on the body is very applicable.

It is in the occupational therapy workshop that the patient will have the first opportunity to come to terms with a disabled or disfigured hand and to re-establish that 'close relationship between hand and brain which will be of such importance' in developing the personal destiny. The longer the period that elapses between the original accident and the first episode of re-establishing this relationship, the more difficult will be the problem.

Here may be the place to describe two women and their reactions to injuries of their hands. The first woman's rehabilitation must be at once acknowledged as not a success. She was a factory worker of about 40 years. Her face was not particularly attractive, but she had beautiful hands, and she had posed these for photographs advertising hand cosmetics. Her right hand was injured at work and a tendon repair was necessary. She was irregular in attendance as an out-patient at hospital and 18 months after the accident she was sent to us for residential rehabilitation. The hand was stiff and showed symptoms of Sudeck's atrophy. She had always been right-handed. Her writing with the right hand was passable, but she preferred to write with her left. In fact she preferred to do all that she could with her left hand, and used the right as little as possible. The scarring and disfigurement were really insignificant, but she had so much adored her hands that she exaggerated the ill looks of the right, and kept it out of sight, and out of mind, as much as she possibly could. Unfortunately she was a lady with a free tongue and other patients, especially the dockers, complained so bitterly about her choice of language that her rehabilitation in residence was short lived. Later she was advised to have psychiatric treatment, but her attendance was again irregular and her attitude unco-operative. She has continued to send Christmas cards and messages of friendliness to the occupational therapist, but the last news of her shows no improvement. She was completely unable to forgive and make friends with her injured hand and this has warped her nature—which may of course have had an innate instability only exaggerated rather than instigated by the accident which disfigured her hand.

The other woman was about 54 years of age. She also worked in a factory, but she was left-handed. A crush accident necessitated the amputation of the terminal joint of her left middle finger. She was sent to us for rehabilitation as an out-patient about 14 weeks after the accident. Her index and ring fingers were limited in movement, she could just move the joints of the remainder of the middle finger. The scars had healed, but the crusts had not yet separated so that she could not start having paraffin wax baths. In occupational therapy we made her a light finger-stall to prevent the crusts catching on her work and so being prematurely torn off. She started basketry at once, and then started making herself a dress on the sewing machine. We found that dressmaking for herself and her young daughter was her main hobby, but she was disappointed that she could not use a thimble as she was accustomed to do on the middle finger of her left hand. This difficulty was overcome by buying a rather large brass thimble and brazing two small loops of brass wire to this, one on each side. Through these loops were threaded fine elastic thread such as is used on a sewing machine for shirring. These were knotted together at knuckle and at wrist level, leaving a loop which could be slipped over the wrist. She could then do handsewing, using her left middle finger with the thimble as she had been accustomed to do. She went back to work in the factory after seven weeks of rehabilitation, and she could also carry on with her leisure interests. This was about six months after the incident of disablement.

It must be stressed when comparing the histories of these women that they were very different in temperament. The first was a loud-voiced rather brassy blonde of 40 years, and the second a quiet sensible woman of 54 years. We did not know either of them before the injuries they had suffered to their master hands. Their reaction to disablement was certainly different, but the difference in the lapse of time, as well as their early treatment, may well have had some influence on their capacities for co-operation and recovery.

Another patient, a young man aged 22 years had gangrene of the right hand following an embolism of the brachial artery. He was found to have a large cervical rib. This was excised and a cervical sympathectomy performed. The excision of dead tissue in the hand left only the proximal phalanges of the thumb and little finger, and these had to have some coverage from abdominal pedicles. Further plastic surgery was required before he was sent for rehabilitation. He was little able to use the rays left on his right hand as the metacarpophalangeal joints were very stiff. It was found also that he could barely read or write, so our social worker arranged for him to go to evening classes to make further training practicable. He was not an easy patient, unco-operative and quarrelsome, and it needed much understanding of his situation to keep him going for the 13 weeks before his surgeon could take him back for further treatment. He was readmitted a month later, at a time when there was another young man with a below-elbow amputation of the right hand. This man had been fitted up with a temporary working prosthesis which enabled him to cut up his own food at table. The patient with the small rays of fingers asked for something like this for himself. We at once fitted him with a similar gadget which, of course, was not ideal because it confined his ray fingers which we wanted him to use in a pincer grip. But we thought and planned. Our occupational therapy technician made him a knife which was built up with Perspex to encourage the pincer grip, but also had a spring clip which went round his wrist to give him some leverage. He was delighted with this, and himself sewed a leather sheath to keep it safe in his pocket between meals. His whole attitude changed and he became courteous and co-operative. He showed the knife to visitors with pride. He not only cut up his own food, but cut up for others more disabled than himself. It was suggested that this young man was very strongly right-handed and the necessity to use his left hand presented great difficulties. Also that the sight of the disinherited master hand was a grave affront which added to his personality change. Inquiries about his education revealed that he had actually been at a school for backward children, but after seven years or more his headmaster remembered him as a reliable, civil and co-operative youngster. His personality was far removed from this description when he first came for rehabilitation, but there was every sign of it returning to its former status after he was enabled to use the right hand again.

The hands in disablement

There are certain differences in the approach of the occupational therapist to the patient when treating disabilities of the master or the slave hand. To begin with, the shock of disfigurement appears to be more severe when the master hand is affected. There is a greater resentment in the conscious mind where its capacity for leadership is diminished. This resentment may be recognized in some highly strung, intelligent patients who react by being interfering and 'bossing about' other patients. Others are plunged into despair out of all proportion to the seriousness of injury or prognosis of recovery. Such patients may need very careful handling and encouragement, but when they have settled down and find that the hand is becoming more agile and powerful they regain confidence and go ahead quickly.

By comparison injury of the slave hand causes less mental affront. But it suffers from being more easily hidden, and may be given less opportunity for activity whilst the master hand becomes greedy for power and the patient uses the excuse of protection of the injured and apparently useless slave hand.

In planning a programme of occupational therapy the patient's normal pattern of movement has been said to be of paramount importance. It has been found however that previous correlated patterns of movement can effectively nullify the therapeutic effect of an occupation when the patient's slave hand is affected. If he is allowed to carry out work which he has habitually done with the master hand leading whilst the slave hand has acted statically to steady the tool or the hand, this treatment will not restore mobility or independence of action to the slave hand. Another problem may be that of accustomed pace which accompanies a well-known pattern of movement. The patient with a disabled slave hand cannot achieve this pace without the discovery and practice of trick movements. These may not only result in making greater demands on the master hand and so increase its dominance but may affect the whole balance of the body and, as already mentioned, lead to skeletal changes in the shoulder girdle and spine. Such trick movements may appear to assist productivity for the moment but this is based on poor foundations. When the patient cannot achieve a true economic pace of productivity he will suffer from discouragement and fear of the future. The disappointment will lead to frustration, making more indelible the scar on the mind. The prevention of such psychological damage is one of the primary objects of treatment.

It is essential for the occupational therapist to know the work by which the patient has earned his living in the past, as well as the hobbies which have given him interest in his leisure hours. Even if the actual work or hobby cannot be used therapeutically, the demands which these would make on the patient's capacity when he is fit should be the goal of treatment, and only by considering these demands from the earliest days of treatment can the therapist plan a programme which will be progressive. Thus did the surgeon who, in arthrodesing a brick-layer's shoulder, as already described, planned the angle of arthrodesis which would make bricklaying possible. The therapist must follow in his wake to achieve the medical direction of the aims of treatment, whilst remembering that it may be neither practical nor therapeutic to follow slavishly the exact patterns of movement which are habitual to the patient's mode of life.

It has previously been mentioned that physiotherapy and occupational therapy must be carried out in close co-ordination and co-operation. In the treatment of hand injuries this point may be again emphasized. An injured hand will often require treatment in physiotherapy with paraffin wax baths, massage with cream, and specific exercises. The occupational therapy carried out immediately after this, whilst the hand is warmer and more supple than before, will be of much more benefit than the same carried out when the hand is cold and stiff. Co-operation between these departments must include careful timing of the programme of treatment, as well as knowledge of each other's work.

A man aged 40 years, right-handed, had a crush injury to his left hand which involved the median nerve and the extensor tendons to index and middle fingers. These appeared to show recovery and he returned to work as a centre-lathe turner. Fourteen months after injury he came for a review, the tendons were freed and a nerve graft performed. After five weeks the plaster was removed and he was sent for rehabilitation. The hand was stiff and unco-ordinated in movement. He was fitted with a median glove to encourage abduction and oppo-sition. At first his great anxiety was to get back his touch on the electric screw-cutting centre-lathe. But in a day or two he realized that this did not make adequate demands for free movements. He still insisted that he was only interested in metalwork, so he was employed using a hacksaw and file on making angle brackets for another patient's ironing board. He soon made further investigations into the capacities of the woodworking and wood-turning sections which he had looked at with little interest on his first tour after admission, and he began to appreciate some of the table-lamps and fruit bowls made by others. He sawed out, planed and roughly shaped with a spokeshave a piece of walnut for a bowl. The handle on the left side of the spokeshave had to be padded for him to get a good grip, but this padding rapidly disappeared when it got in his way. He then turned a bowl on a foot-power lathe, and found that it was a different matter to hold wood-turning chisels firmly with both hands, rather than to screw down the tools in the clamp of an electric centre-lathe. His left hand had to work quite as hard as his right. After four weeks he showed enough improvement to return to work with his own firm who promised to give him work which would necessitate the use of his left hand, as indeed work on a centre-lathe does. The securing of the work in its place, the lifting and fixing of the chuck and gear of a big lathe will make an equal demand for use of both hands. A centre-lathe turner is expected to set up his own work, as opposed to a capstan turner who is a machine operator.

Another patient, an engineer, highly skilled and intelligent, had his left arm drawn in to the end of a jet engine of the aeroplane he was testing. The arm was badly burnt and when he was sent for rehabilitation about nine weeks after the accident the grafted skin was as thin as tissue paper, the elbow, wrist and fingers stiff and unco-ordinated. He was very intelligent and understood at once when the writer explained that his skin would not stand the dirt, oil and minute scraps of metal to which it would be exposed in the engineering section of the occupational therapy workshops. He fancied, when it was suggested, basketry. He could only cut the canes with his right hand, whilst manoeuvring a small vice to help hold them to measure with his left hand. As his range of movement and grip improved he finished one basket-edge tray with help, and did a second unaided. He progressed to woodwork and found that sawing and planing required the use of both hands. His skin toughened up in pace with his capacities for grip and agility. By the time he would have been fit for the engineering section he was discharged, as his firm were most anxious to have him back and promised work on inspection. He said, regretfully, that it would only require the use of a slide rule and micrometer. However he told the writer his father had been a carpenter-joiner; there were repairs and fittings he thought would improve his home and his hand by continuing woodwork, and he had his father's tools stored away in an attic. In a few months he answered his follow-up inquiry saying that he had returned to his own job of fitting and adjusting jet engines.

When the master hand has been affected, we have always tested the patient's capacity to write as soon as possible. At a residential centre, such as Farnham Park, a patient may be far from home and feel acutely the separation from family and friends; the trouble will be less acute if he can write for himself. As well as having this psychological value, writing is an activity which requires little power but a considerable amount of mobility and skill. If a daily exercise is kept up of writing his name and the date, the patient will see for himself how he is improving. Details of the techniques we have used to teach writing are given on page 99.

Complications which may accompany trauma

There are some defects which are apt to occur in the hand itself as a whole when the site of injury is limited to one digit.

Sweating

In our occupational therapy workshops profuse sweating in the hand which has been diagnosed as suffering from Sudeck's atrophy has been more usually noted than the dry and cold condition. Such sweating whilst the skin is already soft from disease has its dangers. Patients easily develop blisters, and sometimes find it difficult to grip tools properly when the handles are slippery with sweat. If the patients are working with materials which are smooth and absorbent, such as leather, they may leave marks on their work which cause some embarrassment. It has been found useful to keep surgical spirit and talcum powder easily available for patients to rub on their hands at reasonable intervals, more especially after washing. This not only gives temporary relief but helps to harden the skin and prevent blistering.

This sweating may be found to decrease rather more quickly than would be expected from the rate of recovery of the primary disability. It is suggested that there is some nervous factor of insecurity present when a patient starts working again. As he becomes accustomed to the atmosphere and personnel of an occupational therapy workshop the sweating becomes less marked. An analogous situation may be found, the writer has been told, when a toolmaker changes his job. At first he will find his work and tools filmed with rust every morning. Other toolmakers recognize this as the ordinary signs of the 'new boy'. When the toolmaker settles down and is at home with his mates, the sweatiness disappears and his work stays bright during the overnight absence. A disabled person learning a new job at a Skill Centre, such as watch repair or instrument work, is always given time to settle down and to see if the sweatiness is or is not a permanent state. If it is, of course training in such work would have to be abandoned and another training advised.

Muscle wasting

Another secondary disability which occurs after the disuse necessary for the treatment of a primary injury of the hands is a marked wasting of the first interosseous muscle which abducts the index finger to serve as a firm pillar against which the thumb can work in opposition and grip. This muscle seems to waste with extraordinary rapidity, and a drift to the ulnar side of all the proximal phalanges may follow. This of course is the position commonly noticed in persons suffering from rheumatoid arthritis of the hands. Occupational therapists treating such patients recognize that the ordinary position of knitting is deleterious to patients suffering from this disease, whilst the habit of holding the needle and twisting the wool round it, used in the Shetland Isles, is beneficial.

Patients who develop this drift of the index finger after trauma present a rather different problem as the muscle can be developed and restored to its original strength fairly quickly. On occasion a soft band of elasticated mesh fabric may be twisted round the index finger, and then round the wrist on the radial side. This makes a simple and comfortable night splint which helps to keep the first interosseous muscle in the position of relaxation which will aid recovery. It has not been found practicable to use this as a working splint, as the elastic mesh is found to wrinkle and slip down on the web between the index and middle fingers where the skin is thin and tender. But careful observation and supervision, accompanied by clear explanation as to the importance of this muscle, has always gained the co-operation of the patient. It has often been found that the teaching of voluntary control of positions of work when this is in any degree possible is more efficacious than splintage, which may be used to its best advantage when conscious control is relaxed during sleep.

Aims and principles of treatment of hand injuries

The aims and principles of treatment of hand injuries may be resolved as follows.

First, a hand that is disabled or disfigured must be regarded with kindness and friendliness. The patient's own attitude is of primary importance. It is often observed that this is one of detachment, if not of resentment and disgust. If the hand is to be reaccepted into its position as the most important tool of conscious thought, the occupational therapist must pave the way by showing the sort of care and and interest that would be equally appropriate in coaxing a lost and frightened puppy back to confidence. As the hand begins to respond in giving better service to conscious thought, the patient will begin to exert and extend the relationship that was natural previous to injury.

It has been found useful on occasion to stress the fact that neatness and smoothness of movement will make disfigurement less noticeable to others. If an old patient returns to visit and shows agility and freedom in gesticulation with a disfigured hand when talking, the repercussions in confidence amongst present patients will readily be observed. Photographs of patients with injured hands at work may be kept as a permanent exhibit. Without drawing attention to these, it will be noticed that present patients study them. This helps to accustom them to the fact that others, worse off in dilapidation of the hands, have faced up to the disability and surmounted it.

Secondly, if the master hand is disabled it must be trained to resume its position of leadership if this is in any way possible. This is particularly important in people of the later age-groups when habit has established a strong dominance. Skills such as writing, which are learnt early in life, are particularly difficult to transfer from the master to the slave hand.

Thirdly, if too gross a dilapidation has occurred, then cerebral control in dominance must be transferred to the slave hand. It will be found easier to do this if the first approach is made through an occupation which is both simple and strange to the patient. The processes of work must be demonstrated by the occupational therapist using, as leader, the hand which corresponds to the patient's slave hand. Some clumsiness on the part of the therapist demonstrating the technique is not necessarily out of place as it shows that difficulties are shared. The abdicating master hand must be employed at the same time in no matter how modest a role. It must learn to take its place as a helpmate, and to do so with grace and efficiency.

Fourthly, if the slave hand is disabled, the master hand must be restrained from becoming too protective or greedy for power. The slave hand must be given new and unaccustomed opportunities to assert its power and value. This again may be achieved by demonstrating work that is strange to the patient, work that demands an equal use of both hands. The good hand must teach the disabled one to regain function and power.

Lastly, to build the foundations of co-ordination, the therapist must learn to observe the feeling and appreciation of texture, position and correlated tensions caused by changes of position either external or internal. Then she must be able to teach these appreciations to the patient by drawing his attention to such dimmed or distant feelings that can be enlisted to help. Perhaps the first contact may be made by explaining to the patient that he must learn to watch his actions so as to avoid the risk of injury to tissues not yet completely healed. Then the patient must be taught the control of position and action by visual appreciation. The sense of touch educated the appreciation of vision in the early days of life. Now the relationship of teacher and pupil is transposed. Vision must be used to re-educate touch, the sense that has been dimmed by injury. Co-ordination of movement, controlled by appreciation of touch as well as by vision, must be learnt, and this is a slow process. Often the patient may be discharged as fit to use his hands 'in commission' long before he has recovered the senses of appreciation and expression, but if the therapist has been able to win understanding and co-operation during the days of treatment, she may be rewarded by the visit of an ex-patient, gesticulating with his injured hand in his account of his work, touching and feeling things with a certainty of appreciation that would have appeared impossible a year or so earlier.

AMPUTATION OF THE THUMB

The thumb of the master hand appears to work in a more vulnerable position than the thumb of the slave hand. Loss of the thumb on the master hand is a major calamity. Patients have come for rehabilitation with no thumb at all, with a floppy pedicle graft taken from the abdomen, with a transplanted big toe and with pollicized index or ring fingers.

One young woman seen in the early days at Farnham Park had had her right thumb torn off in a machine. The wound healed quickly and she was referred for occupational therapy 10 days after the accident. The stimulus of shock had not then passed off and she showed little appreciation of her loss. As well as doing basketry, in five days she could write well holding her pen between the index and middle fingers. She learnt to tool leather which requires more power of grip than writing and then she made a saddle-stitched purse holding a needle in the same way. After five weeks of rehabilitation she could use her right hand so deftly that the loss of her thumb attracted no attention. Her high spirits brooked no difficulties she could not surmount and early rehabilitation was directed to the demonstration of methods of using her hand and not, as so often is the case, to the restoration of confidence.

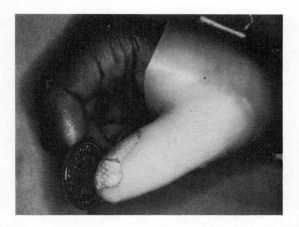

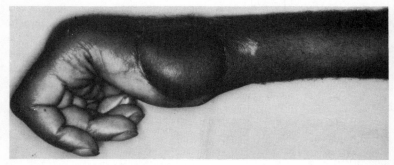

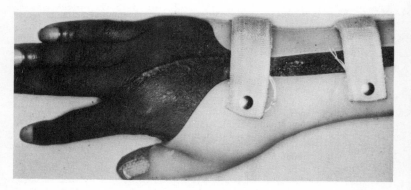

Figure 7.1. – *Thumb prosthesis designed by the occupational therapist and constructed by an orthotist. An adhesive dressing improved the gripping surface*

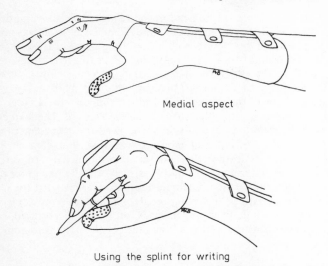

Medial aspect

Using the splint for writing

Figure 7.1. (continued)

A patient who lost his right thumb in a hot press accident was going to have a pollicization. When the surgeon opened up the hand he discovered that there was an insufficient arterial blood supply to make the operation successful. A thumb prosthesis (*Figure 7.1*) was therefore designed by the occupational therapist and made by an orthotist. This was constructed from heavy polythene with webbing and Velcro straps. Initially the tip of the thumb was too slippery for good pinch-grip but an ordinary adhesive dressing, which was easily replaced when worn or dirty, overcame the difficulty.

Patients sent for rehabilitation after partial reconstruction of the thumb by a pedicle graft from the abdomen, but before the final operation for bone insertion, present a difficult rehabilitation problem. When the writer was first confronted with this flabby sausage of flesh it was not easy to see how work could be planned which would assist in mobilization of the hand as a whole and general toughening of the skin. It was found necessary to make a 'corset' finger-stall for external stabilization of the thumb appendage. This corset was made of Perspex moulded to form a tube to contain the thumb, with a flap extending to the wrist to keep it in place with a wrist strap. We roughened the outer sides of the tube and covered it with leather; otherwise it was too slippery to act as a pedestal against which the opposing fingers could work in holding an object. (Nowadays this would have been made from Orthoplast.) As a progression in treatment another method of supporting this floppy thumb was found. The 'corset' stall was made of leather reinforced by spring wire. The thumb-stall was sewn into a glove in the ordinary way but only the index finger required a short stall, as far as the proximal phalanx, and the other fingers were left free. The glove was fitted close to the hand, like the median glove, with a zip fastener down the back. This leather thumb 'corset' was found useful to follow on after the stiffer corset of Perspex. The leather gave some protection to the soft new skin but allowed it to get some pressure. Whichever method of external splintage was used, the whole surface of the 'corset' and its leather fixation was punctured with holes so that the skin could get a free air supply to assist the toughening process.

The patient whose thumb had been replaced by his great toe (*Figure 7.2*) had the advantage of having tough skin available on the working surface of the hand. Even so, the lack of sensation required careful supervision of his work. It takes a long time for the patient to appreciate

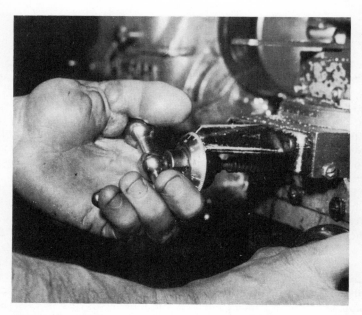

Figure 7.2 — Using handle of screw-cutting lathe to encourage grasp between thumb and other fingers, and mobility of hand and wrist. Patient lost both thumb and index finger in a bomb explosion. The thumb has been replaced by pollicization of the great toe

the secondary joint sensations which may be developed gradually to provide the knowledge of position and activity. This knowledge normal people take for granted, especially in the constant use of their hands. At first the patient must learn to watch position and use and gradually he will learn to notice the feeling induced by the changes of position and muscular contractions.

Many patients have been sent for rehabilitation following pollicization of either the index or the ring finger. Both these operations

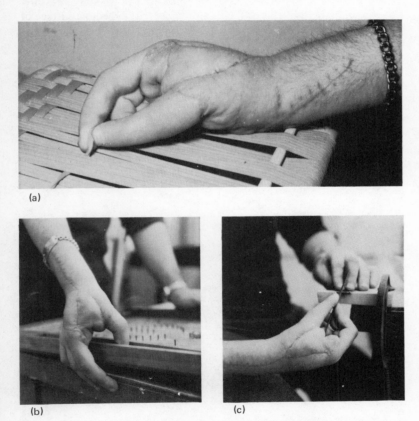

(a)

(b)   (c)

Figure 7.3. – Pollicization of the index finger following traumatic amputation of the right thumb by a circular saw. (a) Stool-seating using light pinch in the early stages of treatment. Any such activity helps to reorientate the sense of position of the pollicized digit. (b) Playing bagatelle, flicking the ball to exercise the extensor muscles of the thumb and mobilize the distal phalanx. (c) Shaping a metal brooch with a needle file using heavy pinch in the later stages of treatment

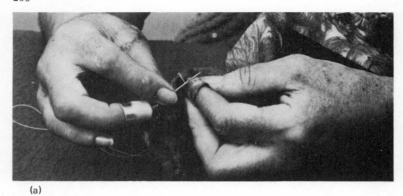

(a)

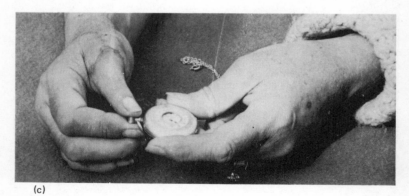

(b)

(c)

Figure 7.4. — Pollicization of the ring finger following avulsion of the terminal joint of the thumb when the mooring rope of a boat twisted round it. (a) Fine pinch — sewing. (b) Span — using large scissors. (c) Precision pinch — winding watch

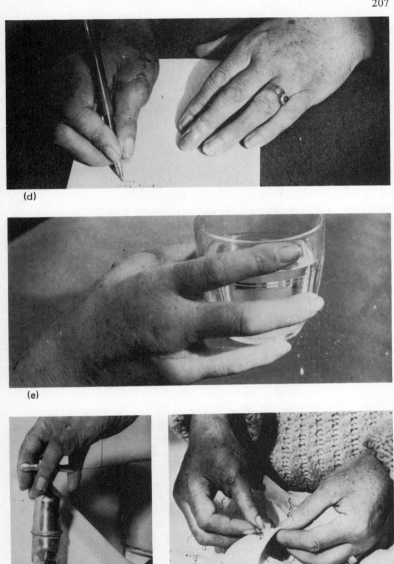

Figure 7.4 (cont.) – *(d) Tripod pinch* – *writing. (e) Co-ordination* – *lifting glass of water. (f) Power* – *turning a tap. (g) Functional activities* – *doing up buttons*

have the great advantage that when the finger to be pollicized is dissected out the nerves and blood supply are transferred intact to the new site. There will also be movement in the terminal joint of the new thumb and a thumb nail. One patient, who had lost the terminal phalanx of his thumb, made an excellent recovery and returned to his job as watch-maker. Without a thumb nail and without a terminal phalanx, however, he was clumsy and slow at work. His surgeon therefore removed the proximal phalanx of the thumb and performed a pollicization. After rehabilitation he was well able to manage his job.

Pollicization of the ring finger produces a better cosmetic effect because the index finger remains intact and therefore that part of the hand is unaffected by the operation. It is also easier to re-educate the hand because only the new thumb is being retrained, not a new index finger as well. Some experts, however, consider that the index finger is less involved in picking up objects than the other fingers, and therefore pollicizing the index and having to use the middle finger as a new 'index' should be little problem.

Retraining the hand after pollicization

The first objective is to re-educate pinch-grip and regain movement in the terminal joint of the new thumb. The thumb stabilizer (*see Figure 8.47a* and *b,* page 337) can be used in the early stages of treatment to block the reconstructed first and second metacarpophalangeal joints and so encourage mobilization of the interphalangeal joint of the new thumb. Initially the patient practises picking up soft objects and using activities requiring little power, then builds up to heavier work incorporating picking up various small objects using the thumb nail.

Perception of the new thumb must be learned and a variety of activities should be used to rebuild body image. In the treatment of any hand injury there is always the danger that by limiting the activities used in treatment the correct use of the hand will also be limited. Everyday activities such as using a knife and fork, writing, winding a watch, striking matches or sewing should be utilized to teach the patient to use the hand automatically in the right way, whatever he may be doing. This also helps to get patients to use accustomed patterns of movement for which there are well laid down patterns in the brain. Sometimes a patient's hobbies can be used to good effect.

It is interesting to watch the patient's adaptation to the new digit. Reorientation of the transposed digit as thumb occurs by stages. Initially, to flex the new thumb the patient needs consciously to flex his ring or index finger. If he tries to flex his 'thumb' nothing happens.

Similarly, when picking things up he still feels he is using a finger. He must be taught to watch what he is doing and so be aware with one of his senses that his 'thumb' is a thumb. After a time, which varies considerably from patient to patient, the tip of the thumb feels normal, perhaps because it is most consciously used, although the interphalangeal joint still feels part of a finger. Gradually this feeling of normality moves proximally until even the scar line at the base of the thumb is reorientated. For some further months unfamiliar deep sensations, such as pain resulting from a hard knock, still feel as if they emanate from a ring finger.

In the final stage of treatment the strength of the hand must be built up and for this industrial outwork has provided excellent repetitive exercise. Although the hand will continue to improve after discharge, sometimes treatment must be developed to suit particular work requirements. An electrician may need to flatten his hand to get it into a narrow space to reach cables. Another worker may need a wide span. Someone who lost his thumb in a machine accident may need to be reaccustomed to moving machinery.

AMPUTATION OF THE FINGERS

Patients who have lost most of their fingers will lack the supporting pedestal against which the thumb can work in gripping any object. This loss can be replaced to some extent by modelling a block of Perspex to form a pillar and fixing it in a position which will encourage the patient to mobilize the thumb and develop a pincer grip.

Figure 7.5 shows an example of the use of this pillar. It must be so attached that it is stable, without interfering with the mobility of the thumb, the remaining metacarpal or carpal joints, or the wrist, as illustrated. For this purpose a leather palm, rather like that used by a sailor for stitching canvas, must be constructed, stitched, stretched and hammered to fit. Hide leather has been used, which is stiff and requires lining with something soft such as chiropodist's felt. It has been found an advantage to cover the top of the Perspex pedestal with a rubber thimble such as used for counting banknotes.

Various gadgets may be attached to this 'sailor's palm' foundation. One patient learnt to use the thumb and opposing pedestal in gripping most things, but was worried that he could not do up the button of his shirt sleeve on the opposite side. He had to be provided with a button-hook which fitted into a slot on the 'sailor's palm' before he felt independent. He also sadly missed the index finger in typing and a spring attachment was made fitting into the back of the 'palm'.

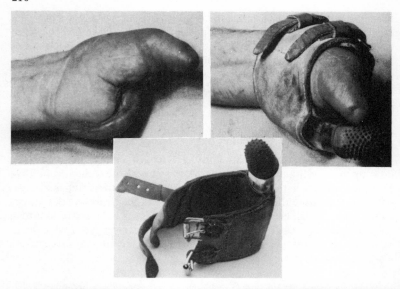

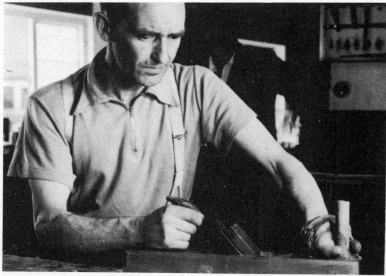

Figure 7.5. – Patient whose left hand was crushed in a revolving door. He had compound fractures of all metacarpals and then developed gangrene. On admission, only the first phalanx of the thumb remained, so we made him a Perspex pillar to give him pinch-grip. He eventually returned to work, skimming pots of molten metal, using both hands and the prosthesis

It would be tedious to relate all the adaptations made for individual patients to help to replace the loss of one or other digit. The patient's own interests and needs form the basis of each gadget. It has often been observed that when the patient is encouraged to help devise and make the tool he wants he will the more willingly use it. In using it he is helped to regain power and mobility of the remaining fingers. Often these remaining fingers will develop in efficiency until the gadget, tool, or adaptation is no longer necessary and the patient is observed to forget to use it. If inquiry is made there is often a rather lordly reply 'Oh, I don't need *that* any more'. This is the right and proper development which should be the aim of rehabilitation, as no gadget can be invented to replace the ingenuity and deftness of movement which man can develop to overcome his own disability.

Some patients who have lost part or whole of the middle and ring fingers show a significant drift of the index finger away from the thumb. The first interosseous muscle which pulls the index finger towards the thumb is, in the normal state, constantly in a state of tone or contraction to give the thumb a firm opposing pedestal. This muscle is observed to waste quickly with disuse, and when the middle and ring fingers are not there to give support to the index finger the weakness becomes more apparent. In occupational therapy it has been found helpful to make handles for various tools with deep grooves to encourage the index finger to work in good alignment. Sometimes a loop of leather may be made to hold the index and little fingers apart with a rubber 'spacing' pad in place. The patient himself must be taught to hold and keep the index finger in such a position that the first interosseous muscle may be encouraged to regain its full strength.

Elderly patients naturally have more difficulty in adapting themselves to new patterns of movement required to make up for the loss of even part of a digit. An example of this problem recurred when treating a man aged 60 years. He had lost the tip of the left index finger, including the nail, in an accident with a circular saw. He was right-handed and at first it was not anticipated that the injury would be a serious disability. But as an expert woodworker, especially in the use of veneer, he was accustomed to picking up small veneer pins using the nail of his index finger against the ball of his thumb. It took about 14 weeks of perseverance for him to learn the reverse movement using his thumbnail against the stump of the index finger. He practised first with nails, then on panel pins until at last he could manage the small veneer pins, whilst he did woodwork for himself and helped others. For long he complained bitterly that he would never regain his speed in tacking on large panels of veneer whilst the glue was hot. At last he learnt the new trick of movement sufficiently to be confident he could return to work.

The value of work in its effect of toughening skin on the hands tender from disuse has already been mentioned, and precautions against damage of the skin in the early stages of toughening have been discussed. For patients with areas of the hand, or whole digits, reconstructed from grafts from abdominal skin, the value of work has been found no less, but the precautions against damage must be intensified. All work with the hands entails contractions of muscles which pull on

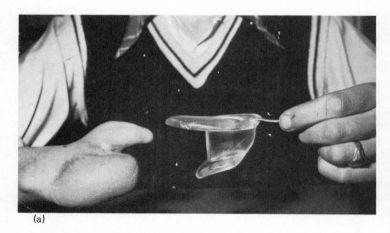

(a)

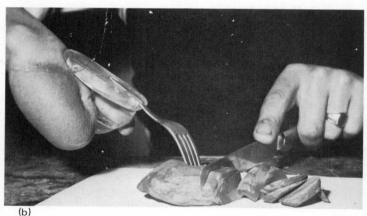

(b)

Figure 7.6. – Patient whose hand was severely mutilated in an accident. A thumb and a pedestal against which it could grip were reconstructed by plastic surgery. (a) A Perspex handle, specially moulded in the workshops, enabled him to hold a fork. (b) Practising using the adapted fork by cutting up plasticine

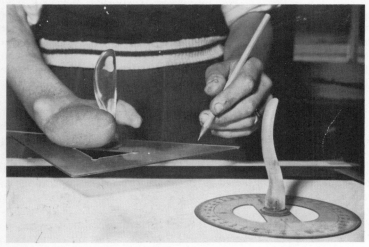

(c)

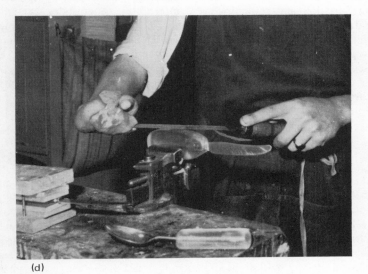

(d)

Figure 7.6 (cont.) — (c) A Handled 'sucker' to help him to lift and move his drawing instruments. (d) Plasticine used to make a shaped hand-hold on a file. This patient is now making an adapted handle for another patient's knife

the skin and cause wrinkles and creases. There must also be pressure and friction from the tools and materials handled in work. The patient cannot be expected to anticipate that the texture of skin transplanted from the abdomen is different from that covering the rest of the hand. This is the responsibility of the therapist and it has often been found advisable at first to request permission for a tender area to be covered with a light dressing during working hours. This dressing not only is a protection but serves to warn the patient against careless movements which so often cause small lesions, which occur quickly and are slow to heal. Some incidents of damage seem to be inevitable until the new skin is really consolidated by the establishment of circulatory and nerve supply, and the general toughening by use. It has been observed that the patient becomes despondent and annoyed by these incidents and is apt to question the value of such long drawn-out operations and treatment. The writer has on such occasions found it useful to show photographs of former patients, such as *Figure 7.6*. The patient shown had most of his hand destroyed in an accident when he was 16 years old. He had been fitted with prosthetic fingers but the skin over the remnants of his hand was insufficient protection against the friction of using the prosthesis. Six years later he had extensive grafts to reconstruct a thumb and a pedestal against which the thumb could grip. Both rehabilitation and retraining were interrupted by episodes when the grafted areas were damaged at work, but eventually he completed training as a draughtsman. Two years later he visited us in the workshops, bringing with him a folio of blueprints showing his work. He used the reconstructed hand easily in gesticulation and in showing off his drawings. He obviously had confidence in his hand as an organ of commission and appreciation. The skin looked healthy and tough and wrinkled freely as he moved the joints.

ASSESSMENT OF HAND FUNCTION

At Farnham Park the occupational therapists, physiotherapists and doctors are all concerned with assessing hand function. Obviously it would be confusing for the patient to have his hand assessed regularly by three different disciplines and, since all the staff meet weekly to discuss the patients' programmes, individual findings will be shared. The assessment methods described here are those used in the occupational therapy workshops and are only a part of the whole assessment of a patient's hand.

Assessment of hand function can be both a testing and a treatment procedure. Isolating movements which are difficult to perform indicates to the therapist the areas in which practice is most needed. Although usually the hand is tested once a week, some practice material, similar to that used for example for testing stereognosis, may be used to provide regular re-education sessions. Tests are structured to assess fairly clearly defined movements but they may also be used to check whether the patient can achieve function by unconventional means. If he cannot pick up a safety pin straight off the table, can he manage it by sliding the pin to the front of the table and grasping it as it reaches the edge, using a different type of pinch? With rheumatoid patients it is particularly appropriate to check whether they can perform a specific task at all and, if so, to analyse how they do it. Some patients will never regain full normal movement; it is one of the functions of an occupational therapist to prove to them how much they can manage to do despite their handicap.

The therapist must record whether the dominant or non-dominant hand is being tested. Some people are strongly right- or left-handed and have less highly developed function in the non-dominant hand. Others have good bilateral function, often because their particular jobs demand this. When comparing the function of the injured hand with the unaffected one these points should be borne in mind. Joint mobility should be the same for both hands but strength, dexterity, co-ordination and sensation are likely to be less developed in even the normal non-dominant hand.

Some of the movements that are tested require stamina as well as range to be useful functionally. A patient may pronate and supinate quite adequately in a test situation but get tired and be unable to use the movement for any length of time. Repetitive movements used in industrial outwork or craftwork will provide both treatment and assessment of function.

Assessment must also encompass the individual's specific needs. What does he find difficult in activities of daily living? Can he push his shirt into his trousers, tie shoelaces, do up shirt buttons? He may admit, 'I get help with so and so' and will then need practice in the department together with encouragement to try and do this for himself at home. He may have got out of the habit of using his injured hand and the therapist may need to take him round the workshop to turn door handles, open windows, use keys, turn taps and get the feel of using the hand normally again. It may even be necessary to get him to put his uninjured hand consciously in his pocket to prevent himself from using it until the normal pattern is re-established. Sometimes it is possible for a patient to bring in some of the materials he normally uses at work to practise on in the workshops. However good an assessment test may be, it is no substitute for getting down to practical work.

Assessment tests should be graded. If a patient cannot use a pencil for writing, he may manage if it is padded. By using it in this way he will be re-educating the movement and the padding can be reduced gradually as finger flexion improves. Similarly, if he cannot grasp small or heavy objects he can begin by picking up larger or lighter ones. Using the test to reassess function in this way will indicate how treatment needs to be adapted to the individual's needs.

To give an assessment test any reliability it must be conducted in exactly the same way each time it is used. This can only be achieved if the items used in the test are always the same. It is best to keep them together in a specially designated box. Items such as a watering can or taps cannot always be kept separately but clear instructions can be put in the test box, to ensure that the same additional items are used each time. The instructions should include specific details, such as whether the watering can should contain water (and how much) and the paint-tin paint; the size of small objects such as paper clips or safety pins should be recorded, so that they can be replaced if lost.

The assessment procedure should be carried out with the patient in the same position each time. He should be sitting comfortably with his

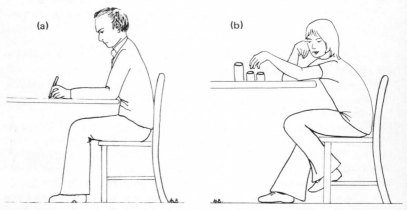

Figure 7.7. – (a) A good position for working when seated. (b) A bad position for working when seated

hips, knees and ankles at right angles. The table top should be just below elbow level, so that he can pick up objects in the best functional position with his elbows at right angles (*Figure 7.7*). Someone in a wheelchair will need a lower table, or the test items can be placed on the wheelchair lap-board. Asking a patient to squeeze a pinch gauge or even open a clothespeg at too high a table will diminish his performance; he will be using shoulder and elbow movement to lift them off the table, instead of concentrating on pinch. Using a different height of table each time will obviously give patchy results.

The therapist's approach to the patient may also affect the test results and should therefore be standardized. If the patient is merely asked to perform the desired action as well as he can, he may not produce his maximum effort. If the therapist allows him to repeat the action two or three times, at the same time encouraging him to try harder and make greater efforts, he may improve on his original performance and achieve a better functional result before beginning to get fatigued by repetition. Even tricks like taking a deep breath before pressing on the pinch gauge, in a similar way to breathing in before a heavy lift, may improve his performance.

If a patient cannot pronate or supinate, or has limited elbow movement, it may be necessary to position items within easy reach. This may mean placing items at an angle rather than flat on the table. A Dycem tray or sheet of Dycem over a board can be tilted sideways to hold the smaller items in an accessible position. The pinch gauge may be placed on its side, or may be better lying at an angle on a cushion. If adjustments such as these are not made, the difficulty of reaching items may prevent the therapist from assessing finger movement.

In addition to checking with the patient the items listed in the test, any other significant details should be recorded. These could include the colour of the hand, temperature, swelling, any superficial cuts, scratches or burns, any pain or discomfort, and the general attitude of the patient.

It is possible to buy standardized tests of hand function designed for use by psychologists. These are expensive and an occupational therapist would need special training to be allowed to used them. These tests are intended to assess hand function at the time of testing and to enable the tester to compare this performance with that of a wider sample of the population. This is not the occupational therapist's primary need. She wants to isolate the areas of inadequate function in order to concentrate the treatment programme on improving the level of function. To fulfil this need the tests described here, provided they are properly used, will be quite adequate. In a research situation, for example, to compare pre- and post-operative function in a series of patients having undergone a particular surgical technique, appropriate standardized tests would be ideal. A test of high validity is testing only what it purports to test, other variables being eliminated; therefore it will give a much truer assessment of that particular function.

The test given in Table 7.1 was devised to provide a breakdown of the different ways in which the hand works and to give several items which can be used to produce each movement. Other functions are listed as a reminder that these should also be checked. This is mainly a diagnostic test to assess those areas where treatment should be concentrated.

TABLE 7.1

Farnham Park
Assessment of hand function

Precision pinch:	picking up pin, pencil, marble
Power pinch:	pulling string, darning, plucking plasticine
Lateral pinch:	turning key in lock
Tripod pinch:	picking up draughts, turning screw cap, tap
Writing:	
Cutting food:	
Small tool grip:	holding screwdriver, knife or fork
Cylinder grip:	holding hammer or chisel
Hook grip:	lifting watering can, 2.5 litre paint can by handle
Span:	opening tailor's scissors, holding large woolly ball, lifting 2.5 litre paint can from above ignoring handle
Release:	throwing ball
Co-ordination:	carrying full glass of water
Strength:	lifting 5.5 kg (12 lb) box with both hands
Flat hand:	taking money out of pocket
Stereognosis:	*Sensation:*
Pronation:	*Supination:*
Elbow:	*Shoulder:*

Table 7.2 presents a more precise test which is used when the patient is first admitted to the Centre, to provide a guide for selecting a suitable occupational therapy activity. It usually takes no more than five minutes. As well as for hand injuries, it has also been found useful in the treatment of those with hemiplegia, disseminated sclerosis, Parkinsonism, disorders of eyesight and, occasionally, head injuries. When used to assess a hand injury it may be repeated weekly. This test can be used to assess pinch between the thumb and one or more injured fingers, or between the thumb and each other finger in turn. The therapist will record the way in which the test has been used.

TABLE 7.2

Farnham Park
Test for assessing pinch

The value of the test is explained to the patient. Each object is then placed in turn on the table surface and the patient is asked to *pick it up* and *put it down*. The patient is *not* encouraged to slide the object to the edge of the table to assist in picking it up but this may be necessary for him to achieve this action. The length of the patient's thumb nail, and finger nail on the index, should be noted, as a longer finger nail makes a considerable difference in picking up the smaller articles. The articles are listed in the order of use. This test would not be used for a patient who was unable to oppose the thumb and index (or middle finger, etc., in the case of an amputee).

1. Stationery Office rubber 38 mm × 19 mm × 8 mm (1½ in × ¾ in × $^1/_3$ in)
2. Metal nut approx. 12 mm wide × 6 mm deep (½ in × ¼ in)
3. Wooden clothespeg (to test power of pinch) — not used when pinch is obviously very weak)
4. Steel screw 25 cm × 5 cm (10 in × 2 in)
5. Large rubber band 6 mm thick × 75 mm long (¼ in × 3 in)
6. Peg-board peg, plastic, 6 mm wide × 25 mm long (¼ in × 1 in)
7. Safety pin. Open and close — only if able to operate clothespeg beforehand
8. Paper clip
9. Wire nail 25 mm (1 in)
10. Drawing pin
11. Small rubber band
12. 2p coin
13. 1p coin
14. ½p coin
15. Panel pin 19 mm (¾ in)
16. Pin, dressmaker's
17. Needle, small
18. Thread needle through a piece of paper, and remove

Measurement of pinch

The Preston pinch gauge (*Figure 7.8*) provides a simple and effective way of measuring the strength of pinch. The dial is set to zero. The patient squeezes the two parts of the gauge together, using the thumb and one finger or the thumb and two fingers. The needle moves around the dial to register maximum pressure, and will only return to zero again when the reset button is pressed.

The gauge is placed at the front of a table with the gripping surface protruding over the edge. The patient is instructed to pinch as hard as possible in one or more of the following ways:

1. Pinch the gauge using only the thumb on one side and the index finger on the other. Only the tips should be in contact with the gauge and the middle finger should not touch the index finger.

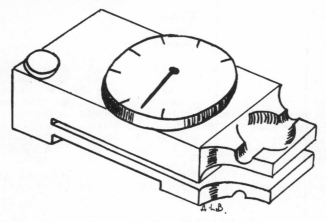

Figure 7.8. – The Preston pinch gauge

2. Pinch the gauge using the thumb tip on one side and the index and middle fingers on the other. The ring finger must not touch the middle finger.
3. Pinch the gauge in any way he can to obtain maximum pressure. The method used by the patient should be recorded.

Great care must be taken to ensure that the patient uses the gauge in the identical way at each testing session. If fingers which are not being tested assist pinch by additional lateral pressure, there will be an inaccurate reading on the gauge. These fingers must be held well out of the way.

A convenient method of recording the measurements is to use a table (Table 7.3).

TABLE 7.3

	Right hand	*Left hand*
Date		
Index		
Middle		
Ring		
Little		

Sensory testing and stereognosis

This is already well covered by C. B. Wynn Parry (1973) and many of the techniques he describes are used at Farnham Park.

It is useful to have a kit of objects of varied shape and texture available for testing. Since the therapist will be assessing whether familiar objects can be recognized it may be necessary to vary the objects according to the patient. Sandpaper or a 7.6 cm (3 in) wood screw will be more familiar to a man, velvet or a small kitchen utensil to a woman. The patient is first shown the test objects and these are identified for him. He is then blindfolded and the objects are handed to him in random order, the results being recorded.

Another way of assessing the ability to recognize different textures is to have a number of blocks of wood each with a sample of a texture, for example a coiled piece of string, mounted on one face. The blind-folded patient is asked to feel the sample on one of the blocks and then identify its equivalent on a masterboard. This entails the retention of feel of the sample while handling other textures. It also eliminates the need for a verbal description.

Device for charting finger flexion and extension

A pictorial method of recording finger movement has been devised at Farnham Park (*Figure 7.9*). A specially shaped piece of Darvic or other rigid plastic sheeting 2.5 mm ($^1/_{10}$ in) thick, or plywood or hardboard 3 mm ($^3/_{16}$ in) thick is mounted on a wooden board. The board must be long enough to extend well above the wrist so that the wrist and the dorsum of the hand will always be in the same starting position. Following some hand injuries, for example a flexor tendon graft, the

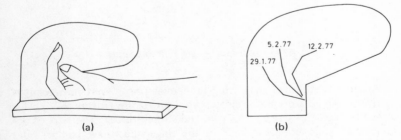

Figure 7.9. – (a) Device for charting finger flexion and extension. (b) Paper pattern which clips to the Darvic material, showing recorded measurements

movements of the wrist, metacarpophalangeal and interphalangeal joints are all interdependent. If the wrist is not stabilized, the measurements of finger movement will not be accurate.

A sheet of paper cut to the shape of the Darvic is attached with paper clips. The hand rests in supination on the board and the Darvic fits between the appropriate fingers. The therapist draws the silhouette of the back of the finger. She can record flexion and extension, both active and passive, using a different colour for each outline. Progressive improvement of just one movement, such as flexion, can be recorded by dating the outline each time. If a patient cannot get his hand into supination the whole board can be turned round. Assistance may be needed to stabilize the forearm in position.

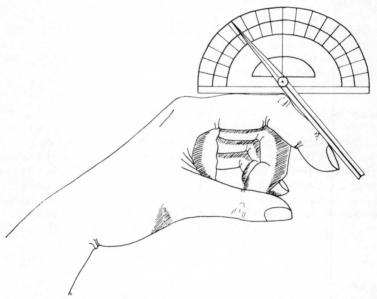

Figure 7.10. – Individual finger joint measuring device

Another method of measuring individual finger joint movement is to rivet a Darvic arm on to a small school protractor (*Figure 7.10*). This device is inexpensive, easy to make and simple to use. The part of the arm which runs along the back of the finger must have parallel sides for accurate measurement; the part across the protractor should be pointed.

Pronation and supination

Another simple measuring device works with the aid of gravity (*Figure 7.11*). A circular protractor, mounted on plywood and with a handle, has a freely swinging measuring arm weighted at one end. As the

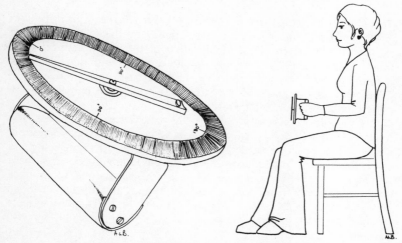

Figure 7.11. – Pronation and supination measuring device

patient pronates or supinates the forearm, the dial rotates but the measuring arm remains vertical. Provided the patient is properly positioned, with his elbow tucked into his side and held at 90 degrees flexion, an accurate reading of pronation and supination will be obtained.

TYPES OF WORK

It has already been observed that the types of work available in any one occupational therapy workshop must be limited by space, and by the amount of staff tuition and supervision which can be afforded by the number of staff taken in relation to the number of patients. Another factor is the preference shown by individual staff for specific skills. An occupational therapist will get more enthusiastic participation from her patients if she enjoys the activity she is teaching. The account which follows gives some idea of the work which has been used at Farnham Park by patients with disabilities of the upper limb. It must be emphasized that even a well chosen activity is not automatically therapeutic.

The occupational therapist must demonstrate the particular movement to be used and then make sure that the patient continues to perform it correctly.

Mosaics

This is a very light activity, it is clean (except for the grouting process at the end) and the work cannot be spoiled by flaking or roughened skin. It is suitable for early mobilization of the hand, requiring gross pinch varying with the size of mosaic used. The amount of work involved varies also, with the size of the articles made which range from ashtrays to coffee tables. Successful results can be achieved by patients with very limited dexterity.

To provide a very easy activity the patient can use mosaics that have been previously taken off the backing mesh. As a progression, stronger pinch will be needed to pull the mosaics off the backing and scrub them clean from glue and mesh. In the later stages of treatment hand-grip can be strengthened by using mosaic cutters to produce shapes to incorporate in more complex patterns. Porcelain and Venetian glass (Smalti) are equally heavy to cut; the latter is more suitable because a rough finish looks better in glass than porcelain (*see also* page 96).

Clay-modelling

Many modern types of clay do not need firing, and articles can be made and decorated by a few simple processes without a kiln. Modelling can be of varying complexity: simple beads, coiled pots, pinched pots, slab, modelled figures made with either finger pressure or with modelling tools.

Clay offers minimal resistance. The skin must be healed but patients who have some tenderness may be comfortable working in this soft medium, although it can be a bit cold. A large variety of movements, both in the hand and wrist, can be incorporated depending on the pottery technique selected. This is one of the few activities which requires extension of the fingers, since they must be extended to roll out coils and to use a rolling pin to roll out slab. It is also a good activity for re-educating a hand with partial loss of sensation. Work can be given which uses all the fingers and the whole palm, not just a part of the hand as in most other activities. By using such a large area, those parts of the skin which lack sensation will, together with the normal skin, be touching the clay. This will help re-education feedback.

Clay-modelling, unlike most other crafts, can be practised without using any grip, for example when rolling out. As grip improves, the size of the lump of clay being worked can be reduced. Eventually pinch-grip can be developed by making smaller and smaller beads. Some irregularities in the shape of modelled clay are quite acceptable. Fine finger movements can be used in the final stages of decorating and varnishing.

Stool-seating

This provides harder work for patients with hand injuries, using tougher material. Non-plastic materials such as seagrass or cord have the advantage that they are relatively soft on the skin and easy to join. Cane and rush are contraindicated because they produce problems similar to those in basketry: working with wet hands, rough textured material and more difficult patterns for the patient to master. Plastic seating materials are suitable for toughening the skin without being too rough.

Stool-seating is self-grading and becomes more physically demanding as the seat becomes tighter on nearing completion. The work can be varied in many ways. The weaving can be done using either a needle or a shuttle. A group of rows in a pattern can be marked with a shed stick, or each row can be woven individually. An open pattern, such as the Spanish pattern, with threads crossing over large sections of the stool will be easier to work than a pattern of close-knit squares or a twill pattern (*see also* page 95).

Cord-knotting

This is a useful minority activity for patients of average and above average intelligence, and is especially suitable for young girls when knotted articles are currently in fashion. It has the advantage of being a bilateral activity, compared with leather-thonging which is unilateral. Macramé is not easily obtained but rayon seating-cord or string can be used. Belts, handbags, shopping bags and dog leads can be made. One young girl with a severe hand injury, who would do nothing else, accepted this craft.

Wire-twisting machine

This is described on pages 24–28. It provides useful exercise in the treatment of hand injuries but some ingenuity is required to make sure that the end-products are salable.

Rug-weaving

This has various uses in the treatment of the injured upper limb.
Weaving gives opportunities to stretch out the arms in pushing and
pulling the shuttles through the shed. Shuttles may be increased in length
as a larger range of movements becomes possible.

All the upright rug looms in the workshops have permanently
raised legs so that they are at a better height for exercising the spinal
extensors and the elevators of the shoulder girdle. This makes them
very suitable for treating patients who need to be encouraged to raise
the arms high, as they must do this to reach the beater, and who require
development of the muscles of the shoulder. The exercise can be increased by changing the shed by hand rather than with the feet.

Some patients should only raise their arms to just below shoulder
level. They include those who have had operations for recurrent dislocation of the shoulder and those who have frozen shoulders, for
whom a repetitive work involving a greater range of movement would
be so acutely painful as to cause spasm. Formerly these patients were
treated on a horizontal loom but this had to be removed because it
took up far too much room in the workshops. Instead of lowering an
upright loom a raised chair is used, with a foot-rest to support the feet
and with the loom pedals tied shorter than normal.

Beating down the weft with the hands widely separated on the
beater, and using a firm pressing-down movement rather than the
common bump-bump action, develops the muscles of the back and
shoulder girdle. If the hands are placed close together in front, the
pectorals will do most of the work.

The outspread fingers may be used to comb down the weft between
the strands of the warp. If this is done with upturned palms it provides
exercise for the finger extensors; with the palm downwards it can
provide traction on joints that will not fully extend. Combing down
can also require active abduction in a hand where the fingers have
stiffened in adduction.

Knobs and handles of various designs can be attached to the beaters
as required to gain a variety of movements in the hand and wrist.

The 38.1 cm (15 in) long springs originally designed for the Guthrie
Smith exercises are used on the beater to encourage the equal use of
both arms and shoulders. If one side is stronger than the other then a
full and comfortable resistance is afforded to that side to pull back the
beater into place. On the weaker side, a spring resistance is afforded that
is within the range of power, and this resistance is gradually increased
until equal on both sides. It is necessary to experiment to get the right
amount of resistance. When the patient can pull the beater down

evenly it is correct. The poundage will usually vary between 10 lb and 30 lb.

The work carried out on an upright rug loom depends to some extent on prevailing fashion. Usually it consists of a flat woven material in tabby using a shuttle. This could be a rug, or a shoulder bag finished off with a twisted or plaited shoulder strap in matching wool. Sometimes one loom is used to make a tufted rug. This provides good pinch-grip, and the tufts can be trimmed later if necessary. Two people can work together on this type of rug.

Machine-sewing

This is mainly used for patients with neurological conditions, the aim being to increase upper limb co-ordination in the later stages of treatment. The work usually consists of making straps for splints or webbing slings. Sometimes, if patients have a special interest, they may do dressmaking.

Basketry

This craft is no longer used at Farnham Park because there are too many contraindications. Cane is both wet and abrasive. It can blister even fit hands and is therefore unsuitable for vulnerable skin. Two good hands are needed to produce a well-shaped basket. It is a difficult craft and needs too much teaching time to produce work of an acceptable standard, and lack of success is discouraging for the patient.

Although a good pinch movement is involved, this is not a powerful pinch; there is no need to pull on the cane and, therefore, there is not enough resistance to build up muscle strength. Just as good a pinch is involved in tufting but the material is gentler, and there is the added advantage of the need to pull the tuft.

Basketry is hard to grade. It has been superseded by mosaics, macramé, remedial games and industrial outwork.

Leatherwork

This is another activity that is seldom used at Farnham Park. Thonging is too quickly finished and therefore production becomes expensive. Complicated thonging, which takes longer, is beyond the scope of most patients.

Saddle-stitching is very difficult to sew evenly and requires a much stronger pinch-grip than most patients can manage. Link belts provide good finger movements but again they can be made very quickly and therefore become expensive to repeat.

Printing

This is mainly used with patients who can cope with a fairly difficult activity requiring patience and at least average intelligence.

The small hand-printing-press is used without adaptations, partly because there is not sufficient staff time to set these up. It is also because in the Centre the physiotherapists and remedial gymnasts co-operate very closely with the occupational therapists on the patients' programmes; when a particular movement can be better achieved in another department, this is done. Also, there is a large number of machines in the workshops. Some of these, especially in industrial outwork, are kept permanently adapted for specific movements, and together they offer a wide range of therapeutic possibilities. It is not necessary, therefore, to make special adaptations for individual patients on the printing press.

Operating the Adana hand-press requires gross grasp together with active depression of the shoulder girdle. The other hand uses pinch-grip and a certain amount of accuracy in placing the paper correctly in the press.

Compositing is one of the few activities where extremely fine pinch can be used. Although the correct working method is to use tweezers, a more delicate pinch will be needed if they are discarded. Graded, resisted pinch can be achieved by using tweezers of varied size and strength.

Typing

This can be used to provide light, gentle mobilization of the metacarpophalangeal and wrist joints using one or more fingers. It can also be an alternative general hand activity for someone who does not want to do crafts. Sometimes a patient with a mutilated hand is loth to use it and must be persuaded to try whichever activity appears least uninviting, which might well be typewriting. Patients with severe disability may need to learn to type, even with one finger, as an alternative to writing.

Clerical work

A variety of simple, repetitive clerical jobs which do not require too great accuracy are used to provide fine movement of the fingers. They are particularly useful for patients who are mentally slow or unable to achieve good results with a craft.

The work mainly consists of jobs for the Centre, such as collating, stapling, rubber stamping, packing envelopes with follow-up forms for discharged patients, and guillotining duplicated slips.

Remedial games

These games need to be simple so that there is the maximum of movement and the minimum of thinking time. A wide variety is useful so that patients can achieve similar movements with different games and still remain interested. Those used at Farnham Park are described on pages 100—108.

Industrial outwork

This is used extensively for specific treatment for a variety of upper limb conditions and is described in detail in Chapter 3, pages 59—64.

Bench woodwork

The term 'bench woodwork' covers a vast variety of methods to make, out of wood, many of the articles we use in our homes. The kind of wood used must be chosen in relation to the article to be made. The use of different textures of wood, from light plywood to medium hard wood and on to really hard wood such as oak, affords an opportunity for progression in the demand for skill and power. This makes bench woodwork a valuable medium for the treatment of disabilities of the upper limb. Some woods must be avoided in an occupational therapy workshop. Teak and other hard woods may occasionally cause dermatitis even in healthy people who are allergic to its contact. To buy teak is very expensive, and its use blunts woodwork tools in any but highly skilled hands. There are many new types of wood now on the market and it is worth while to study the texture and effect of various woods for therapeutic use.

We have found that a supply of plywood 3 mm–12 mm ($^3/_{16}$ in to ½ in) in thickness, some birch ply, some sapele or oak, gives us a fair range of material with which to make shelves, racks, table tops and wooden toys. This plywood is easy to saw and requires only the use of a Surform tool to smooth the edges. It gives opportunity for the use of sanding blocks with various grips to encourage flexion and extension of the fingers.

The finger extension sanding block (*see Figure 10.7*, page 386) has been used to assist in the correction of contractures of the palmar fascia including patients who have been operated on for Dupuytren's contracture. It has also been used in treating a patient with a paretic upper limb following a brachial plexus lesion. The unaffected hand placed on top of the paretic hand will take the affected limb through the required range of movement. This will help to build up a recognized picture of position and movement which must be re-established before such movement can be instigated or brought under control. It has been found that the picture of movement may be dimmed by disuse due to peripheral or central nerve lesion. This dimness would appear in long-standing cases to approach the various degrees of loss of imagined position and movement encountered in those with cortical damage.

Sanding down or polishing a surface may appear to be a monotonous occupation, but the rhythmic and repetitive action that is required makes this type of work a very satisfactory medium for the treatment of the disabilities affecting the co-ordination and control of the upper limb, as well as the development of muscle power and range of joint movement. Sanding is more interesting if it is done as an integral part of a project such as a coffee table. The therapist should be able to guide the patient to select an article which requires sufficient sanding and polishing to be therapeutic but not boring.

The use of white deal to make frames for laundry boxes, or small cupboards which can be covered with more decorative forms of veneer plywood, will give progressive activities. The tools used, rip or panel saws, wooden jack-planes or iron smoothing-planes, all have handles which can be adapted to suit the needs of various grips. We have made saw handles in beech that are up to 13 cm (5 in) round instead of the usual 7.5 cm (3 in). The space for the knuckles has been widened proportionately to allow for swollen or stiff fingers which cannot bend round effectively. Wooden jack-planes can have their handles built up, or new and larger handles fitted (*Figure 7.12*). These handles we have made of beech, cut out roughly to shape with a pad-saw or scroll saw, the edges rasped down, and sandpapered to follow contours which are comfortable to hold. If the therapist is directed to develop

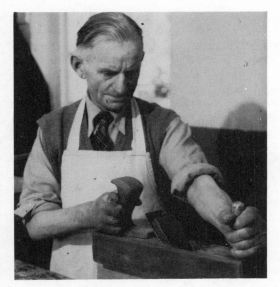

(a)

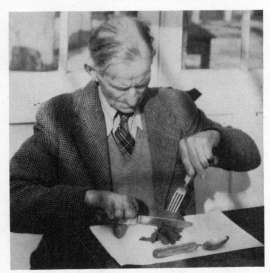

(b)

*Figure 7.12. – (a) The handle of this jack-plane is en-
larged because of this patient's limited finger flexion.
The additional front peg helps him to guide the plane.
(b) Practising cutting up food using plasticine and an
enlarged Perspex-handled knife*

grip in the slave hand, a post about 37 mm (1½ in) thick may be let into the far end of the jack-plane. To this may be fixed a Terry hand grip which encourages the slave hand to grip on the forward push when using the plane.

When a patient has had an injury with loss or damage to the middle or ring finger, it has been observed that there will often be stiffness between the heads of the metacarpals leading to destruction of the palmar arch. The palmar surface of the hand appears almost convex

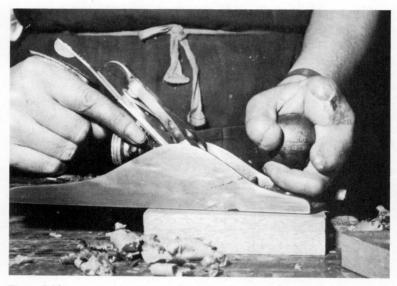

Figure 7.13. – Large knob on a smoothing plane to help restore the palmar arch

instead of concave. It is impossible to approach the treatment of stiffness in the metacarpophalangeal joints until the palmar arch is restored. In such a case the iron smoothing-plane may be used. It is furnished with a ball-handle grip for the slave hand (*Figure 7.13*) normally about 37–50 mm (1½–2 in) in diameter, screwed through, but which may be replaced with others up to 75–100 mm (3–4 in) in diameter. The restoration of the palmar arch will be encouraged by the grip of this ball handle, which should be changed as the joints giving the palmar curve become more mobile. It will be found as the palmar arch improves, the flexion of the metacarpophalangeal joints will also improve.

The grooving-plane used in making a tongue-and-groove joint between planks for a table top is another tool which makes considerable demands on control and power of the slave hand. This is usually manufactured for the right-handed carpenter, who holds the handle at the back, driving forward the grooving-plane. The left hand controls a side handle, thumb in opposition and adduction, and fingers bent at the metacarpophalangeal joints but straightened at the interphalangeal joints. In this way the outstretched finger-tips press against the flat surface of the wood and keep the narrow plane blade level as it ploughs through the edge of the plank.

The spokeshave demands equal use of both hands, and so does the router-plane (commonly called the old woman's tooth). This last tool is usefully employed in making a bookcase, or a pair of steps, when grooves must be cut in the surface of the wood.

The progression to hard wood such as oak to make a bookcase or coffee table will increase the resistance in material and make more demands for skill as well as power in controlling the tool. The final finish using a cabinet scraper is also very useful in treatment. This tool must be held firmly in both hands and requires power in the fingers whilst the hands are flexed at the metacarpophalangeal joints. The thumbs are worked strongly in opposition and adduction, whilst the wrists, elbow and shoulders are all brought into activity in extension with alternate flexion to prepare for the next stroke forward. The bench-scraper gives a much finer surface on hard wood for taking polish than does sandpaper.

These are but a few of the many tools used in bench woodwork. Their ordinary use and adaptation must be common knowledge amongst those who have studied bench woodwork from the therapeutic angle. The use of bit and brace, hand drills of various shapes, and screw-drivers may make the therapist wish that screws figured more largely than is usually necessary in bench woodwork. But some sharing out of the work available, with the appeal to one patient to allow another to do part of a job, will often increase the opportunities to obtain these specific movements of pronation and supination. These movements are not easy to segregate from others for special emphasis in bench wood-work. It is too easy to use compensatory movements of the shoulder and shoulder girdle.

Woodcarving

This uses traditional woodcarving tools and the work is held in a vice. The master hand holds the mallet in a static grip. There is some combined flexion, extension, ulnar and radial deviation, in other words circumduction, at the wrist but not much movement at the elbow and shoulder. This is good exercise for building up power in the wrist and hand in the later stages of treatment. The slave hand, holding the chisel or gouge, is mainly static which helps to build up power in the whole limb but particularly statically in the shoulder girdle.

Woodcarving involves jolting movements and is therefore contra-indicated for patients with inflammation of any of the joints of the upper limb, and also for anyone with a fracture that is not fully consolidated. The work is very useful in the later stages of treatment for finger amputees of either hand who still have pain. The indirect percussion helps to reduce hypersensitivity, increases circulation and reduces oedema. Gripping a tool that is vibrating will mean gentle pulling of the tender skin over the finger-tips.

A progression of this activity is stonecarving. One of our patients made a bird bath. He was a stonemason and at an earlier stage of treatment had made his own mallet.

Woodshaping

This can be done with Surform tools, using soft or hard wood to vary the resistance and grade the work. There are several different Surform tools, and either a plane or a chisel handle can be chosen to suit the therapeutic requirement. Woodshaping produces good, quick results with a high rate of success. The Stanley Surform tool book, *Sculpture with Surform,* outlines the techniques.

Woodshaping is much less jolting than woodcarving and can be used as an activity on its own, or to start an article which is to be finished with woodcarving tools. This would be appropriate for a patient whose fracture was not consolidated when first referred for treatment.

Wood-turning

On occasion it may be found necessary to allow a patient who is limited in his interests to start working on either something he knows how to do, or is particularly interested in learning how to do. The craft chosen by this type of patient may be one that produces an article which he has noticed and admired as the outcome of the efforts of another patient. Such a craft may be wood-turning. It is not ideal for the treatment of hand injuries as the major activity for the hands is the firm holding of the tool, and the changes of position of the hands are few and do not give the fluidity of movement which the therapist seeks as a treatment for stiff or paretic hands.

As has been described in the treatment of disabilities of the lower limb, turning on the foot-power lathe demands considerable activity of the lower limb, but usually fixation of the hands. If agility of the hands is already present and the power of grip and steadiness are to be encouraged together with an improvement in co-ordination between upper and lower limbs, then turning on the foot-power lathe can be considered a well-chosen therapeutic activity. It should be stressed that this co-ordination cannot be achieved by the use of an electric lathe.

Wood-turning should be taught with either hand holding the handle of the chisel well up the shaft, whilst the other hand, pressing the tool on the tool-rest, manipulates the chisel or gouge to form the desired contours of perhaps a table-lamp or bowl. The sanding and polishing of wood that has been turned also takes place on the foot-power lathe. All these processes will encourage the patient to develop a firm grip. Provided this is the aim, wood-turning need not be a shut door to the patient with an inadequate hand. Other work may be used for part of the time to improve the range of movement in the upper limb. Wood-turning on the foot-power lathe produces so many articles of beauty and utility that as a craft it has many attractions for the patient and thereby entices him to make a considerable effort.

Metal-work and engineering

Filing, fitting and bending of metal has been found to provide more or less the same range of activities as woodwork. Metal interests some patients more than wood. But more precautions must be observed in metal-work than in woodwork. Metal filings will be smaller and more abrasive than wood shavings or even wood splinters. The skin of the hands must be in good condition to stand up to the wear and tear of metal-work. On the other hand the use of the electric screw-cutting lathe only entails touching and holding with the finger-tips round the wheels that move the tool carriage. This has been found to be an advantage when the medical directions include the warning that during work no pressure must be exerted on the palm of the hand whilst the fingers should be mobilized to encourage flexion and extension. Work on the electric lathe fulfils these directions, and patients learn to turn down metal bars to make spindles for workshop machines and nail punches.

For patients interested in metal-work who have flexion contractures of the hand caused by local scarring or a cerebral episode resulting in hemiplegia, various handles can be made to fix on drilling machines. The only trouble is in finding an adequate need for holes to be drilled.

This has been found difficult in occupational therapy workshops. One solution is to make solitaire boards. Drilling the holes and the circular groove round the outside of the board to take the discarded marbles entails using three different sizes of bit to produce the curved indentations required.

The metal-work and engineering section of the workshops at Farnham Park has produced a curious selection of work. Some patients like to bring in bits of motorcycle to repair whilst they themselves regain function in their injured hands. Rehabilitation in such cases has appeared to have a dual purpose. A few have made models of aeroplanes complete with engine. Others interested in machinery have assisted in the making of equipment for occupational therapy. Repair of working parts of bench vices and foot-power lathes forms a never-ending succession of jobs as well as the repair of household equipment for the residential part of the Centre. Not only has new-fangled machinery for occupational therapy been constructed but splints made for some patients, and calipers or back-braces repaired and adjusted for others. Wrought-iron work (*see* page 75) is used in the later stages of the treatment of hand and upper limb injuries for final toughening of skin and for building up strength. Patients whose hands need to redevelop fine movement have found interest in sawing out and filing dress jewellery. Engraving has been found to develop power and strength in a slave hand, when the master hand was rendered useless by a brachial plexus lesion.

GIVING SUPPORT TO THE ARM

Sling arm-supports

There are now several overhead arm supports on the market (*Figure 7.14*). These are used at Farnham Park for any patient who cannot hold his arm up to the bench, for example, following a brachial plexus lesion, paretic deltoid or biceps, or motor neurone disease. Before this apparatus was commercially available, swing arm-supports were designed and constructed in the workshops.

Arm-slings for the ambulant patient

Many patients dislike wearing the large white arm-slings so often provided. These triangular slings are not only conspicuous but tend to pull on the patient's neck. An adjustable sling made from carpet webbing, usually in a dark colour, has been found useful in the early stages of

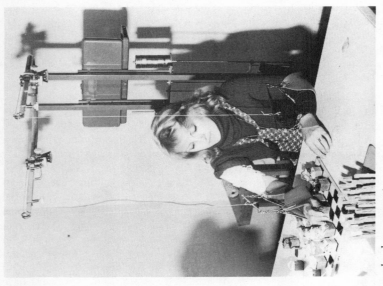

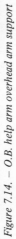

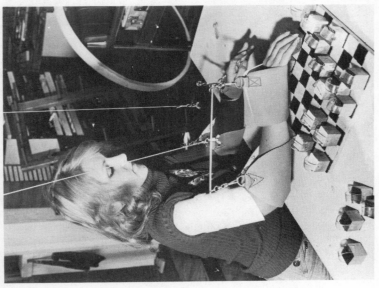

Figure 7.14. – O.B. help arm overhead arm support

all hand injuries to reduce oedema, and also for flail arm conditions including hemiplegia. The sling is worn diagonally across the back (*Figure 7.15*) so that there is no pressure on the back of the neck. The loop which goes round the hand should be positioned on the patient's wrist or forearm because the wrist may be pulled into radial deviation

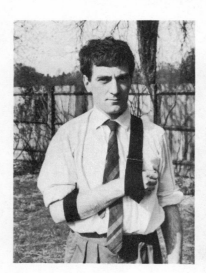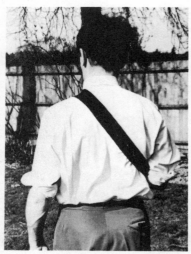

Figure 7.15. – Maudsley webbing arm sling

if it is fitted round the hand. The buckle can be adjusted to alter the height of the hand and the angle of the elbow. This not only helps venous return but also gives the relief of a change of position. It is possible to wear this sling under the sleeve of a jacket so that in public the hand and sling may remain discreetly hidden.

One woman, who had a paralysed arm, made herself a number of slings using wide corded ribbon of different colours to match her clothes. Sometimes she used the same material as her frocks so that all was in keeping. The effect was very decorative.

These webbing slings can be made as part of an industrial outwork project to supply not only the Centre but other hospitals as well. The four different sizes (*Figure 7.16*) can be colour-coded—for example, navy, brown and dark green for adults, red for children—and can be folded and packed in clear plastic bags.

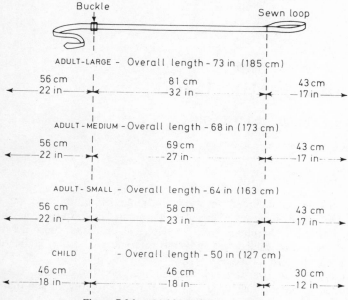

Figure 7.16. – Webbing slings, size chart

REFERENCES

Boyes, Joseph H. (1970). *Bunnell's Surgery of the Hand*, pp. 20–23, 25. 5th Edition. Philadelphia and Toronto; Lippincott

Jones, M. S. (1955). 'Occupational therapy for the upper limb.' *Br. J. phys. Med.* **18,** 119

Lord Chief Justice (1957). In 'Medicine and the law—a hand is an organ' by G. D. Black, *Lancet* **2,** 99

Wood Jones, F. (1920). *Principles of Anatomy as seen in the Hand*. London; Churchill

Wynn Parry, C. B. (1973). *Rehabilitation of the Hand*, pp. 21, 113–119. 3rd Edition. London; Butterworths

FURTHER READING

Cailliet, R. (1971). *Hand Pain and Impairment*. Philadelphia; F. A. Davis Co.

Wynn Parry, C. B. (1973). *Rehabilitation of the Hand*. 3rd Edition. London; Butterworths

8

Splinting the Hand

by Lynn Cheshire, MBAOT, SROT

This chapter is intended to show the range of splints used and the scope of splint-making practised at Farnham Park. Splints that have been devised at Farnham Park are described in detail; those designed elsewhere are described less fully but references to other publications are given whenever possible.

It cannot be over-stressed that all the splinting described here is intended to be an integral part of the patient's treatment, and that the best results cannot be obtained by splinting alone. The combination of all forms of treatment — corrective surgery, chemotherapy, occupational therapy, physiotherapy and remedial gymnastics — is vital to good rehabilitation. For those patients who return home or to work with a resting splint or a working splint it is essential that continued activity and exercises are encouraged.

The splints described in this chapter are as follows:

Farnham Park modular splints
Metacarpophalangeal ulnar drift (MUD) splints
Paddle splint
Wrist extension splint
Oppenheimer (lively wrist extension) splints
Ulnar wrist support
Rigid opponens splint
Soft opponens splint
Chessington median nerve splint
Farnham Park median glove
Thumb stabilizer
Thumb web spreader
Finger bands
Driving splint for a quadriplegic

These splints have each been developed to serve a particular function for a patient suffering from a commonly occurring condition. Each embodies some of the basic principles of splint-making. The occupational therapist, having learned how they are made and fitted, must be able to modify them to suit the requirements of individual patients. Not only does injury or disease affect different hands in different ways, but varying lifestyles affect the way in which patients use their hands.

The occupational therapist is in a better position than the orthotist and the physiotherapist to assess the way in which a patient's hand is employed in everyday activities, and so to choose the most suitable splint. It may not be sufficient to make the one most suitable for the patient's clinical condition; there are other factors to be taken into account.

A housewife will not be able to wear a splint which loses its shape in the washing-up water or while she is stirring a hot pan on the stove. A person who has arthritic hands and lives alone will not wear his splint if he cannot manipulate the fastenings. A young man may not wear one which is too obtrusive and likely to affect his social life.

Every splint should be assessed not solely for its effect on the clinical function of the hand but also for its performance in a working situation. A patient will not wear a splint if it gets in the way. A splint which provides excellent pinch but takes up so much space on the palm that it prevents the patient from holding a knife is not satisfactory.

Sometimes the solution is to give the patient two splints: one which is corrective but unavoidably cumbersome, to be worn during the less active part of the day, the other less restrictive for use during the more active hours. A further reason for providing two splints is that one worn constantly gets dirty and it may be difficult for the patient to scrub it clean without wearing another splint; the wet splint, too, may take some time to dry.

Sometimes the therapist receives a referral for splinting which requires an unusual solution or combination of features. This presents a problem-solving exercise where previous experience and skill in handling materials will be utilized to the full. The driving splint for a quadriplegic, described on page 345, is an example.

Dynamic splints

Few lively, or dynamic, splints are described here because prescription at Farnham Park during the past few years has been largely limited to static, or statically adjustable, splints. This is a result of local medical doubts concerning the measurement of forces applied to the hand by splinting, and the counteracting forces which the body itself provides. Even if these forces are accurately measured they are subject to variations. For instance, a muscle will alter in tone and adapt to stretching; a soft tissue contracture will release to a degree when force is applied; and the tension in a spring or wire alters under force. These changes, which occur during the time that a splint is worn, are difficult to measure and such measurement is often impractical in an ordinary treatment programme. The author considers that there are persuasive arguments both for and against dynamic splints but believes that the most important criterion for successful splinting is that the result is the desired improvement in the patient's function. Such a result appears to be gained as much by dynamic as by static splints, when used with discretion.

Splinting for burns

The majority of burns patients who come to Farnham Park arrive a few months after their accidents. Most have already been given splints if their hands are affected but in some cases there are considerable contractures because previous treatment has been aimed largely at securing healing of the skin. It is quite common for mobility of the joints and the maintenance of good hand positioning, leading ultimately to good function, to be given secondary attention.

Visits were made by the writer in 1972, by means of a Churchill Fellowship, to the occupational therapists at Shriners Burns Institute, Galveston, Texas, and to West Pennsylvania Hospital and Harmarville Rehabilitation Centre at Pittsburgh, Pennsylvania, to study splinting for burns (Malick, 1975). These units use the methods of treatment that originated at Shriners Burns Institute and which are now used at Farnham Park.

The Shriners methods (Larson, 1973) place considerable importance on the prevention and treatment of contractures which occur because of hypertrophic scarring, or after grafting. The treatment involves the use of splints and Jobst anti-burnscar pressure garments. The splints prevent or rectify joint deformities by correct positioning, and the garments apply pressure to the hypertrophic scars to prevent their contraction. The splints are made from Orthoplast (or could be made from San-Splint). The pressure garments are of elasticized fabric which are made to measure by the Jobst Institute, Cleveland, Ohio.

History

Splinting has been considered important for good treatment at Farnham Park since the Centre opened in 1947, and the successive methods described in previous editions of this book reflect the interesting history of splinting over the years. During these three decades, splinting has been transformed by developments in the plastics industry. Considerable time and skill were formerly needed to mould leather and metal to the shape of a limb by beating, soaking, preparing moulds, sawing and filing, to say nothing of the time given to stitching. Now it is possible to prepare a plastic splint within a fraction of the time, and to mould it directly on to the patient.

The first plastic to be used at Farnham Park was Perspex in the 1950s. In the 1960s Flovic was found to be more pliable in moulding and less brittle in wear. Continuing guidance was given by ICI Ltd, who manufacture these materials, and Darvic was found to possess the most suitable properties for our purpose. It was used mainly to replace metal and plaster-of-Paris. It had a rigidity, strength and durability comparable with the metals, and was sufficiently malleable to replace many of the plaster splints. In addition, Darvic was easy to alter, easy to keep clean, smooth and comfortable for the wearer, and was cosmetically acceptable. Synthetic leathers have now largely replaced real leather for those splint parts which need to be soft.

The moulding technique was much improved by the discovery of a method of applying hot plastic directly to the patient. Very thin polystyrene sheeting (extruded, expanded polystyrene sheet, 0.5 mm thick) is glued temporarily to the inner surface of the splint. The splint is then heated and softened, and the polystyrene insulates the patient from the hot plastic while it is moulded firmly on the limb. This method is described in greater detail on pages 261–262.

Splinting facilities and equipment

The ADL kitchen and the engineering section of the workshops originally provided the most convenient space and equipment for splint-making but when the use of Darvic developed, it became obvious that a specially designed area should be planned (*Figure 8.1*). An old cottage kitchen in the grounds of Farnham Park, and a short walk from the occupational therapy department, was selected. Access was not ideal and much refitting was necessary but no rebuilding was needed. A detailed plan was made and then a group of 'pre-work project' patients stripped down the walls, removed an old fireplace, replastered and repainted until a pleasant clinical room was created. Modern flooring, cupboards, lighting and electrical fittings were professionally installed with the help of the funds donated by ICI Ltd and by the British Rheumatism and Arthritis Council.

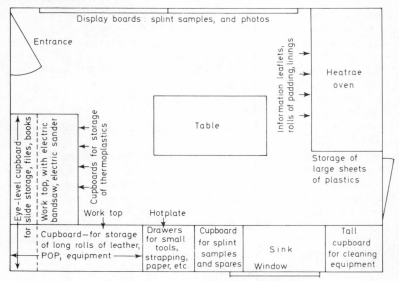

Figure 8.1. – Plan of the splints laboratory

Splints laboratory equipment

Furniture and fittings

Standing cupboards with laminate-topped working surfaces, all wide and deep, for storage of sheet plastics, rolls of paddings and linings
Wall cupboards, for literature, records and photographic slides
Unit of four drawers for tools and smaller items
Working table
Two chairs
Two stools
Ceramic sink, hot and cold water
Display boards on walls, for photographs and splints
Racks, for leaflets on splint materials, duplicated information for students and visitors
Waste bin

Electrical equipment

Heatrae oven, large size, on stand
Pair of electric hotplates (together wide enough to take safely a large dish of hot water for softening Orthoplast)
Burgess BBS 20 Bandsaw, fitted with general-purpose blade
Sanding machine, fitted with medium/fine grit carbon sanding disc, and a rigid (not rubber) sanding plate

Other equipment
  (*see also* Appendix)

  Long-bladed stainless steel scissors (for Orthoplast)
  Curved surgical scissors (for Orthoplast)
  Small scissors
  Tape measure
  Selection of needle files, half-round, flat, and rat-tail (for Darvic)
  Blunted scriber
  Pens and markers
  Paper, aluminium foil, Aloplast (for pattern-making)
  Cotton gloves, aprons, overalls
  Sewing threads, various needles
  Non-rusting tongs
  Large, shallow, stainless steel dish (for Orthoplast)
  Tea towels
  Metal funnel
  Knives, various
  Punches
  Cryogel cold packs (for Orthoplast)

Safety equipment

  Telephone
  Fire extinguishers, for both electrical and chemical fires
  Adequate ventilation, required to remove fumes, especially from adhesives
  Dust extractor, for sanding/buffing

Splint materials
  (*see also* Table, page 246, Appendix and relevant text)

  Selection of thermoplastics, and plaster-of-Paris
  Selection of paddings and linings
  Selection of adhesives, including double-sided adhesive tape
  Selection of ready-prepared straps, sizes from 300 mm to 1800 mm (11 in to 71 in)

Literature

  Splint manuals and reference books
  Suppliers' publicity leaflets on splint products
  Duplicated book lists, materials and equipment lists

TABLE
Splint materials

Name	DARVIC; FORMASPLINT	ORTHOPLAST ISOPRENE	SIN SPLINT	VITRATHENE	PLASTAZOTE	PLASTER-OF-PARIS BANDAGE
Manufacturer	(These are both the same material) Imperial Chemical Industries Ltd.	Johnson and Johnson (USA)	Smith and Nephew (Canada)	Stanley Smith and Co.	Bakelite Xylonite	Various manufacturers
Description	Polyvinyl chloride (PVC) Thermoplastic	Isoprene rubber (Transpolyisoprene) Thermoplastic	As for Orthoplast	Polythene Thermoplastic	Expanded cross-linked polyethylene Closed-cell construction Thermoplastic	Plaster-of-Paris impregnated gauze bandage
Specifications	As Darvic: Sheets: 8 ft × 4 ft and 6 ft × 4 ft Thickness: Wide range from thin foils upwards For splinting 2.5 mm and 1 mm are used Colour/Grade: White opaque standard grade. Colourless transparent security grade (extra strong) Surface: Polished (resists dirt best). Matt (less suitable) As Formasplint: Sheets: 916 mm × 610 mm × 2.5 mm thick Colours: White, opaque. Colourless, transparent Surface: Polished	White opaque Sheets: 450 mm × 700 mm × 3 mm thick plain Sheets: 910 mm × 700 mm × 3mm thick perforated Surface: Smooth matt	Pink opaque Sheets: 450 mm × 600 mm × 3 mm thick Surface: Smooth, very slightly grained	Colour/Grade: Pink, low density 2 SSAO White, low density Grade 2 Sheet: 3050 mm × 1525 mm × 3 mm or 1.5 mm thick Sheet: 1525 mm × 1525 mm × 3 mm or 1.5 mm thick Sheet: 762 mm × 1525 mm × 3 mm or 1.5 mm thick Also available 4.5 mm and 6 mm thickness Surface: Smooth	Colour: Pink or white, standard density Sheet: 900 mm × 600 mm × 3 mm thick perforated or unperforated 900 mm × 600 mm × 6 mm thick perforated 900 mm × 600 mm × 12 mm thick perforated Surface: Firm cut foam (Greater variety of colours, thicknesses and densities also available – see under Suppliers)	Rolls of bandage: From 5 cm to 15 cm wide and 294 cm (3 yards) long (Wider and longer sizes available)
Rigidity and malleability	Rigid Good malleability Is not elastic	Semi-rigid Exceptionally malleable High elasticity	Semi-rigid Good malleability Good elasticity	Semi-rigid Good malleability Good elasticity	Low rigidity Medium elasticity Good malleability	Very high malleability Conforms faithfully to fine, complex contours Very rigid

Advantageous properties	Durable Non-inflammable, self-extinguishing Easily cleaned Sets quickly Withstands hot water Resistant to most chemicals Non-toxic Non-allergenic Transparent to X-rays Suitable for strong, narrow splint components Resists dirt Neat, clean, pleasant appearance Smooth to the skin Light, non-bulky	Extremely faithful in moulding Very elastic Easy to mould Sets slowly Self-adherent (dry heat method) Self-straps and self-hinges possible Durable Will not crack Very versatile, as combines high rigidity/malleability Transparent to X-rays Reasonably easy to clean Non-allergenic Sympathetic surface Unaffected by most chemicals (see disadvantages) No special preparation equipment needed Pleasant in appearance	Moulds well to complex contours Durable Washable Resistant to chemicals Transparent to X-rays Non-inflammable (melts) Withstands hot water Light Self-adherent	Very light Durable Washable Keeps fairly clean Transparent to X-rays Sets quickly Soft to skin Comfortable, warm Buoyant, useful in hydrotherapy Self-bonding, in oven Laminates well Resilient under pressure Resists chemicals	Quick and easy to mould Requires minimum equipment Non-toxic Non-allergenic Rigid Non-inflammable
Disadvantageous properties	Moulds poorly to small contours Insufficiently elastic for some enclosed splints Sets quickly Hard Preparation time-consuming without electric saw Non-resistant to ethyl, acetone and some benzine preparations Swarf produced when sanding/finishing; therefore goggles should be worn	Inflammable, non-self-extinguishing Self-adherent, can tangle permanently Soils fairly quickly Deforms in hot sunlight, hot water Dissolves in benzine, carbon-tetrachloride, trichlorethylene, toluene, etc. Sets slowly without coolants	Slightly bulky, as lining incorporated Insufficiently rigid for narrow components Warm to wear Requires lining for moulding technique Must not be applied to patient without insulating lining	Inflammable, melts or burns Lacks rigidity Bulky Sometimes too warm	Not waterproof Tends to be rough Very hard Soils easily Cannot be adjusted Heavy, if thick Long setting time Tends to crack
Forming temperature / *Application to patient*	Softens above 70°C (158°F), over hot-plate, in oven, under infrared lamp Must be insulated (polystyrene sheet) to apply to patient	Softens at 65°C (150°F) Use dry-heat or wet-heat Dry-heating: heat-gun, oven, infrared lamp Dry-heat maintains self-adherence Wet-heating in water destroys self-adherence Applied direct to patient's skin	Softens at 140°C (in 10–15 min) in oven Applied direct to patient, with lining	Softens at 140°C, in oven Applied direct to patient Sets quickly	Softens in cool water No heat required Sets at room temperature Moulded direct to patient, separated by layer of petroleum jelly or stockinette to prevent sticking
Alteration / *Reuse* / *Spot-heating*	Easy to alter Reusable, remouldable Spot-heats	Alters extremely easily Spot-heats well Minimally reusable, does not return completely to flat Fairly remouldable	Remouldable, not reusable Difficult to spot-heat Difficult to alter in part only	Reusable, remouldable, in total Alterable, in total Spot-heating difficult	Unsuitable for alteration Should be completely remade Not reusable

Table (cont.)

	DARVIC/ FORMASPLINT (cont.)	ORTHOPLAST ISOPRENE (cont.)	SAN-SPLINT (cont.)	VITRATHENE (cont.)	PLASTAZOTE (cont.)	PLASTER-OF-PARIS BANDAGE (cont.)
Suggestions on use	Suitable for rigid resting splints Durable and clean for work splints Best for splints covering one aspect of hand only, e.g. paddle, wrist extension	Excellent for intricate/reverse contours; enclosed splints; thumb splints Manufacturer's pack contains pattern suggestions		For semi-rigid splints More rigid if totally enclosed Highly suitable for gauntlets	Bulky for working splints Best for resting splints, especially of enclosed type, e.g. gauntlet Good as padding	Best for resting or serial splints Not very suitable for working splints Requires lining Provides excellent rigidity
Economics	Inexpensive material May be expensive in labour		Expensive material Inexpensive in labour Inexpensive equipment	Reasonably inexpensive Inexpensive in labour Requires suitable oven	Inexpensive material Inexpensive in labour Requires suitable oven	Inexpensive Requires little equipment
Suppliers	*Darvic* ICI Ltd. (Offices and agents worldwide) G. H. Bloore, Ltd 480 Honeypot Lane, Stanmore, Middlesex *Formasplint:* Nottingham Handcraft Co., Nottingham, England (Agents' addresses supplied worldwide) J. A. Preston Corporation (North America)	Johnson & Johnson Slough, Berks, England and New Brunswick, New Jersey, USA (Offices worldwide)	Nottingham Handcraft Co., West Bridgford, Nottingham, England Smith & Nephew Ltd (Worldwide)	Stanley Smith & Co., Isleworth, Middlesex, England	Smith & Nephew Ltd, Alum Rock Road, Birmingham B8 3DY, (Offices in other countries) Hinders-Leslies Ltd, Higham Hill Road, London, E17 (Supply a greater variety of types of Plastazote)	Smith & Nephew Ltd, Alum Rock Road, Birmingham B8 3DY, (Offices in other countries) Also various other orthopaedic suppliers

Terminology used for splinting

Apart from the nomenclature commonly used when describing the hand, there is some terminology, becoming well-used for surface characteristics of the hand, which needs to be clarified when describing methods of splinting. Whenever possible terminology is used which is

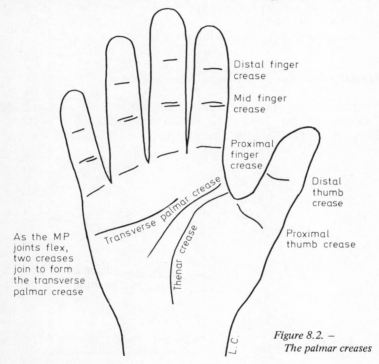

Distal finger crease

Mid finger crease

Proximal finger crease

Distal thumb crease

Transverse palmar crease

Thenar crease

As the MP joints flex, two creases join to form the transverse palmar crease

Proximal thumb crease

Figure 8.2. –
The palmar creases

understood internationally. The terms 'radial' and 'ulnar' are preferred to 'lateral' and 'medial', while 'palmar' is used in preference to 'volar', as it is often better understood by assisting staff who may have limited medical knowledge.

For the fingers, numerical labelling, for example '2nd digit', has been abandoned and the terms 'thumb', 'index finger', 'middle finger', 'ring finger' and 'little finger' are now used. Numerical labelling is still used, however, for the metacarpals.

The palmar creases map out the palm of the hand in functional terms and are useful in the designing of splints. A system of nomenclature is given in *Figure 8.2.*

GENERAL PRINCIPLES

Optimum positions

It should be stressed that each patient must be carefully assessed for splinting. The optimum position may vary considerably with the principles of the particular treatment being applied to the patient and with the length of the periods of immobilization.

As a general rule only, the following are used:

Optimum position for prolonged immobilization

The dangers of immobilization should not be underestimated and a suitable splinting position for a hand undergoing active mobilization can be most unsuitable for an immobilized hand (James, 1970).

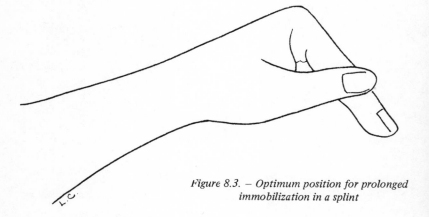

Figure 8.3. — Optimum position for prolonged immobilization in a splint

For a hand which is completely immobilized for 24 hours or more after surgery or trauma, a suitable optimum position (*Figure 8.3*) is:

Wrist: Neutral or a few degrees of extension. Slight ulnar deviation.
Thumb CMC joint: Some abduction and some opposition.
Thumb MP joint: Extension.
Thumb IP joint: Extension.
MP joints: In 60–90 degrees of flexion – most important (*Figure 8.4*).
IP joints: In extension.
Metacarpal arch: Concave, not flattened.

This positioning of the metacarpophalangeal joints will prevent the disabling contractures of the collateral ligaments which so often occur if the hand is immobilized with these joints in less flexion. When they

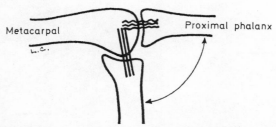

Metacarpal

Proximal phalanx

L.C.

Figure 8.4. – Lateral view of a metacarpophalangeal joint. Diagram to show that the collateral ligaments are slack when the joint is extended, and taut when the joint is in 60–90 degrees of flexion. Thus, if metacarpophalangeal joints are to be immobilized for a prolonged period, they should be held in at least 60 degrees of flexion to prevent contractures of these ligaments which can result in a disabling loss of flexion

are held in 90 degrees flexion the collateral ligaments are fully on stretch. The less flexion there is, the more slack the collateral ligaments become and, if they contract, the result may be a severe reduction of mobility and function at the MP joints.

Optimum position for splinting during active treatment

Wrist: 20–30 degrees extension. Slight ulnar deviation.
Thumb CMC joint: Abduction and some opposition.
Thumb MP joint: Slight flexion.
Thumb IP joint: Slight flexion.
MP joints: 45 degrees flexion.
PIP joints: 30 degrees flexion, more or less.
DIP joints: 10 degrees flexion, or less.
Metacarpal arch: Concave, not flattened.

The hand is almost in a position looking as though it is about to pinch an object (*Figure 8.5*). It is in this position that the minimum increase in mobility will enable the patient to pick up and put down a small object; thus the hand can quickly become *functional*, even if only minimally so. A hand that is stiff in a more extended position will take longer to become functional, as there is so great a distance between the thumb and fingers. The metacarpal arch (or transverse palmar arch) should always be maintained in a concave position during splinting, not flattened out. Thus a normal functional position is encouraged. It

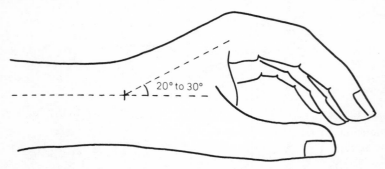

Figure 8.5. – Optimum position for splinting during active treatment

should not be forgotten that in flexion the tips of the fingers converge on the scaphoid. Therefore, any splint which is assisting in the increase of flexion, or extension, should follow this rule of convergence, or divergence, to achieve true function.

Sensation

Sensation is considered by many to be of as great importance as mobility in the hand, since few patients will use a hand that has impaired sensation, particularly of the palmar surface. It is important, therefore, to leave as much of the palmar surface as possible free from splinting. This applies particularly to the finger-tips, especially those of the index finger and thumb, and to the ulnar border of the hand, that is, the little finger and the hypothenar eminence, which are used in writing as a pivot for the rest of the hand and also in many skills involving fine pinch, such as watch- and clock-making. A working or functional splint must therefore be considered in relation to the amount of skin surface which should be unencumbered in order to undertake an activity effectively, as well as to the disability for which it is prescribed.

The skin

Apart from sensation, the palmar skin should be left as free as possible for satisfactory prehension. The patient will be unwilling to use a hand that is too encumbered.

The palmar creases are most useful in designing and fitting splints, as they indicate in functional terms the points on the palmar surface where movements take place. Thus if a splint covers the transverse palmer crease, even fractionally, some of the movements of the meta-carpophalangeal joints will be obstructed and, conversely, if a splint covers the thenar crease it will be partly or wholly immobilizing the carpometacarpal joint of the thumb.

Leverage and forces

In splinting, leverage and forces must be carefully thought out so that the splint is efficient without being cumbersome. Pressure should not be applied on a joint but, whenever possible, to the natural padding of the hand, for example, the fleshy hypothenar eminence. The palmar

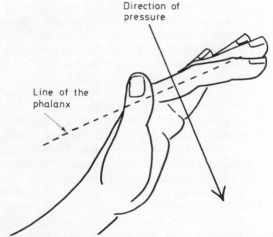

Direction of
pressure

Line of the
phalanx

Figure 8.6. — Diagram to illustrate the principle of applying pressure at a right angle to a phalanx, in this case the proximal phalanx of the index finger

surface is naturally well equipped to bear pressure but the advantages of this must be weighed against the disadvantages of covering this specialized sensory area. Splints should either push or pull at right angles to the bone on which the pressure is being applied (*Figure 8.6*). This subject is well covered by Barr (1975).

Cosmesis

The appearance of the hands has deep subconscious significance. The sensory images of one's hands stem from early childhood interaction with the environment through the learning processes of touch and manipulation which were largely made by the hands. Thus the hands are visually and sensorily the extension of the self, and it is true to say that our self-image is more closely linked to our hands than to our faces. We rarely look at our faces or see ourselves as others see us but we frequently, and usually subconsciously, look at and feel our hands as we work. These effects must be borne in mind when splinting. It has often been found helpful to explain this hand imagery to patients, to give them insight into the disturbing psychological effects that they experience with their disability.

Patients vary considerably in accepting or rejecting their splints because of appearance. Given the choice of a white or a flesh-coloured material, the majority of a small sample of patients chose white. Their preference may well have been due to the neat, clean and clinical appearance of the white material. The flesh-coloured alternative was of different material which produced bulkier-looking splints. Some flesh-coloured materials are of a pleasing shade but few are a good match to human skin. This is especially a problem with a black or brown skin. Transparent materials may provide a satisfactory answer but they sometimes give an unwholesome appearance as the flesh is compressed under the splint and looks squashed and pale.

Few people choose to have the encumbrance of any kind of appliance on their hands — many loathe wearing gloves even in bitter weather — since sensation and dexterity are always reduced, resulting in annoying hindrances to manual activity. However willingly a patient accepts such hindrances with a splint, in addition to the disturbances he is already experiencing with his disability, the therapist must ensure that bulkiness, protrusions and ugliness are reduced to a minimum. Obviously the splint must be large enough to provide the necessary support and leverage but often, with extra thought, the appearance can be much improved by trimming off unnecessary bulk from corners and borders. It has often been found that this produces an almost beautiful-looking splint, as the contours at their most economical have a sculptured appearance. There is no excuse for corners or protrusions that have no therapeutic function and that catch on the patient's clothing and bed-clothes. Splints should be properly finished to a good standard of craftsmanship, with smooth edges, neat straps, clean contours and clean materials. It is most unprofessional to fit a patient with a splint that is badly finished.

Most patients are anxious lest the abnormal appearance of their hand and splint will disturb others, especially at meals or social functions. It may often be wise to compromise by giving a patient two splints, one highly effective but perhaps inelegant, and one less effective, but cosmetic, for social use. A young patient was to be best man at a wedding, so a very small and unobtrusive wrist extension splint was made solely for this occasion, in lieu of his larger but more effective splint as this was psychologically important.

Comfort

The comfort of the patient is of paramount importance. No patient should be expected to wear an uncomfortable splint, and he certainly

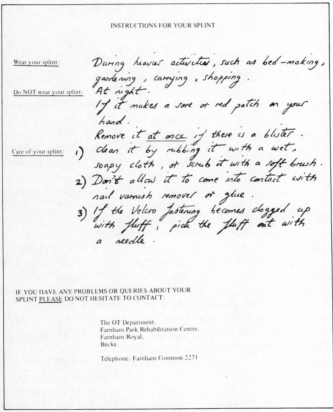

Figure 8.7.—Sample of an instruction sheet given to a patient with a splint

will not do so when out of sight of the therapist or doctor unless he is highly motivated. Too many splints are 'hidden' in patients' lockers or left at home 'by mistake'. Even the most comfortable splint is a hindrance to the human hand, and patients must be given careful instruction, attention and encouragement to induce them to use their splints correctly.

It has been found helpful to involve patients in all stages of the fabrication of their splints, even though they may have to sit and watch for several hours; this time can be used to explain the purpose of the splint, and to give repeated instructions on its use. When the splint is ready the patient should practise getting it on and off correctly under the supervision of the occupational therapist. Written instructions (*Figure 8.7*) should be given to the patient who does not attend for treatment every day, with a note on the cleaning and care of his splint.

PATTERN-MAKING

A good pattern is the basis for a good splint. As in dressmaking, it is the pattern, and the skill with which it is made, that determines the fit and fitness of the final article. There are a number of techniques and many helpful suggestions worth remembering, especially for patients with severe deformities and contractures.

The patterns which have been found most useful at Farnham Park are described below. They may be adapted or combined to suit individual patients and also to suit the technique and the material chosen for the splint itself. A rigid material that does not stretch during moulding will usually need a pattern made from paper, which also will not stretch. If the pattern fits the patient's hand well, then the splint will also fit. Conversely, when making a splint in a stretchable material such as Orthoplast, a paper pattern will be inappropriate. It is difficult to wrap paper accurately around the hand without creasing or tearing, and a stretchable pattern medium is more effective in this case.

The first consideration when making a pattern is to position the patient correctly. The patient's total posture should be relaxed and he should be well supported. He should be seated on a comfortable chair, alongside a table close to the affected side. The chair should have a cushion to give comfort and relaxation, especially for a patient who is in pain or has an arthritic condition. The table top should be at approximately elbow level, so that the patient's elbow, forearm and hand can rest there with the shoulder relaxed and tension in the arm reduced. A soft pad can be placed under the elbow if it is painful, has nodules or is subject to pressure sores. If the arm as a whole is not correctly positioned and supported, the patient will be tense and may assume an awkward, stiff posture of the hand, making it difficult for the therapist to manipulate and control.

Having got the patient comfortably settled, the therapist can now work facing him, and can both observe and control his limb during pattern-making, moulding or fitting of the splint. The hand can be lifted so that the elbow is flexed but still resting on the table, and the forearm can easily be turned into supination and pronation. If the patient has loss of range of these movements, the position of the seat or table can be altered until the most efficient working arrangement is found.

The patient should be handled gently but firmly, so that he feels secure and thus remains relaxed. Rheumatoid patients, in particular, should be handled on muscle areas, so avoiding painful joints and, conversely, those with Guillain-Barrè Syndrome (acute infective poly-neuritis) should be handled on the joints, as their muscles may be excruciatingly tender. In the latter case the hand is lifted by a wide pinch-grip, using the thumb and index-finger tip at either side of the wrist joint like a pair of tongs, and at the metacarpophalangeal joints in a similar way.

For the patient who has severe spasticity, or where minimal handling of the limb is prescribed, for example in the case of burns or when dressings should not be disturbed, the pattern can be made on the unaffected hand and reversed to fit the affected one.

Therapists are often reluctant to mark the patient's skin but this is one of the most reliable ways of planning, designing and matching a splint, and few patients object to having temporary marks made on them. Several of the methods described below incorporate useful marking techniques and show how these facilitate pattern-making.

Paper pattern – flat method

A sheet of thick typing paper or yellow X-ray packing paper, long enough to reach from the patient's finger-tips to his elbow, is placed flat on the table. The patient's hand and forearm are placed on the paper and positioned as required. For example, when constructing a wrist extension splint, the wrist is placed in a little ulnar deviation to allow for the correct functional position. Keeping the patient's hand in place, an outline is drawn on the paper closely round the hand and forearm, holding the pencil or pen absolutely vertical throughout. If the pencil slants there will be distortion of the width. The positions of relevant joints are marked precisely on this outline, and also those of any creases to be used, for example, the position of the transverse palmar crease, which will determine the distal border of the splint.

The desired pattern for the splint is drawn over the outline. This is then traced on to a second piece of paper. The original pattern is kept as a record, and also as a reference in case the cut-out pattern does not fit and has to be radically altered. The cut-out pattern is fitted to the patient's hand, which is held in the required position. Any adjustments are made by trimming or adding to the pattern, or by gluing a small tuck in the paper. The pattern is then traced on to the splint material. To achieve accurate positioning of the splint on the patient, small lines can be marked on the edges of the pattern and on to the patient's hand. These are transferred to the splint material, ready to be matched to the skin marks during moulding.

Paper pattern — block method

Instead of placing the paper flat on the table, a pattern is taken round a block. The pattern will then more readily follow the dimensions of the hand when it is in a functional position, or when the patient is unable to hold his fingers in sufficient extension for the flat pattern method. This block method is particularly useful when treating a patient with rheumatoid arthritis or spasticity, or post-traumatically when the hand is stiff, swollen and painful.

One end of a large sheet of paper is wrapped around the block, which can be a solid cylindrical object such as a jar or a tight roll of bandage, or a cone or a block of firm foam of suitable dimensions for comfortable grip (Barr, 1975). The patient's hand is then placed over the paper-covered block, the thumb lying in some opposition and abduction round one end of it, and the forearm supported on the table top. An outline of the hand is then drawn on the paper.

Paper pattern — strip-and-glue method

This is used for a splint which needs to be small as well as accurate, and which will be moulded to encircle the hand rather than lying on the palmar or dorsal aspect alone. Several narrow strips of paper, approximately 2 cm wide, are wrapped round the positioned hand, stuck in place on the skin and joined to each other with tiny dabs of Copydex adhesive. This allows the pattern to be easily peeled off without harm to the patient. The paper strips thus form a patchwork of pieces which make up a correctly angulated pattern. A good example of the use of this technique is the rigid opponens splint (*see* page 331).

Measured method

Circumferential and longitudinal measurements of the patient's hand are taken, using a tape measure. These are transferred either to a sheet of paper to make a pattern, or directly to the splint material. This method is usually employed for splint patterns which do not need to be absolutely accurate, for example, for a Vitrathene gauntlet which will stretch to fit during moulding.

Details of the measurements needed and a suitable method are shown in the gauntlet for the Farnham Park modular splint (*see Figure 8.18*, page 296), the measurements in this case being combined with an outline drawing of the hand. Measurements alone are useful for a Plastazote gauntlet, the dimensions being drawn directly on the material, which is cut out and wrapped round the patient's hand, so that minor trimming and alterations can be made before moulding.

Skin pattern method

Some patterns seem to defy accuracy and are difficult to fit to severely deformed hands. In such cases it is often best to draw the outline of the splint directly on the patient's skin and trace or transfer this to paper, aluminium foil or Aloplast (*see below*). This is a suitable method for the thumb stabilizer (*see Figure 8.47*, page 337), and is especially helpful in achieving a good fit round the thumb and the thumb web. It is also satisfactory and quick when making a simple splint like the ulnar wrist support (*see Figure 8.40*, page 328).

Aluminium foil

The advantage of aluminium foil is that it can be wrapped closely round the hand and will then hold its creases and shape, particularly round contours. When trimmed, adjusted, removed from the hand and flattened a little, its outline can be traced directly on to the splint material. This method is useful for splints made from a stretchable material like Orthoplast.

Aloplast

This is children's non-toxic, plastic modelling clay, similar to Plasticine but odourless. For pattern-making it is rolled out until thin, cut to a rough shape and wrapped round the patient's hand. The desired outline of the splint is inscribed on it and the surplus trimmed off. The remaining pattern is flattened out and the outline traced on to the splint material. This is also a suitable pattern method for Orthoplast, as it has a similar stretching property.

Soft wire

This is used solely for spring wire splints such as the Oppenheimer splints (*see Figure 8.39*, page 325). Very malleable wire, for example soldering wire, thick fuse wire or floristry wire, is shaped round the patient's hand in the position in which the final splint is to be made, and then copied exactly in spring wire.

MATERIALS FOR SPLINTING

This section describes the use and the fabrication techniques of the materials which have been found practical for splint-making at Farnham Park. More detailed descriptions are given of those materials which may be less familiar to the reader, and particularly of the Darvic/Formasplint technique as this was developed at this Centre. It must be stressed, however, that all materials have their advantages and disadvantages, and that different materials will be of value to different therapists in different situations.

The Table on pages 246–248 compares those materials which are in common use. It is often found that the very property which makes a material suitable for one splint contraindicates it for another. For example, Plastazote is a semi-rigid material that is soft to the skin and makes a comfortable resting gauntlet. If the patient has a strongly contracted hand, however, Plastazote alone would not provide sufficient rigidity and control. Such a problem may be overcome by combining two materials. The Plastazote could be reinforced with strips of Vitrathene, or the splint could be constructed in Vitrathene and lined with Plastazote.

The value of each material is due to its particular combination of properties. A material only appears valueless if it is being used incorrectly and if the therapist has not studied and assessed its properties. Nevertheless, it is rarely practicable or economical to carry the full range of splint materials in an occupational therapy department, and it is unlikely that the therapist would build up the skill to use each and every material successfully.

Some experts recommend that a stock that fulfils all needs should include three splint materials: one rigid, one semi-rigid and one soft. It is most important that the therapist should be practised in the use of each of her chosen materials because competence in moulding, positioning and finishing are acquired skills. This accounts for the fact that many therapists have their favourite materials from which they produce a wide variety of splints but which other therapists find difficult to use, and vice versa. Sheer practice is the basis of successful splint-making.

A selection of paddings and linings is also necessary, plus a variety of straps, preferably ready-made and of various sizes. Attachments such as rivets, hooks, Velcro fastener, metal rings and loops, and an assortment of elastics are all invaluable, and may provide inspiration for solving problems.

Metric sizes and measurements are usually given in this book. They are not necessarily direct conversions from British measures but are those which are, or will be, used by manufacturers and suppliers, depending on the materials which are being described. Metals remain in imperial measures, in accordance with the current recommendations of the Metrication Board.

DARVIC/FORMASPLINT

Darvic and Formasplint are the two names given to the same material; for convenience, the name Darvic is used throughout this book. It is a PVC sheet material of good strength and rigidity, and for splinting it is obtained to the following specifications:

> White, opaque, 2.5 mm thick
> White, opaque, 1.0 mm thick
> Transparent, 2.5 mm thick

Further notes on the properties and uses of Darvic are to be found in the Table on pages 246–248. In general it is suitable for splints where strength and rigidity are required and in particular for those which must incorporate strong, narrow areas, for example, the metacarpophalangeal ulnar drift splint (*see* page 302). A high temperature is required to soften Darvic for moulding. The relevant temperatures for each of the different heating methods are given below. They vary accordingly, but the Darvic itself has to reach a temperature of 70°C (158°F) for softening.

If the splint is to be moulded directly on to the patient whilst it is hot, insulation is essential. The method of insulation developed at

Farnham Park is simple and quick, and, above all, allows close moulding as it is not bulky. A very thin lining of extruded, expanded polystyrene sheeting, 0.5 mm thick, is glued temporarily to the inside of the splint immediately before the moulding process. It is important to ensure that the polystyrene sheeting is of the correct *density* to provide the patient with sufficient protection against the heat of the splint during moulding. The therapist's hands must also be protected and the simplest method is to wear thin cotton gloves that fit well, such as dermatological or soft household gloves.

Pattern-making

Darvic is a strong material but lacks elasticity. It is therefore advisable to ensure that those parts of a splint which are to be moulded in very acute contours should be made as narrow as possible. For instance, on a paddle or wrist extension splint it is best to 'waist' the wrist area, in order to achieve close moulding and to prevent buckling and an untidy appearance. Suitable shaping is shown in *Figures 8.35* and *8.38*.

The patient's hand is placed palm down on a sheet of paper, with the joints in the desired positions, and the outline traced closely round with a pencil which is held constantly vertical. The pattern is cut out, fitted to the patient and adjusted where necessary.

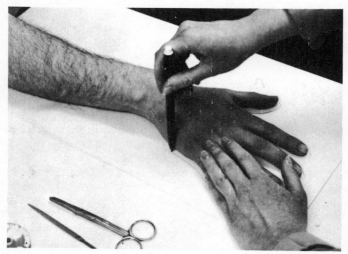

Figure 8.8. – Preparation of a Darvic splint. (a) The outline of the patient's hand is drawn on paper

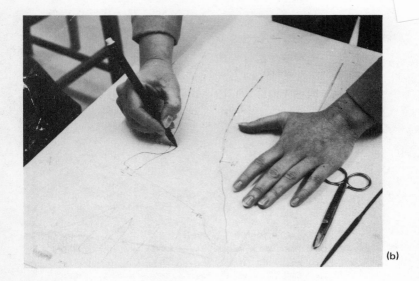

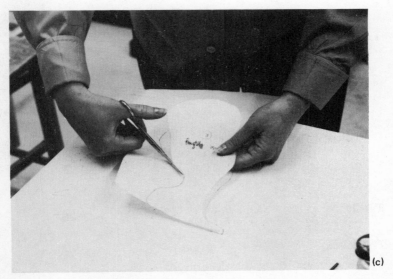

Figure 8.8 (cont.) – (b) A pattern is drawn on the outline. (c) The pattern is cut for fitting to the patient

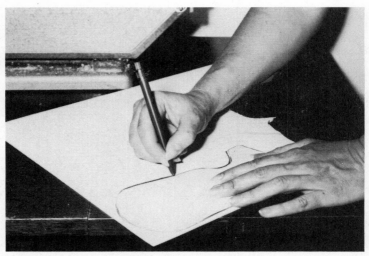

Figure 8.8 (cont.) − (d) The outline of the splint is transferred to the Darvic by tracing round the paper pattern with a wax pencil

Marking out

The pattern is transferred to the sheet of Darvic with a wax pencil.

Cutting

The sheet is then cut in one of the following ways:

1. By a fine-toothed electric bandsaw (*Figure 8.9a* and *see* equipment list, page 244). This is the most efficient method.
2. By using tin-snips or plaster cutters. This method is slower and requires strength.
3. By coping-saw or fretsaw.

The thinner Darvic, 1.0 mm thick, can be cut with strong scissors.

Preparation

The rough edges are smoothed a little, by:

sanding on an electric sanding-wheel (*Figure 8.9b*); or
filing with fine engineers' files (a half-round file is best, using the convex surface); or

using a flexible drive tool with a filing and/or felt buffing head as used by dentists and jewellers; or
scraping with a sharp knife blade.

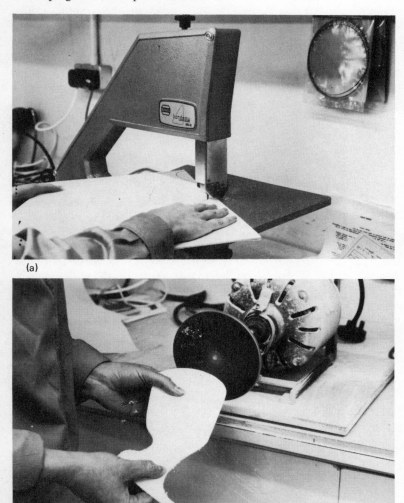

(a)

(b)

Figure 8.9. – (a) The Darvic is cut to shape on an electric bandsaw. (b) The edges of the splint are smoothed and bevelled on an electric sander fitted with a rigid sanding-plate

Insulation

The inside surface of the Darvic splint is brushed with a thin coat of
Copydex rubber solution and the splint is pressed down on to a sheet
of polystyrene until it has adhered. The polystyrene is trimmed with
scissors so that it overlaps the splint by 2 to 3 mm all round (*Figure
8.10c*). This border will curl round the edges of the splint when heated
and thus protect the patient's skin.

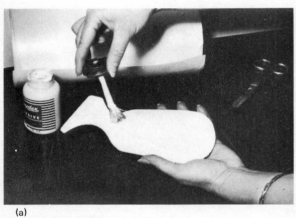

(a)

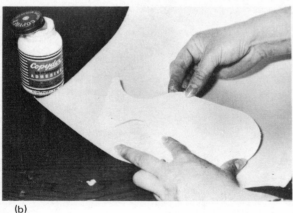

(b)

*Figure 8.10. − (a) Copydex latex rubber solution is applied
to the inner surface of the splint. (b) Very thin extruded
expanded polystyrene sheet is stuck on with Copydex. This
will provide insulation for the patient during moulding*

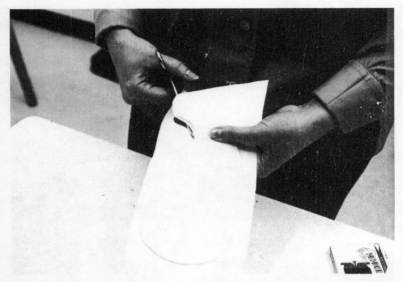

Figure 8.10 (cont.) — (c) The polystyrene sheet is neatly trimmed, leaving a narrow protruding border of 2–3 mm

The Copydex is not allowed to dry hard but is left in a semi-dry, tacky state during moulding so that the polystyrene can be removed when no longer required. Other types of adhesive are not suitable as their solvents may destroy the polystyrene or form too permanent a bond.

Softening and moulding

The therapist wears thin cotton gloves to protect her against the heat, as Darvic must reach 70°C (158°F) before it softens. The splint is held a few inches above an ordinary electric hotplate set at a high temperature, for approximately two minutes until it becomes pliable (*Figure 8.11a*). The outer side of the splint must be towards the hotplate and the insulated inner side away from the heat. If this is not done correctly the polystyrene lining will shrink and shrivel. It is also possible for the splint to be heated in a splint oven set at 140°C (275°F) for two minutes; any longer than this will cause deterioration of the polystyrene lining. This method, however, does not allow parts of the

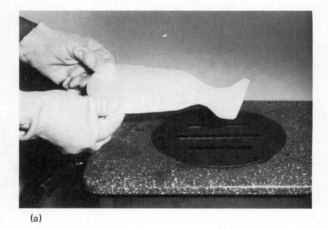

(a)

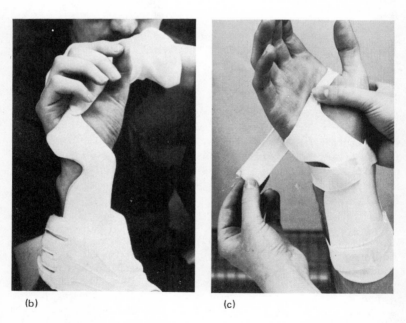

(b)   (c)

Figure 8.11. — (a) The outer surface of the splint is heated a few inches above the electric hotplate until it becomes pliable. The therapist wears light cotton gloves as a protection from the heat. (b) The splint is moulded to the patient. (c) The straps are fitted

splint to be moulded separately (*see below*) as does the hotplate method. Other methods of heating are an infrared lamp, which takes longer but may be useful where large areas are to be moulded; a heat-gun; an upturned domestic iron, which can be used when no other source of heat is available, though even hot coals have been used in Bangladesh!

Immediately before moulding, the insulated side of the splint is temperature-tested by pressing it *firmly* on to the inside of the therapist's own wrist to ensure that it is not too hot for safe application to the patient. It is then quickly applied to the patient's limb and moulded to the desired shape (*Figure 8.11b*). The Darvic will cool and set rigid in approximately one minute.

It has been found best to heat and mould most splints in two or more stages, the most complex part of the splint being moulded first and the less crucial part second. When moulding a paddle splint, for instance, the thumb and palm are shaped first and allowed to set; then the wrist and forearm parts are heated and moulded second. This allows each part to be carefully and accurately fitted. When moulding is completed, the polystyrene lining is peeled off and discarded.

Finishing

Any surplus material is trimmed off, and the edges bevelled and smoothed by any of the methods listed under Preparation (*see* pages 264–265).

Remoulding

If a satisfactory fit has not been obtained, the splint may be reheated, flattened and cooled, and the moulding procedure begun again. Remoulding may be undertaken several times without loss of the malleability or durability of the Darvic. Remoulding of a small part can be done by spot-heating.

Spot-heating

An upturned metal funnel is placed on the hotplate and the splint held over the aperture. This is a useful method for making adjustments to the splint during initial moulding, and also for serial splinting.

Reinforcement

This is seldom necessary but small strips of Darvic can be heated and moulded to the splint. When cool they are glued on with an impact adhesive such as Evo-Stik.

Attachments

Holes can be drilled in Darvic to take rivets or stitches for straps. Velcro and various other fabrics, including synthetic leather, can be glued on with Evo-Stik impact adhesive or with Croid Solvent Adhesive No. 6143.

Cleaning

Darvic is easily washed with warm water, and soap or detergent. Removable straps (*see* Strapping, page 292) will make it easier to keep the whole splint clean.

Ventilation

Holes can be drilled in the Darvic. Alternatively, 'windows', which are really more effective, can be made by drilling and sawing out areas in the centre of the forearm and palm of the splint, leaving at least 6 mm width of surrounding splint to maintain adequate strength.

Orthoplast Isoprene and San-Splint

These two materials have almost identical characteristics, except that Orthoplast Isoprene (usually known as Orthoplast) is white and San-Splint is flesh-coloured. Both materials are supplied in sheets, either perforated or unperforated, in the following sizes:

Orthoplast, unperforated: 450 mm × 700 mm × 3 mm thick
Orthoplast, perforated: 910 mm × 700 mm × 3 mm thick
San-Splint, unperforated: 450 mm × 600 mm × 3 mm thick
San-Splint, perforated: 450 mm × 600 mm × 3 mm thick

They are materials which combine very high malleability when soft with good rigidity when set and so have a very wide application for hand-splinting. They are suitable both for large, simple splints such as a paddle, and for small intricately-contoured thumb splints. One of the most useful properties is that an integral hinge can be made by simply grooving the splint surface (*see* Hinge-forming, page 277). A very high temperature is not required for softening and these materials can be applied directly to the patient's skin without insulation.

Pattern-making

A pattern can be made in paper but where this is difficult, say, for a splint with several contours such as a thumb stabilizer, a successful pattern can be made from a thin piece of children's plastic modelling putty, such as Aloplast, which can be fitted more closely to the hand.

Areas where extra strength is required should be left a little wide to allow additional guttering, so that the edge may be folded back. This is particularly applicable to the wrist area (*see Figures 8.35* and *8.38*).

Marking out

The outline of the pattern is inscribed firmly on to the material using a blunted scriber or other blunt-pointed instrument. Pens or coloured markers should not be used since they cannot be eradicated and spoil the appearance of the splint.

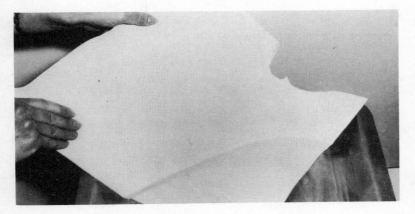

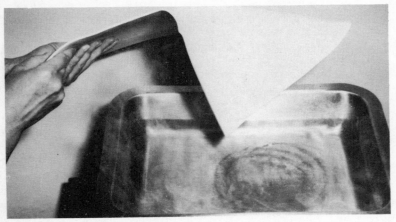

Figure 8.12. – Preparation of an Orthoplast splint. (a) and (b) The sheet of Orthoplast is softened in a shallow dish of hot water

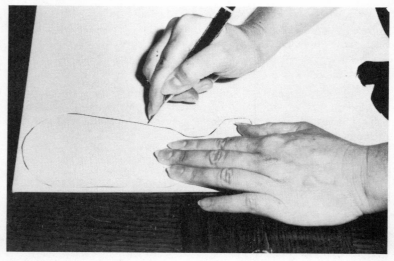

Figure 8.12 (cont.) – (c) Whilst the Orthoplast is soft, the shape of the splint is transferred by inscribing the outline around the paper pattern. This is done with a blunt-pointed instrument, because pen or pencil marks cannot be removed from Orthoplast and would spoil the appearance of the finished splint

Cutting

The material is heated until soft, when it can easily be cut with scissors. A sharp pair with long blades is best, as long, steady cutting strokes produce a neatly bevelled edge. Small, curved surgical scissors are useful for acute contours. This method eliminates any finishing process on the edges of the splint and thus saves time. The material can be cut with tin-snips when cold, provided it is held well down into the jaws of the cutters to obtain maximum leverage. This method does not produce a smoothly bevelled edge, however, and smooth edge finishing is then difficult.

Softening

There are a number of softening methods:

Hot water   A large, shallow, non-rusting metal dish is necessary and should be almost full of very clean water heated to 70°C–78°C (150°F–170°F), that is, a little below simmering temperature. Cleanliness is

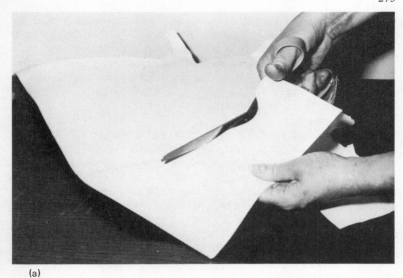

(a)

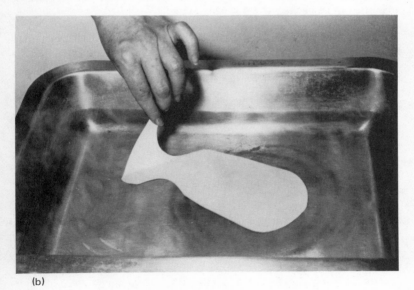

(b)

Figure 8.13. – (a) The Orthoplast is cut whilst soft with a good pair of scissors. Careful cutting will produce a smoothly bevelled edge, eliminating the need for further finishing. (b) The splint is reheated in the hot water immediately before being moulded on the patient's hand

necessary as any particles in the water may stick to the surface of the splint. The temperature should not be above 78°C. The Orthoplast is immersed for approximately one minute and then dried lightly on a smooth cloth before being applied to the patient. It should be noted that Orthoplast and San-Splint lose their self-adhesive quality after immersion in water. This can only be restored by carefully cleaning the material with dry-cleaning fluid.

Heat gun   An industrial heat gun or a hair-dryer set at a low temperature can be used, preferably with a stand for support on the table. By this dry method the material retains its self-adhesive quality and will bond immediately on contact. This is a useful property but care must be taken during moulding, as any folding may result in the splint sticking to itself. It is then impossible to separate.

Oven   The material may also be heated in an oven at 72°C–80°C (160°F–175°F) for about four minutes. During heating the splint should be placed on a flat surface to prevent sagging and on silicone release paper to prevent sticking. The separating sheets provided in the manufacturer's packaging are usually suitable.

Infrared lamp   The material is placed on a clean, dry surface under the lamp until it becomes sufficiently pliable. The pliability should be tested at frequent intervals to ensure that the material does not overheat.

Dry-heating using hot water   If dry-heating is required and only hot water is available, a piece of the material can be put in a water-tight, boilable plastic bag and immersed in hot water.

Moulding

Once heated, Orthoplast and San-Splint will stay soft for approximately three to five minutes, allowing adequate working time. Both can be applied directly to the patient's skin, after testing the temperature by pressing the hot material *firmly* on to the inside of the therapist's forearm. A light application test is not sufficient, as most splints are wrapped firmly and closely to the patient and will thus produce a higher contact temperature. If using the hot water method of softening, the material must be dried before being applied to the patient. It should be laid flat on a clean smooth towel (a linen tea-towel is suitable) and patted dry on both sides.

The material should be moulded firmly on the patient, and pulled and stretched where necessary so that it conforms faithfully. While setting it can be held in position manually or by a crêpe bandage. The edges can be rolled back to provide a more gently bevelled edge against the patient's skin or to give greater rigidity to the splint.

To speed up setting, which is slow at normal room temperature, the following methods are suitable:

1. Cold-retaining jelly in sealed plastic packs, such as Cryogel or those used for picnic boxes, is applied after cooling in a refrigerator or in a box of ice-cubes. This is an excellent method as the packs are easy to handle, are not messy, conform easily to the surface of the splint and can be pushed into awkward contours, such as between the fingers.

2. Ice-cubes in a plastic bag are applied to the splint for a few minutes but, being lumpy, they may make dents in the splint surface, so method (1) above is preferable.

3. If suitable, the patient wears the splint and his hand is plunged into a bowl of cold water containing ice, or held under a running cold tap.

4. The splint is removed when half-set and held under a running cold tap, or left for 20 minutes in a domestic refrigerator, or 10 minutes in a deep freezer.

5. Cold spray in a pressurized container, as used for first aid in sports, may be applied but care must be taken, as cooling sprays may cause skin burns.

Remoulding

A splint can be softened and remoulded several times but the material will not return fully to its original flatness, especially if it has been stretched.

Spot-heating

The edges of the splint can be selectively dipped in hot water, or small areas can be held over the spout of an upturned metal funnel on a hotplate. Some heat-guns and hair-dryers have nozzles suitable for spot-heating.

Reinforcement

One of the neatest ways of reinforcing Orthoplast is to roll or fold the edges of the splint. Alternatively a strip of the material can be moulded and bonded on to the cooled splint (*see* Attachments and bonding, below). To make a stronger reinforcement the strip can be twisted like a strip of pastry, pinched into a ridge or moulded over a drinking straw, plastic tube or metal rod to form a stiff tunnel.

Finishing

The edges need no treatment provided the splint has been cut out when warm. If finishing is necessary, a leatherwork tool intended for bevelling leather edges may be used. The surface can be made more dirt-resistant by coating with a light lacquer but this should be non-toxic, non-allergenic and waterproof.

Attachments and bonding

Attachments such as hooks, loops and straps can be sandwiched between two layers of the material and bonded into place, or fitted into a pocket made between layers. Self-bonding, that is without an adhesive, will occur only if the dry-heat methods of softening are used, and the material has not been soiled or previously put in water. The material can be bonded to itself by the application of a solvent, such as tri-chlorethylene (household dry-cleaning preparations, for example Dab-It-Off). This should be rubbed firmly on both surfaces and the material bonded whilst soft. For a stronger bond, contact adhesives such as Evo-Stik work well.

Velcro is most securely glued on if Evo-Stik is used, and webbing and plastic straps are also firmest with this adhesive. Webbing and synthetic leather straps can be satisfactorily attached with double-sided pressure-sensitive tape, provided the straps are the circumferential type.

Riveting or sewing may be used and for this holes can easily be drilled or punched (*see* Holes and ventilation, below).

Self-straps

Self-straps can be formed by firmly pulling small strips of the material until they have stretched to about three times their original length, and are fairly thin. Such a strap is incorporated in the splint itself and extra material should be allowed for this when cutting out the pattern.

Hinge-forming

This is one of the most useful and unusual properties of Orthoplast. A self-hinge is formed by making a deep straight groove with a blunt-pointed instrument in the softened material. Another groove should be exactly matched to it on the reverse surface, and as the material cools this hinge should be flexed several times until supple. If the hinge is found to be insufficiently supple, the grooves should be made deeper.

A hinge of this type is helpful in a splint which encloses the limb, so that it is easier to remove. This will be appreciated by a patient with a weak grip.

Holes and ventilation

Holes are very easy to make with a leather punch or by pushing through the material with an awl or blunt-pointed instrument. Suitably shaped leather punching tools can be used for forming slots. Drilling is not a suitable method for making holes, as the heat which is created causes gumming.

Cleaning

The surface of the splint is rubbed firmly with a cloth or a cotton-wool pad soaked in surgical spirit or methylated spirits. If very soiled, it may be scrubbed with a soft brush, soap and *cold* water. Hot water must *not* be used as it can result in deformation of the splint.

Instructions to patients

Patients should be instructed in cleaning the splint as above and carefully warned against over-heating it. It should not be worn in the bath, whilst cooking or whilst sunbathing, and should not be dried on a radiator or left in a car on a hot day. Splints made from Orthoplast or San-Splint are not suitable for wear in a warm treatment pool or during any other heat treatment, as they may become distorted.

VITRATHENE AND PLASTAZOTE

Vitrathene and Plastazote are described separately on the following pages, so that their individual characteristics may be understood, but most experts frequently use the two materials together. This is because Vitrathene can provide rigidity and reinforcement for Plastazote, while Plastazote can give resilience and softness to Vitrathene. For instance, a gauntlet of Plastazote requiring extra support to hold the wrist in the desired position will have a strip of Vitrathene bonded to the outside of the splint, over the dorsum of the palm, wrist and forearm. Alternatively, the gauntlet can be made of two layers of Plastazote with the piece of Vitrathene sandwiched between them. Conversely, a Vitrathene gauntlet may be too hard and uncomfortable to be in direct contact with the patient's skin, and a Plastazote lining can then be incorporated during moulding.

VITRATHENE

Vitrathene is polythene, supplied for splinting in sheet form, in pink or white, as follows:

> Sheet: 3050 mm × 1525 mm × 2.5 mm thick
> Sheet: 3050 mm × 1525 mm × 1.5 mm thick
> *Note:* Smaller sheet sizes are also supplied (*see* Table of splint materials, p. 246)
> Density: Pink, low density 2SSAO. White, low density, Grade 2.

Vitrathene can also be supplied in other thicknesses and densities, and in rod, block and tube form. It is light, strong and suitable for splints that do not have to be completely rigid. Most therapists use it for splints which enclose or almost enclose the limb, such as gauntlets or arm cylinders. It is also suitable for leg cylinders and for cervical and lumbar supports. Vitrathene cannot be applied directly to the patient's skin as it remains at a high temperature when soft. It is therefore insulated by a cellular lining which is permanently bonded to the splint for comfort. This lining may be made from either Plastazote or polyurethane foam sheet 6 mm thick.

Pattern-making

A pattern can be made in paper from a tracing of the patient's limb, with circumferential measurements if an enclosed splint is required.

Marking out

The pattern is transferred to the Vitrathene using a ball-point pen.

Cutting

The material is cut with shears, a fine knife or a fine-toothed fretsaw. If reasonably even, the edge does not require finishing as it will melt a little and become smooth when heated.

The lining is cut to the same shape but is made 3 mm wider than the Vitrathene, all round, to protect the patient.

Softening

Vitrathene softens at 130°C (263°F). A Plastazote oven, or similar hot-air type of oven, is used, preheated to 140°C (275°F). The oven tray is covered with a sheet of silicone-treated release paper. The lining is put on this paper, then the Vitrathene is positioned accurately on top of the lining and left in the oven for 10—15 minutes, or longer, until the Vitrathene has become transparent. During the heating process the lining and the Vitrathene will bond together.

Moulding

When heating is completed, a piece of stockinette is stretched over the Vitrathene and pressed gently on to the surface. The stockinette adheres lightly and is used to lift the Vitrathene. Within a few seconds the lining loses most of its heat and the lined surface is then temperature-tested, by firmly pressing on to the therapist's skin, and applied to the patient. On no account must the Vitrathene itself be allowed to touch the patient as it is extremely hot. The splint is wrapped round the limb and bandaged firmly in place until cooling and setting occurs after five to ten minutes. The limb must be maintained in the required position during this time, and undue pressure should not be applied since this may compress the lining to such an extent that the patient may be burnt. If great pressure is necessary for accurate positioning, the patient should be additionally insulated by bandaging *before* the hot splint is applied. When fairly cool the splint is removed from the patient and allowed to cool completely. Any trimming is then done with large scissors. Curved surgical scissors are useful for contours.

Remoulding

The whole splint may be returned to the oven but it will not return completely to the original flat state.

Spot-heating

This is difficult, as a high temperature throughout the depth of the material is necessary. Spot-heating can be done with a heat-gun but requires considerable skill.

Reinforcement

Additional pieces of Vitrathene may be added by placing them on the top of the main splint during the heating process. They will bond in the oven and do not require adhesive.

Finishing

The edges will have become smooth during heating but if the splint needs trimming after this, they can be scraped smooth again with a sharp-bladed knife. They do not need to be very finely bevelled because the soft lining cushions the edges.

Attachments and bonding

Bonding can be difficult on Vitrathene due to its high chemical resistance. A flexible impact adhesive such as Evo-Stik is satisfactory for circumferential straps, or they may be fixed with double-sided pressure-sensitive tape for short-term wear. Various attachments and types of straps can be riveted or sewn on through holes, or sandwiched between two layers of Vitrathene before heating in the oven. If the latter method is used, the straps must be of materials that will withstand a high temperature, for example cotton webbing.

Holes and ventilation

Holes may be made with a leather punch, or drilled at a low speed. Gumming will occur if a high speed drill is used. For ventilation they should be approximately 5 cm (2 in) apart. Small holes may be pierced in the material by means of a hot awl.

Cleaning

Both the Vitrathene and the linings are washable in warm water and soap.

PLASTAZOTE

Plastazote is a polythene material of closed-cell construction. In appearance it is a firm, resilient foam sheet. It is usually obtained perforated, in white or flesh pink, in sheets of the following sizes:

900 mm × 600 mm × 3 mm thick
900 mm × 600 mm × 6 mm thick
900 mm × 600 mm × 12 mm thick

Other sizes and colours may be obtained for special requirements and the 3 mm thickness given above is also commonly supplied unperforated. Plastazote can be applied directly to the patient's skin during moulding and does not require insulation. It is not very suitable, however, for working splints since it is bulky and hot, and is best used for totally enclosed resting splints such as gauntlets, and arm and leg cylinders, which are not required to be very rigid. It is soft enough to be suitable for applying to delicate or damaged skin for which it will also provide protection against bruising, for example, for an incoordinated patient. It can be made more rigid by laminating two layers together with a stiffening of polythene between, though this further increases its bulkiness. In its thinner forms, especially 3 mm thicknesses, Plastazote makes a durable and resilient lining or padding for splints made from harder materials.

Pattern-making

A paper pattern can be made or circumference measurements can be taken. The pattern does not have to be very precise in size, as trimming is simple.

Marking out

The pattern is traced on to the material with a ball-point or felt-tip pen.

Cutting

A large pair of scissors or a sharp knife is satisfactory. It can also be cut on an electric band-saw.

Softening

A hot-air oven is preheated to 140°C (275°F), never less than 135°C (270°F) or more than 145°C (285°F). Silicone-treated release paper, which is supplied with Plastazote sheets, should be placed on the oven grid. The Plastazote is then laid flat on this while softening. Small thin splints should be heated for about one minute, laminated smaller splints for two to three minutes, a gauntlet for four to five minutes and leg splints for six to seven minutes. Plastazote will fuse to itself when heated at 140°C, and the layers which are to be laminated should therefore be placed accurately together in the oven. When polythene sheeting reinforcement is to be added, either on the outer side of the splint or between two layers of Plastazote, it is positioned as required on the Plastazote and both materials heated together for about 15 minutes. During heating the polythene will bond to the Plastazote.

Warning: On no account must the hot polythene be allowed to come into contact with patients' skin as it will readily cause burns.

Moulding

The material is removed from the oven, allowed to cool momentarily until tolerable to the patient, and stretched gently around the patient's limb. It is usually sufficient to maintain it in position by hand until it sets in about three or four minutes. A larger splint may require two pairs of hands or the assistance of bandaging.

Remoulding

If remoulding is necessary, the splint should be returned to the oven, taking care that it does not fold over or adhere to itself.

Spot-heating

This has not been found suitable with Plastazote.

Reinforcement

Solid low-density polythene sheeting, 3 mm thick, is most commonly used. It can be fused in strips to one side of the Plastazote or sandwiched in between two layers during heating in the oven; several layers of polythene strips may be used to increase the reinforcement.

(Again, do not let the hot polythene touch the patient's skin.) Aluminium or Cramer wire may also be sandwiched between two layers of Plastazote to provide a more rigid splint.

Finishing

This is not necessary before application to the patient. During heating the edges will melt slightly and become smooth but if any trimming is required, a very sharp knife or No. 1 glass paper can be used. A fine electric sander is very effective for a smooth bevelled edge but no sanding should be done until the material is cool, or it will drag.

Attachments and bonding

Rigid attachments tend to pull away or tear the Plastazote, and metal rivets may escape unless they are tightly fastened to a strip of polythene reinforcement. Plastic rivets, available from Plastazote suppliers, have large heads and washers and are simple to apply and excellent for attaching straps. After fitting, the excess length of the rivet stem is trimmed off and can be lightly heat-sealed with a soldering iron.

Straps can be attached with these rivets, with double-sided pressure-sensitive tape, or with Evo-Stik adhesive. Slots can also be cut in Plastazote to allow for removable strapping, or spaces may be left between layers of the material by including straps during heating. Velcro is best attached to circumferential straps rather than directly to the plastic as it tends to pull away if bonded with an adhesive. Sewing with long stitches is also fairly strong.

For self-bonding and sandwiching (laminating) *see under* Softening on page 00. For other types of bonding, Evo-Stik is a secure and sufficiently flexible adhesive.

Cleaning

Plastazote can be washed in hot water and soap, or lightly scrubbed with a soft brush. Tubular cotton stockinette may be worn under the splint and changed frequently if greater hygiene is required.

METALS

Metals are now used at Farnham Park only for specially engineered attachments or for reinforcement of a splint when extra strength is required. A reinforcement of 12 mm D-section half-round aluminium, taken from a discarded caliper, can be attached by rivets to the length of a wrist extension splint. This was once done for a patient whose job involved unloading heavy crates from lorries and who was required to catch the crates as they were lowered.

Spring wire (also called piano wire) of various gauges is used for lively wrist extension splints (*see* page 327). It can be made to look more attractive by covering the wire with 2.5 mm hollow plastic tubing, usually white, such as that sold as plastic cane and obtained from craft suppliers.

Other metals are described, along with the construction of modular splints, on pages 294–301.

LEATHER AND SYNTHETIC LEATHER

Corfam is a synthetic leather originally designed for shoe-making. It is a poromeric material, that is, porous and permeable to water and air, and is exceptionally durable. It is supplied in various 'leather' finishes, 'suede' being the most supple, and has a soft, brushed, white inner surface which patients find very comfortable. It is washable, can be worn in water and most chemical substances, and resists dirt and grease well. Like leather, it will stretch in one direction so that when cut correctly it can be both supple and firm. Velcro can easily be sewn on to it by hand or by machine. Corfam is used for flexible splints, such as the soft opponens splint (*see* page 335), and for straps.

Very soft surgical leather or gloving leather is used for small finger-splints such as finger bands (*see* page 344). When soiled, a new splint must be made unless washable gloving leather has been used.

PADDINGS AND LININGS

To provide effective lining to splints it is necessary to appreciate the properties of the materials available, and thus avoid wasteful and sometimes harmful mistakes. Lining or padding should be used only when essential to the comfort and good treatment of the patient. If not used with care it may reduce the accuracy of the fit of a splint, increase its bulk, give a less attractive and acceptable appearance, and make the splint unhygienic.

Paddings may be divided into two main types, fibre and foam. The fibre paddings are made of wool, cotton or synthetic material, and are felted or woven. The felted types are usually manufactured in different densities and degrees of compression, and the woven materials in different thicknesses, some being brushed for extra surface softness. The degree of compression, combined with thickness, will provide the choice of resilience to suit the needs of the patient. The foam types are of plastic or rubber and will be either open or closed cell. The term 'cell' refers to the type of bubbles in the foam, either partially broken bubbles which interconnect with each other, or completely enclosed ones which do not connect. The open cells permit air, water and particles of dirt to travel through them and therefore have reduced resilience. They are compressible, absorb moisture, are not waterproof and are not hygienic unless the foam has a sealed outer skin. They do however allow some ventilation. The closed cells are more resilient, more hygienic, waterproof, provide no ventilation unless the foam is perforated, but do provide insulation.

Wool has excellent natural resilience but it is difficult to keep clean, and may be too warm for some uses as it does not absorb moisture readily. Cotton is highly absorbent, and therefore helpful when a cool lining is required. It is easily washed but has poor resilience. All the synthetic materials tend to feel hotter than the natural fibres but many of them have good resilience and are usually easier to wash than natural materials. Rubber also feels hot but is more resilient than most plastics and keeps its resilience longer. Many plastic foams gradually become more compressed in use and may lose their resilience altogether after a time, but they resist grease and human contact better than rubber, which may eventually rot.

To fulfil certain requirements, some linings are supplied in a combined form, for example, foam rubber with a cotton fabric surface. Sometimes a sandwich of thin materials like this can be made in the department but it is necessary to bond the layers correctly. For instance, a layer of waterproof adhesive may prevent ventilation or absorbency, and instead it may be best to join the materials at intervals with spots of adhesive to prevent the loss of these properties.

Some linings, like Plastazote, when used on Vitrathene, can be permanently bonded by heating. Others are supplied with an adhesive backing which allows for quick application; with these it is best to wet the scissors or knife before cutting to prevent the adhesive from sticking to the tools. Various adhesives may be used but with plastic and synthetic linings it is best to test a small piece first, as some adhesives contain chemicals such as acetone or ethyl preparations which dissolve certain man-made fibres.

It is often wise to provide more than one removable lining for some splints, so that they may be washed and dried, or replaced. A simple way to attach these is to use several strips of double-sided adhesive tape so that the lining can be peeled off.

Padding materials may also be valuably used during the moulding of a splint to prevent pressure areas. A fairly thick, rounded piece of resilient padding is lightly fixed with a strip of adhesive tape over the area to be protected, for instance, over the ulnar styloid. The splint is then moulded over the padding, thus leaving a space when the padding is discarded.

List of paddings and linings

The main list starting on page 287 describes a wide variety of paddings and linings to cover almost every need. It is not necessary to hold such a comprehensive stock, although the initial outlay would not be too great and the materials themselves have a good shelf life if kept clean and cool. It is suggested that a smaller stock would be adequate for most departments and the following materials would provide a suitable selection:

Plastazote, 6 mm thick, to provide a resilient padding for a gauntlet which exerts pressure on the patient's skin and which needs to be washable and hygienic.

White wool felt, 3 mm and 6 mm thick, to provide softness combined with high resilience, for example, where pressure is being applied to correct contractures and where the skin is frail.

Formatex, 3 mm thick, to provide softness and good hygiene in a situation not requiring a high degree of resilience.

Moleskin, to provide a little softness without any resilience, or for comfort for excessive sweating.

Warning   It is advisable to obtain all paddings and linings from reputable suppliers who, preferably, have experience of the medical application of their products. This is especially applicable when using plastic and synthetic materials, many of which are allergenic. They may also be inflammable or may melt, or they may emit dangerous fumes or gases when heated, for example, during alteration of a splint.

Resilience   The resilience of a padding or lining may be graded as follows:

Low resilience:	Squashes flat under light pressure.
Reasonable resilience:	Does not squash except under medium pressure.
Good resilience:	Does not squash flat except under high pressure.
High resilience:	Retains most of its resilience. Does not squash flat even under high pressure.

White wool felt

Also called chiropodial felt. Made from real wool. Supplied in thicknesses from 2 mm to 10 mm in sheet form, in densities described as compressed, semi-compressed and soft, with or without adhesive backing. All densities have good resilience, compressed has very high resilience, semi-compressed is generally the most useful. Firm but kind to the skin. Hard-wearing but after long usage may pack down to a hard block. Not washable, replaced when dirty.

Other felts

Some also known as chiropodial felts. Cheaper alternative to pure wool; made from synthetic and wool mixtures. Usually off-white, supplied 5 mm or 7 mm thick in sheet form, of semi-compressed density, with adhesive backing. Are a little less satisfactory in every respect than wool but still have good resilience and density, though may pack down more quickly. Not washable.

Moleskin or Swansdown

Good quality thin cotton fabric with a soft, raised fleece on one side. White or pale pink, supplied less than 1 mm thick in sheet form, with adhesive backing. No resilience. Very gentle to the skin, and absorbent. Particularly useful as it takes up little space and is suitable for patients who complain of sweating. Reasonably durable. Not washable, replaced when dirty.

Fleecy web

Loosely woven fabric with a very soft, thick, raised fleece. White or pale pink, supplied 3 mm thick (approximately) in sheet form, with adhesive backing. Low resilience. A heavy grade is also available, which is thicker. Very soft to the skin. Reasonably durable. Not washable. Slightly higher resilience than above materials.

Terry towelling

As obtainable from fabric departments of large stores. Thin towelling is preferable and should be of pure cotton. Low resilience. Comfortable for the patient who has severe sweating, as it is highly absorbent. Durable. Washable. May also be available with adhesive backing from sports suppliers.

Stockinette (Tubinette)

Tubular knitted fabric, usually of cotton and rayon mixture. Off-white, supplied in a continuous length in various widths, some especially to fit hands. No resilience. Reasonably soft to skin. Reasonably durable. Useful slipped over hand and arm, inside splint, with a hole cut to allow for the thumb, if patient complains of discomfort or sweating. Also bondable to inner surface of enclosed splint. Suitable covering for plaster-of-Paris slab. Provides insulation for hot splint-moulding, thicker grade being preferable for this, but is not adequate for safety with high-temperature moulding.

Foam rubber – open cell

Also known as sponge rubber because of its open-cell structure. Usually of foamed latex rubber. Various shades available, pale grey common. Supplied in thicknesses of 3 mm, 7 mm, 10 mm and upwards to 25 mm, in sheet form, with or without adhesive backing. Reasonably resilient but much less so than closed-cell rubber (*see below*) of the same thickness and type. Reasonably soft to the skin, rubbery texture. Absorbent, but not cooling, for sweating problems. Reasonably durable, though may rot in oily conditions, and crumble with friction. Reasonably washable.

Foam rubber – closed cell

Various types available with differing resilience and durability, colour and thickness. Generally have high resilience, are non-absorbent and easy to clean. Tend to be warm or hot to wear but usually have a smooth, comfortable surface. Very durable except under some oily conditions. Washable. Two useful types are:

Zopla flesh foamed latex   Closed-cell latex foam. Pink, supplied 5 mm or 7 mm thick in sheet form, with adhesive backing. Soft, warm, with very pleasant smooth surface. Non-absorbent. Reasonably durable except as above. Washable.

Wet-suit rubber As used for underwater diving suits. Closed-cell rubber, one side covered with synthetic stockinette fabric. Usually black, supplied 4 mm thick, in sheet form. Either side comfortable to the skin. Good resilience. Non-absorbent. Durable. Washable. Can be sewn.

Foam plastics – open cell

Obtainable in various forms, made from different plastics (*see* Warning, page 286). A useful type is:

Polyfoam or Silcofoam A polyurethane polyester foam. White, supplied 5 mm and 7 mm thick, in sheet form with adhesive backing, or as Plain Polyfoam without adhesive. Low resilience. Light, soft, warm. Absorbent but not cooling. Reasonably durable. Washable if without adhesive backing.

Foam plastics – closed cell

Cross-linked, expanded polyethylene foam of closed-cell construction (*see* Warning, page 286). Useful types are:

Plastazote (*see also* pages 281–283) Thermoplastic. Supplied in thicknesses of 1.5 mm, 3 mm, 4.5 mm, 6 mm and upwards to 24 mm, in sheet form, perforated or unperforated. Standard density suitable for padding splints. High resilience. Firm to the skin, warm or hot. Non-absorbent. Durable. Washable. Heavy density has very high resilience but available 6 mm thick and in black only.

Formatex and Velvotex White, supplied 3 mm thick, in sheet form with adhesive backing. Also useful, if obtainable, in thicker sheets without adhesive. Soft and cosy, very gentle to the skin. Reasonable resilience. Can deform under strong pressure, and resilience tends to break down. Reasonably durable under light pressure. Washable.

Silicone foam elastomer (Dow Corning Silastic Elastomer, Medical Grade 386) Supplied in the form of two tins of chemicals which are mixed thoroughly, foam up, expand and set in about two minutes. Before setting, the liquid foam is spread on the splint, preferably on a base of thin open-cell foam to which it can anchor. The patient's hand is pressed into it, thus moulding the foam accurately to the fingers.

Good resilience. Reasonably durable. Washable. Is extremely expensive but may be the only method of supporting a very deformed hand.

Extruded expanded polystyrene   Like very thick rice-paper. White, supplied 0.5 mm thick, in sheet form. Used only for insulation of very hot splint materials to protect the patient during moulding (*see* page 261).

Combination materials

These are useful to gain advantages which cannot be obtained by using one material alone. Combinations other than the commercial ones given below can be devised by the therapist to suit her own requirements.

White wool felt/closed-cell foam latex   (Zopla Foam-o-Felt) Combines the resilience and durability of white wool felt with the surface washability and non-absorbency of the latex foam. These sheet materials are bonded together, the latex side being worn next to the skin, and supplied 5 mm and 7 mm thick. Pink latex, white felt, with self-adhesive backing on the felt.

Cotton fleece fabric/closed-cell foam latex rubber   (Zopla Swanfoam) Combines the absorbency and softness of the cotton with the resilience of the latex. Retains resilience well. Cotton layer worn next to skin. Supplied in 5 mm and 7 mm thicknesses, in sheet form. Pink cotton, pink latex. Self-adhesive backing. Reasonably durable. Not washable.

STRAPPING AND METHODS OF FASTENING

For the majority of straps which are for temporary use, 2.5 mm cotton webbing is used. The straps are usually of the circumferential type, that is, they fit round the splint, with Velcro sewn at either end. Only one free end is left, as it is almost impossible for even the most dexterous person to fasten a splint on himself if both ends of a strap are hanging loose. The other end is always fixed close to the splint.

For long-term use Corfam (synthetic leather) straps are preferred (*see* page 284). Corfam stretches in one direction, like leather, and should be cut so that the length of the strap is in the non-stretch direction.

If the patient's skin is particularly delicate, very soft surgical leather or gloving leather is used.

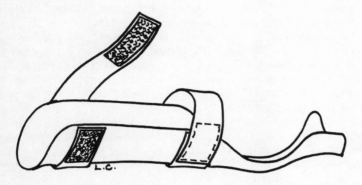

Figure 8.14. — Two circumferential straps with Velcro fastenings, suitable for a wrist extension splint

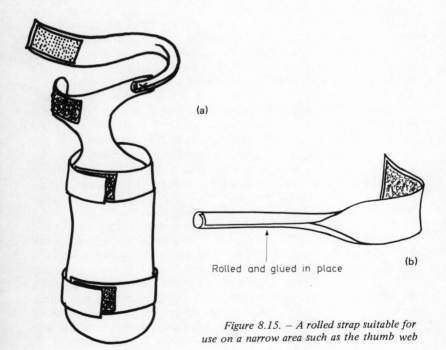

(a)

Rolled and glued in place

(b)

Figure 8.15. — A rolled strap suitable for use on a narrow area such as the thumb web

Straps may need padding when extra pressure against the skin is necessary, for example, to counteract contractures. Plastazote, Velfoam or chiropodial felt, 3 mm thick, are most often used for this.

Removable straps, as used with Darvic splints, are attached with double-sided adhesive tape. These straps should be circumferential, so that when they are fastened the tension comes on the strap itself and not on the adhesive tape. Circumferential straps which are not removable can be bonded to the splint or, with suitable splint materials, sandwiched between two layers.

Some splints, because of their shape, cannot have circumferential straps. In this case, the straps are attached by stitching, riveting or bonding, as appropriate.

Some patients with arthritic hands must wear two resting splints at night and may find it impossible to do up the fastenings on the second one. One solution is to provide self-hinged Orthoplast or San-Splint gauntlets; with a little practice these can be eased open and will then spring closed round the arms without the aids of straps.

The Velcro touch-and-close fastener has solved many of the problems encountered by patients when putting on or taking off their splints. It is therefore now used on most of the splints made at Farnham Park. Velcro requires less dexterity and strength than buckles, can even replace hooks and is soft and therefore less likely to damage the skin. It can be sewn, glued or riveted on to a splint or a strap. Two pieces of Velcro, one of loop and one of hook pile, may be joined to form a whole strap. Velcro does not fray after cutting and is washable in water at a temperature below boiling point. The hook pile, however, can damage or snag delicate fabrics such as underwear or hosiery, and become tangled in pile fabrics such as woollens, blankets and brushed nylon, and also on a hairy arm. To avoid this, sufficient loop pile should be provided on the splint to cover the hook pile completely. The hook pile may also become clogged with fluff and fine fibres which should be picked out with a thin awl or a pin to restore efficiency. The loop pile has a more delicate surface than the hook pile and after some time will tend to fray out and should be replaced.

To enable a weak patient to open a Velcro closure more easily, some of the pile at the end of the strap may be shaved off to leave a small tab. Alternatively, the end of the strap can be sewn into a loop big enough for one or more fingers to hook into.

Cinch-type fastenings (*Figure 8.16*) provide extra leverage, allow accurate adjustment and are particularly suitable for a patient with a weak grip or for a splint that must fit tightly. Various types of special 'rings' are available which, despite their name, are rectangular with rounded corners and come in different widths. It may be difficult to thread a strap through too narrow a ring, so the correct width must be chosen. A roller buckle with the prong removed is good for some arthritic patients who find that the roller makes tightening the strap easier. D-rings are not suitable because they tend to pucker the strap, which will then be both uncomfortable and more difficult to tighten.

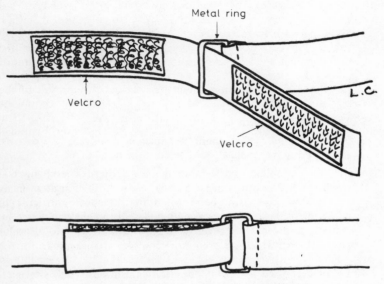

Figure 8.16. – Cinch-type fastening, with Velcro

All 'rings' are best sewn on tightly so that they do not flop when the patient is manipulating the strap. An excellent plastic ring, available from North America, will stand up and hold its position while being threaded; the long sides of this rectangular ring curve inwards to grip the middle of the strap so that the ring stays firmly where it is placed.

All metal fastenings should be nickel-plated to retain their smooth surface, resist corrosion and prevent discoloration of the patient's skin. It is best to position metal fastenings well on to the splint, so that they will not touch the patient's skin as they tend to be uncomfortably hard.

In addition to Velcro and 'rings' it is useful to keep a small stock of items that have been used successfully to solve fastening problems. These should include dressmaker's hooks, tubular rivets, eyelets, plastic rivets and paper clips for hook-making (Malick, 1974).

FARNHAM PARK MODULAR SPLINTS

These splints were originally designed at Farnham Park Rehabilitation Centre, by the occupational therapy technical instructor in collaboration with the head occupational therapist, to overcome the problems encountered in reducing deformities of the hand in juvenile rheumatoid arthritis (Still's Disease). The main problems were:

1. Splinting each finger correctly in relation to the degree of contracture, that is,
   (a) the angle of flexion/extension which had occurred as a result of the contracture;
   (b) the angle of rotation which had occurred as a result of the contracture.
2. The force or strength of the contracture.
3. Providing a splint that could be adjusted reliably by the patient, so that correct splintage could be continued at home.
4. Providing a splint that did not involve springs. The changes in tension which occur during a given time, both within a spring and within an elastic band when extended, are difficult to measure. If these tensions are applied to a patient's fingers they are counteracted by changes in tension in muscles, joint capsules and ligaments which are even more complex to measure.

The problems were solved by the use of push-rods. Each is a small metal rod with a U-shaped cup at one end, joined to the rod with a hinge which allows the cup to fit snugly against the finger. The rods slide into holes in a carrier attached to the splint and each is held by a small terminal screw (*Figure 8.17*). Each finger is controlled by its own push-rod, and adjusted separately. The push-rods can slide back or forth within the carrier to increase flexion or extension of a finger joint. They can also be rotated in the carrier to correct, or match, rotation of a metacarpophalangeal joint. Many patients with juvenile rheumatoid arthritis have exaggerated deformity of these joints, particularly of the little finger.

In use, each push-rod is adjusted to its maximum tolerable pressure against each finger and is locked by the terminal screw. It will usually be found that after a short time the contracture will have adapted to this pressure and the push-rod can be moved to a new position. Adjustments may be made at any time if the patient feels he can tolerate a little more pressure, or, if he feels too uncomfortable, the pressure can quickly be reduced.

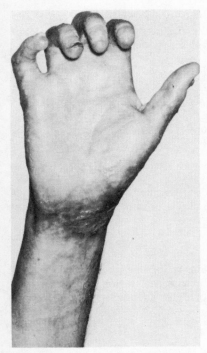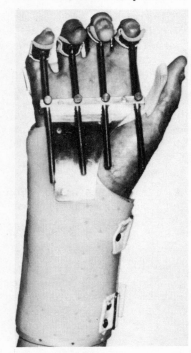

Figure 8.17. – This Farnham Park modular splint is used to increase extension of the interphalangeal joints of a patient with contractures following burns

It has been found that most patients, even as young as 12 years, can be relied on to adjust the splint satisfactorily themselves. Perhaps this is due to the freedom of choice they are given, or because they know they can relieve discomfort themselves. They realize that it is their own responsibility to achieve improvement.

Further indications for use

Modular splints can also be used for contractures of the finger joints, but only those which show radiographically that alteration of the joint position is possible. A medical opinion on the X-ray is therefore requested before accepting a referral for a modular splint. These contractures may be the result of rheumatoid arthritis in adults, of Dupuytren's contracture, or of contractures following burns or trauma.

The modular system is used to give precise individual control of each finger, where a splint like the paddle splint is considered unsuitable to achieve the desired result. The modular splint is worn between treatments or when the patient is resting, and many patients have found the best time is during television viewing. As a rule, a paddle splint is used whilst the patient is sleeping, as the modular splints tend to catch in the bed-clothes but, if the patient is comfortable, the modular splint may be used during sleep also. During active treatment sessions the patient may wear a gauntlet or other supportive splint for the wrist, if necessary, but usually the hand is left as free as possible.

Contraindications

A patient with loss of sensation is not supplied with a modular splint unless he is exceptionally reliable and will examine the skin frequently for pressure areas.

Construction and materials

There are two main types of modular splint, the interphalangeal joint extension model and the metacarpophalangeal flexion model. The two may be combined in one splint, or other adaptations of the system

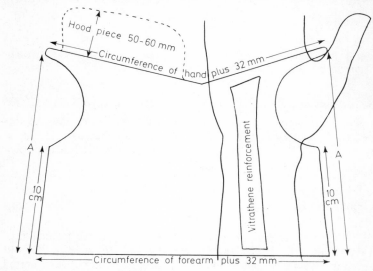

Figure 8.18. – *Pattern for the Vitrathene gauntlet. The hood piece is added to the interphalangeal extension model, and may be reinforced with a strip of Vitrathene, to hold the metacarpophalangeal joints in the desired degree of flexion ('A' is the measurement from mid-forearm to palmar crease)*

may be made to suit a particular patient. For both types of splint the gauntlet part is made in the same way, to a pattern designed at another hospital (Ansell *et al.*, 1972) (*Figure 8.18*). It is made of 1.5 mm Vitra-thene lined with 6 mm Plastazote, and moulded to the patient's forearm

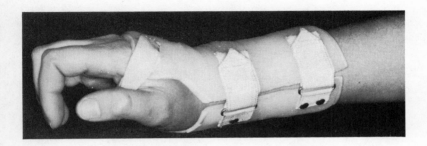

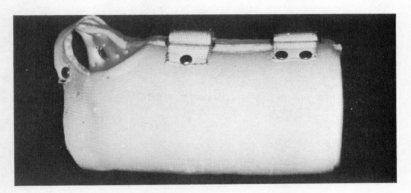

Figure 8.19. — The Vitrathene gauntlet, lined with Plastazote, having the opening on the radial side to allow room for the attachments

and hand, extending from mid-forearm to the transverse palmar crease; the thumb is usually left free (*Figure 8.19*). For the interphalangeal joint extension model the gauntlet is continued as a hood over the dorsum of the metacarpophalangeal joints, holding them in 30 degrees of flexion, to prevent hyperextension when pressure is applied by the push-rods. A transverse bar can be used as an alternative to the hood (*Figure 8.20*).

The opening is usually made along the radial side of the splint so that it allows the maximum area for the attachments to be secured, and is easy for the patient to put on. The wrist is positioned in 5 to 10 degrees of extension. Straps are cinch-type, made of cotton webbing with Velcro fastenings. They are riveted to the splint and, on the inside of the splint, each rivet is covered with a small disc of synthetic leather, to prevent damage to the patient's skin.

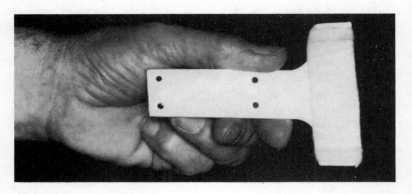

Figure 8.20. – *Transverse bar, to maintain the position of the metacarpophalangeal joints, made from Darvic and lined with white wool felt. This is used as an alternative to the hood. It is attached to the dorsum of the splint and can be used to prevent hyperextension of the metacarpophalangeal joints on the interphalangeal joint extension model of the splint*

The interphalangeal joint extension model

The carrier

Aluminium bar, $^5/_8$ in by $^1/_4$ in (15 mm by 6 mm) is cut to the width of the palm at the metacarpal heads, less $^1/_4$ in (6 mm). A $^3/_{16}$ in (5 mm) hole for each finger rod is drilled on the $^5/_8$ in (15 mm) face of the bar. To determine the position of the holes, the bar is placed on the transverse palmar crease of the hand, and points in line with the centre of each finger are marked (*Figure 8.21*). The holes are drilled at these points. On the $^1/_4$ in (6 mm) face of the bar, holes are drilled and tapped for the locking screws which are 8 BA terminal screws.

The bracket to hold the bar is made of 20 s.w.g. aluminium. Its distal edge is cut straight, to lie along the line of the transverse palmar crease. At the thumb it is curved to clear the thenar eminence (*see Figure 8.17*).

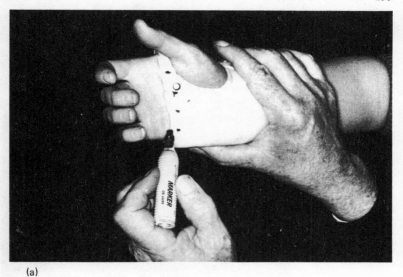

(a)

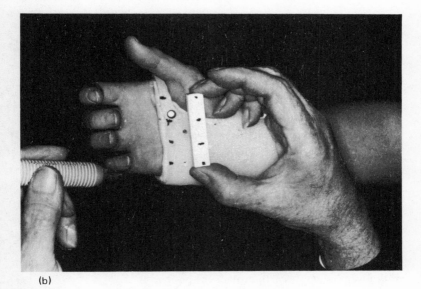

(b)

Figure 8.21. – (a) Marking out the positions at which the push-rods will be fitted to the splint. Note the holes in the Vitrathene for attaching the carrier. (b) The aluminium carrier is marked in preparation for drilling the holes which will take the push-rods

The push-rods

Each push-rod is made from $^3/_{16}$ in (5 mm) stainless steel rod which is cut out to the required length, usually about 74 mm (3 in) long, with any unnecessary surplus trimmed after fitting. Across the centre of one end of each rod a slot is cut 6 mm deep and 1 mm wide to take the finger cup. A hole is drilled at right angles to the slot to take the hinge-pin which is cut from steel wire.

The finger cup is constructed from 21 s.w.g. brass. This is cut to a small rectangle, the length being approximately one-third of the circumference of the patient's finger, and the width being the distance between the middle and distal finger creases when the patient's finger is flexed.

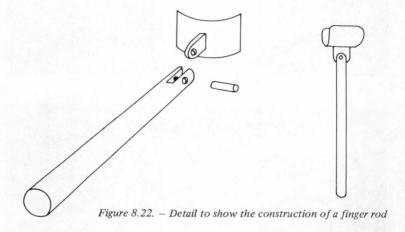

Figure 8.22. – Detail to show the construction of a finger rod

The size will thus vary, the middle finger cup, for instance, being considerably larger than the little finger cup. This rectangle of brass is then curved longitudinally to fit against the patient's finger. A tiny D-shaped piece of brass is then cut, approximately 6 mm wide by 7 mm long, and a hole to take the hinge-pin is drilled in it. This hole should be large enough to allow free rotation of the hinge-pin. It is then brazed at right angles to the cup in the position shown in *Figure 8.22.* The hinge-pin is fitted and secured, and the cup is covered in Corfam or thin synthetic leather to protect the patient's skin.

The push-rods are assembled in the carrier, adjusted on the patient and locked in place with the terminal screws.

The patient is carefully instructed in the method of adjustment of the push-rods and is required to demonstrate his ability to follow these instructions. He is told to release slightly the pressure of the push-rods on his fingers whenever he feels he cannot tolerate it and to increase the pressure when he feels he can take a little more. It is explained to him that he will usually be able to increase the pressure at intervals, as his fingers will adapt to the pressure, especially within half an hour of first putting on the splint. Initially, frequent checks are made to ensure that there is no breakdown of the skin due to the pressure. When the patient has learnt to adjust the splint correctly, less frequent checks are made by the therapist.

The metacarpophalangeal joint flexion model

Individual finger rods are only used when the positions of the meta-carpophalangeal joints are so varied that pressure from a transverse bar alone would not provide correction for all the fingers. The push-rods

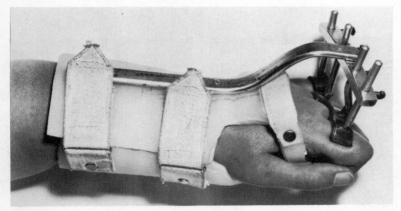

Figure 8.23. – The Farnham Park modular splint – metacarpophalangeal joint flexion model

are made in the same way as for the interphalangeal joint extension model but the carrier is fitted with an outrigger on the dorsum of the gauntlet (*Figure 8.23*).

For many patients a transverse bar is sufficient to achieve correction (*see Figure 8.20*). This is made from a strip of Darvic, lined with white wool felt, 5 mm thick, or with Plastazote, 3 mm thick, and is moulded across the proximal phalanges. It is mounted on the gauntlet by a shaped metal rod, which is hinged to allow for adjustment. A screw system is used to adjust the position of the bar which applies pressure to the dorsum of the proximal phalanges and thus increases flexion of the metacarpophalangeal joints.

METACARPOPHALANGEAL ULNAR DRIFT SPLINTS (MUD SPLINTS)

The aetiology of ulnar drift is not known. Ulnar deviation occurs in the normal hand during normal use, due to the anatomical shape of the metacarpal heads and the length of the collateral ligaments. When there is synovitis present, however, as in rheumatoid arthritis, the metacarpophalangeal joint capsules become distended and, following this, the ligaments weaken. Thus, whenever the hand is used for grasping, the normal tendency to ulnar deviation is increased to an abnormal

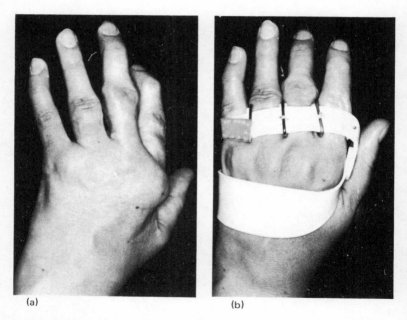

(a)   (b)

Figure 8.24. – The metacarpophalangeal ulnar drift splint. (a) Patient with severe ulnar drift of the metacarpophalangeal joints. (b) The same patient wearing the ulnar drift splint, showing the amount of correction obtained

degree, and the metacarpophalangeal joints are described as being in ulnar drift (*Figure 8.24a*). There is abnormal angulation at the affected metacarpophalangeal joints and the patient finds he is unable to correct the position voluntarily. Fine pinch is impaired and there is loss of power when grasping. Added to this there may also be considerable pain in the metacarpophalangeal joints and in the rest of the hand.

In addition to synovitis, there are also other factors which are thought to contribute to ulnar drift and these are:

1. The relocation or slipping of the extensor tendons in a more ulnar direction.

2. The detachment of the collateral ligaments so that the intrinsic muscles tend to cause subluxation. This subluxation is further increased by the destruction of the metacarpal heads themselves.

3. Radial deviation of the wrist which occurs as a result of disease of the ulnar styloid process, and which subsequently disturbs the alignment of the hand in relation to the forearm, a condition known as Z-deformity.

Bearing all these factors in mind, it was deduced that a suitable splint for ulnar drift should be designed to hold the metacarpophalangeal joints in normal alignment and, *at the same time,* allow full flexion and extension so that function is both maintained and improved (*Figure 8.24b*). The first objective was achieved by a rigid plastic splint and, simultaneously, the second objective by incorporating a hinge. This hinge was constructed to match the axial movement of the patient's second metacarpophalangeal joint.

The values of splinting for ulnar drift are numerous, the most significant aims being:

to reduce pain;

to prevent strain and further functional damage to the joint capsules and to the extensor tendons;

to improve function, particularly pinch;

to maintain and increase power in the hand, including the forearm muscles, by enabling the patient to function with greater ease and less pain.

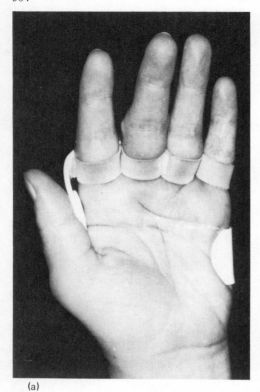

(a)

Figure 8.25. – (a) Palmar view of the MUD splint. (b) Radial view, showing how the hinge allows flexion at the metacarpo-phalangeal joints

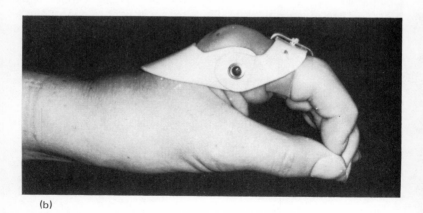

(b)

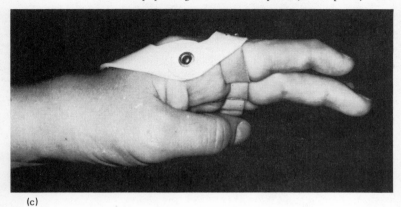

(c)

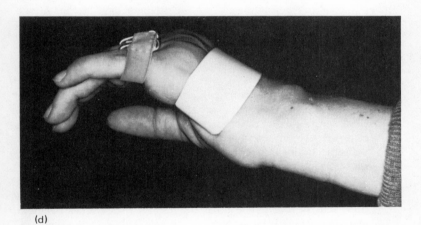

(d)

Figure 8.25 (cont.) – (c) Radial view showing how the hinge allows extension at the metacarpophalangeal joints. (d) Ulnar view

Indications and contraindications for use

1. It is used in rheumatoid arthritis of the metacarpophalangeal joints where ulnar deviation is already established and the deformity, therefore, cannot be permanently corrected by splinting. Usually at this stage the stability of the index finger is disturbed and this has a serious effect, particularly on precision handling, because pinch becomes increasingly hampered.

Selection of this splint is determined by examination of the metacarpophalangeal joints. Ulnar drift is clearly evident and there is usually slipping of one or more of the extensor tendons. When there is ulnar drift of the little finger alone, a smaller splint is made on the same principles (*see Figure 8.31*, pages 312 and 313).

2. The splint is worn as a working splint during the day, especially during heavier activities, so that the metacarpophalangeal joints and surrounding structures are protected from as much strain as possible. As the splint is designed to be durable, heatproof and waterproof, it can be worn during activities such as cooking, laundering, driving, gardening and carpentry as well as during normal employment. Patients report that the splint relieves discomfort and pain, and that their hand feels stronger. They usually regulate for themselves the amount of time that they wear the splint, which may be anything from three to nine hours a day, either continuously or for periods of one to three hours. The therapist must instruct the patient to wear the splint whenever *heavy* activities are being done.

3. The splint is *not* used if there is either ulnar drift or anterior subluxation present which cannot be corrected manually by the therapist.

4. This splint is also unlikely to work well if the patient no longer has reasonable extension of the metacarpophalangeal joints. Once severe flexion deformities have occurred, palliative splinting can give very limited benefit, although for some patients a splint without a hinge may be helpful in improving function (*see Figure 8.33*, page 315).

5. This splint is *not* used in the very early stage of onset of ulnar drift. More support is required for the hand and wrist at this time and the preventive ulnar drift splint is essential to achieve real prevention of the deformity (*see* page 314).

Construction of the MUD splint

A paper pattern is made on an outline drawing of the hand and forearm (*Figure 8.26*) with the wrist held in slight ulnar deviation, the fingers adducted and the metacarpophalangeal joints corrected to as much radial deviation as possible. Care must be taken to mark the exact point of the 2nd metacarpophalangeal joint, over which the hinge will be made. The finger bar is designed to lie over the proximal phalanges and must be sufficiently narrow to avoid contact with either the metacarpophalangeal or proximal interphalangeal joints.

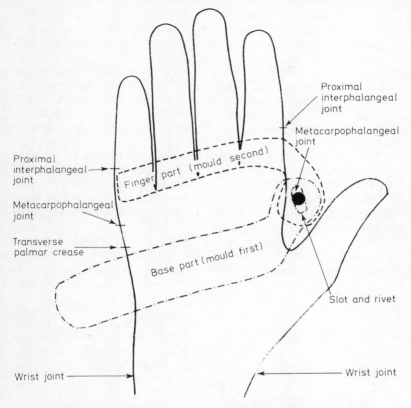

Figure 8.26. – Pattern for the metacarpophalangeal ulnar drift splint

The pattern is fitted carefully to the patient while the fingers are held in the corrected position. The patient's metacarpophalangeal joints are moved passively to ensure that the hinge areas of the splint will coincide. It has been found easier to stick the pattern to the patient's hand for this procedure, using a few tiny dabs of Copydex adhesive. The two parts of the splint are then cut out in Darvic and heated as described on pages 264–269.

The base part is moulded on to the patient first, with the hand held in the functional position (*see* page 252). It is fitted snugly and firmly round the ulnar border of the hand and into the palm, just proximal to the transverse palmar crease. The hinge area must be kept flat. The hinge area should sit alongside the 2nd metacarpophalangeal joint at the required angle of correction, that is, parallel to the 3rd metacarpal and at a right angle to the plane of the palm. It should protrude dorsally a little, so that the edge of the splint does not dig into the 2nd metacarpophalangeal joint.

Any pressure is borne on the first dorsal interosseus muscle and on the hypothenar eminence. The base part should grip round the metacarpals; it is important to fit the splint in this way and to avoid applying pressure to the 2nd metacarpophalangeal joint. If the splint obstructs full flexion of the little finger, a little of the plastic in the palm is trimmed off.

The position of the fingers is corrected by drawing them gently out of ulnar drift. The finger part of the splint is then moulded over the base part. The finger bar should lie comfortably over the proximal phalanges without touching the joints. It should also be slightly arched. The hinge area must be absolutely flush with that of the base part so that the hinge will work smoothly.

Maintaining the fingers in the corrected position, the patient is asked to flex and extend the metacarpophalangeal joints fully. A point is marked on the outside of the hinge area which appears to move the

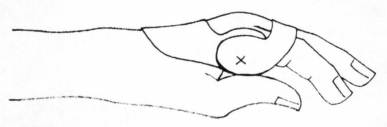

Figure 8.27. – Drawing to show the point X where the hole is drilled on the finger part when making the hinge

shortest distance (*Figure 8.27*). This point should be just below, that is just palmar to, the metacarpophalangeal joint. This is the axis of the 2nd metacarpophalangeal joint. A hole, 3 mm in diameter, is drilled in the finger part on this point.

A short, straight slot is now drilled in the base part in the following way. Maintaining correction of the hand position, a wax pencil is held in the hole already drilled, and the patient is asked to flex and extend the metacarpophalangeal joints again. The pencil will inscribe a short arc on the base part of the splint, and the two limits of this arc are then joined by drawing a straight line. A *straight* slot is made on this line; a curved slot would not move smoothly when made into a hinge. The two parts are joined together using a 7 mm nickel-plated tubular rivet (speedy rivet) (*Figure 8.28*). The smooth head of the rivet should be on the inside, against the patient's skin. It is important to ensure that the rivet is not too tight to allow free movement of the hinge.

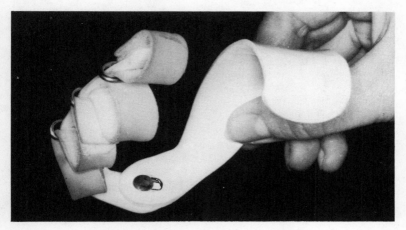

Figure 8.28. – The inner side of the hinge, showing the head of the rivet and the straight slot in which it slides and rotates

Keeping the patient's fingers corrected, the position of the finger straps is marked and small holes are drilled for the sewing process (*see Figure 8.24b*). Three nickel-plated loops, each 18 mm long by 8 mm wide, are sewn in place using heavy nylon thread or fine braided fishing line. The thread is heat-sealed at the knots using a match flame. It should be noted that the nickel-plated loops are oval-ended and narrow (*Figure 8.29*). Rectangular loops will dig into the sensitive finger webs, as will loops that are too wide.

Two narrow strips are cut from non-stretching synthetic leather, preferably Corfam. Velcro fastenings are sewn on these, one strap having two pieces of Velcro and the other one piece (*Figure 8.30*). Another piece of Velcro loop pile is glued to the splint at the little finger. The straps should be measured so that they fit firmly on the patient. They are sewn on with nylon thread using the same method as for the metal rings.

Any necessary adjustments are made, and the patient is taught how to take the splint on and off by himself. Patients have found it easier

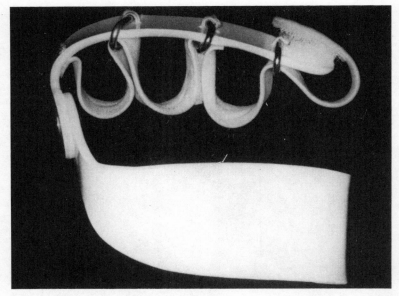

Figure 8.29. – Dorsal view showing the arrangement of the two straps

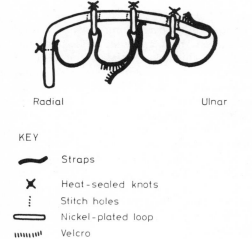

Radial   Ulnar

KEY

⟋ Straps

✖ Heat-sealed knots

⋮ Stitch holes

▭ Nickel-plated loop

ınıııtıtı Velcro

Figure 8.30. – Detail to show the fitting of the two straps

to do this by first fitting their fingers correctly into the finger bar and straps, and then pulling the base part on, and round the hypothenar eminence. For removal, the base part is hinged up from the hand first, and the finger part is then drawn off.

Modifying a MUD splint

One patient, a woman with quite severe rheumatoid arthritis of her dominant right hand, was nevertheless very active and very determined to remain so. She ran her home, nursed her elderly bed-ridden mother, did most of the gardening and in her spare time indulged in crochet work. The results of her remarkable determination were a set of deteriorating metacarpophalangeal joints but an exceptionally strong hand. She succeeded in breaking the finger bar of her first ulnar drift splint, so a more durable version was attempted. It appeared that she had broken the splint while repeatedly doing activities requiring strong grip. The new splint was made, as usual, from Darvic to provide a firm hinge section but this meant that it was rigid where it crossed the back of the fingers. In this patient's case the splint did not curve sufficiently to match her well-developed gripping position, and broke under the strain.

Most of the Darvic finger bar was therefore discarded, leaving only the hinge area intact. A new finger bar was formed from Orthoplast and attached to the remaining hinge piece. The Orthoplast was more flexible than the Darvic had been but was not sufficiently rigid to be able to replace Darvic at the hinge part. To achieve additional flexibility of grasp, a small self-hinge was formed in the Orthoplast, just radial to the index finger. Thus the patient was able to achieve full grasp, as well as full extension of the metacarpophalangeal joints, without loss of the correction of her ulnar drift.

This was a valuable adaptation for this particular patient but it would only be of value for a minority of rheumatoid cases, as few have such a high degree of mobility.

Ulnar drift splint for the little finger only (*Figure 8.31*)

The hinge for this splint is constructed in the same way as the hinge for the metacarpophalangeal ulnar drift splint previously described. The strap is made entirely of Velcro.

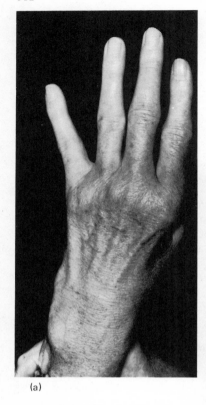

(a)

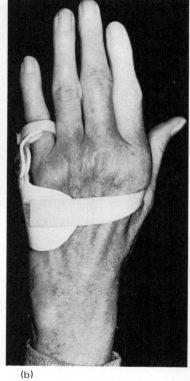

(b)

Figure 8.31. – Ulnar drift splint for the little finger only. (a) Patient with ulnar drift of the metacarpophalangeal joint of the little finger. Note the slipping of the extensor tendon. She was unable to correct the deformity voluntarily and complained of difficulty in dressing, putting on gloves, and delving into her pockets and handbag. (b) Dorsal view, when fitted with the splint

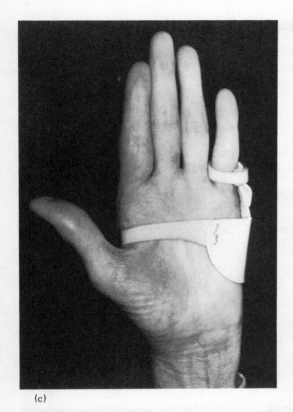

(c)

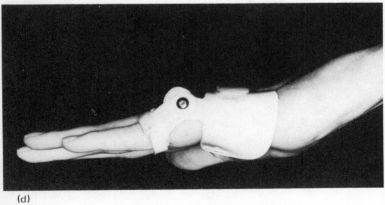

(d)

Figure 8.31 (cont.) — (c) Palmar view. (d) Ulnar view

Preventive ulnar drift splint

This was designed by Lawton (1974). The aim of this splint is to achieve permanent correction of ulnar drift. There is little hope of this if the splint is not prescribed early enough, and it is useful only if synovitis of the metacarpophalangeal joints is controlled by medication. If not, the splint should be discarded after a total trial of approximately nine months.

It is used in the very early stages of rheumatoid arthritis where there is prolific synovitis of the metacarpophalangeal joints and before the extensor tendons slip. The splint is usually worn for not more than

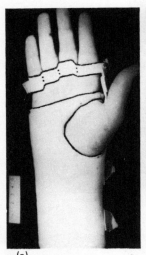

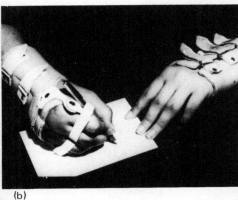

(b)

(a)

Figure 8.32. – Preventive ulnar drift splint. (a) Palmar view. (b) The splint used by a young male patient who has early signs of prolific synovitis of the metacarpophalangeal joints

six months, and all day during normal light activities except for two exercise sessions. It is used as an integral part of the treatment programme while the patient is receiving suitable medication, such as gold or penicillamine. The patient is expected to continue with all feeding, personal toilet, dressing, housework, shopping, writing and light leisure activities and to carry on with his or her normal occupation whenever generally fit enough.

The gauntlet is moulded in Vitrathene lined with Plastazote, and the base part of the hinge and the finger part are made in Darvic. The finger bar is worn on the palmar aspect of the fingers, and the hinge is constructed by the method described for the metacarpophalangeal ulnar drift splint (*see* page 308).

Non-hinged ulnar drift splints

There is a variety of similar designs based on those published by Quest and Cordery (1971) and by Malick (1975). These splints have been found useful at Farnham Park for patients who are unsuitable for hinged splints because of subluxation or severe loss of flexion at the

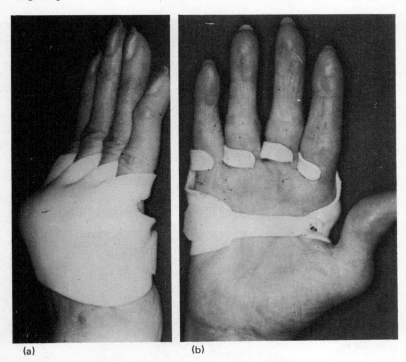

(a)   (b)

Figure 8.33. – Non-hinged ulnar drift splint. One variation of this type of splint which is used when there is subluxation and severe loss of mobility of the meta-carpophalangeal joints. (a) Ulnar view. (b) Palmar view

metacarpophalangeal joints. Patients find that they have improved function with a non-hinged splint (*Figure 8.33*), due to the stabilization and support provided at the metacarpophalangeal joints, and that pinch is improved.

A pattern is usually made by using children's plastic modelling putty, preferably of the non-toxic type such as Aloplast, rolled out thinly with a rolling pin. A temporary pad of 10 mm thick wadding or cotton wool is put over the dorsum of the metacarpophalangeal joints, and the splint is then moulded over this in Orthoplast, since accurate and varied contours are required. When the splint has set the pad is removed, leaving a space over the patient's joints which prevents painful pressure from the splint. A soft webbing strap with Velcro fastening is usually suitable, or the strap can be stretched from the splint material white it is warm (*see* page 276).

PADDLE SPLINTS

These splints (*Figure 8.34*) are used as a treatment in hand injuries, rheumatoid arthritis, flaccid or spastic paralysis, burns and peripheral nerve lesions. Their purpose is threefold:

1. To maintain the hand and wrist in the required position at night, at rest or during intervals between treatment periods.
2. To maintain, at night or at rest, the progress which has been gained during the day's treatment.
3. To increase joint range gradually, that is, as a serial splint.

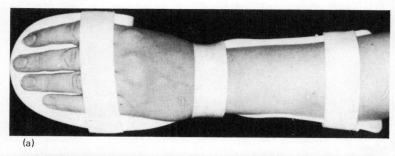

(a)

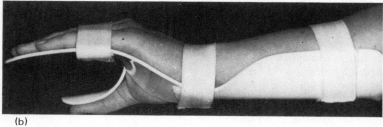

(b)

Figure 8.34. – Paddle splint, made from Darvic. (a) Dorsal view. (b) Ulnar view

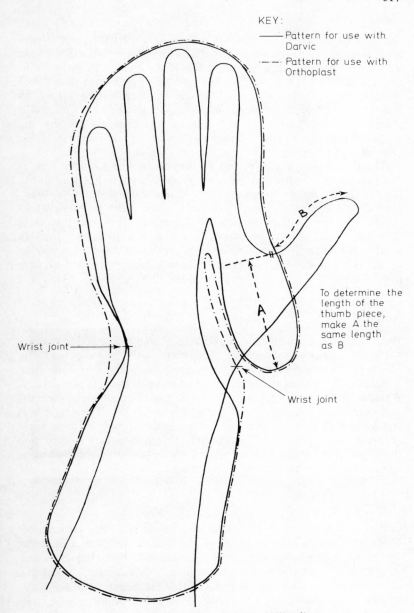

KEY:

———— Pattern for use with Darvic

·—·— Pattern for use with Orthoplast

B

To determine the length of the thumb piece, make A the same length as B

A

Wrist joint

Wrist joint

Figure 8.35. – Patterns for the paddle splint

Construction

The pattern (*Figure 8.35*) will vary a little in shape with the materials used, as suggested below under Materials. The splint should extend from a point two-thirds of the way up the inside of the forearm to about 5 mm beyond the tips of the fingers. The patient's finger nails should not protrude beyond the splint, as they may be injured if caught in the bed-clothes or knocked against furniture. As a general rule the hand is placed in a functional position but many variations are possible, depending upon the condition being treated and the preferences of the medical staff.

The thumb part, the palm and the finger areas are moulded first, as these require the most accurate positioning. When a satisfactory fit has been obtained, the wrist and forearm section is completed. The thumb part should be gutter-shaped, especially when there is paralysis, to prevent the thumb from slipping off the splint. This thumb section, however, should only apply anterior pressure, and should not forcibly press along either side of the thumb as this could cause deformity of the metacarpophalangeal and the interphalangeal joints. If thumb support is unnecessary it is often best to have no thumb piece at all.

Materials

Paddle splints are usually made in Darvic, 2.5 mm thick, as this provides sufficient rigidity to control the hand, particularly for the patient who has increased muscle tone or contractures. Occasionally a reinforcement is added over the wrist area of the splint when extra strength is necessary. When using Darvic, the pattern should be narrowed a little at the wrist and thumb-base to facilitate moulding (*Figure 8.35*). If less rigidity is required, Orthoplast or San-Splint, 3 mm thick, may be used but a generally wider pattern is then required to gain adequate rigidity, and the edges of the splint can be folded back for strength, or turned up as an edge round the hand for added comfort.

Strapping

Cotton webbing straps, 24 mm wide, with Velcro fastenings are suitable. Three straps are usually fitted, at mid-forearm, at the wrist and across the proximal phalanges, and may be padded with thin Plastazote. The wrist strap is most effective if placed directly over the wrist but, if this is not entirely comfortable, it can be fitted just proximal to the ulnar styloid. If the thumb has a tendency to slip off the splint, a small strap is used. A thumb-holder of elasticated fabric may be easier for the patient, so that fastening is eliminated.

Modifying the paddle splint for rheumatoid arthritis

Various adaptations to the paddle splint are made to suit rheumatoid patients (*Figure 8.36; see also* Lawton, 1974).

The wrist is held in 20 degrees of extension or as much extension as is comfortable for the patient. Where radial deviation is present, this is corrected within the patient's tolerance, usually by applying a strap

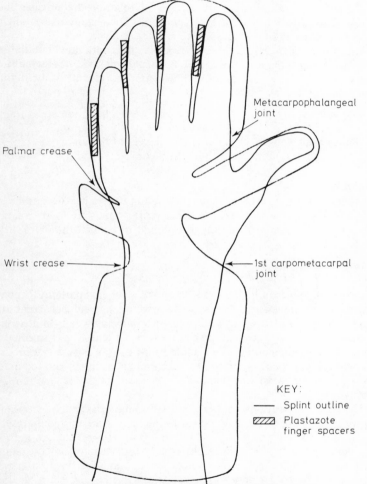

Metacarpophalangeal
joint

Palmar crease

Wrist crease

1st carpometacarpal
joint

KEY:
—— Splint outline
▨▨ Plastazote
finger spacers

Figure 8.36. — Pattern for a paddle splint for rheumatoid arthritis (By courtesy of the Canadian Red Cross Memorial Hospital, Taplow)

across the metacarpals and round the palm (excluding the thumb). This should not be forced, as the radial deviation is usually due to disease of the ulnar styloid and force may encourage subluxation.

Where possible, the metacarpophalangeal joints are held in about 20–30 degrees of flexion to discourage anterior subluxation. Where ulnar drift is present, this is held in a corrected or partially corrected position by forming a supporting lipped edge on the splint against the little finger and gluing small wedges of foam plastic between the fingers. The foam must be of the type that is firm enough to produce correction; thus, Plastazote is suitable.

The interphalangeal joints are held in the optimum functional position of slight flexion. The thumb is usually splinted but may be left free where no correction or support is required. It is held in the following position, if possible:

Carpometacarpal joint: Midway between abduction and adduction and in partial opposition.
Metacarpophalangeal joint: In a few degrees of flexion.
Interphalangeal joint: In slight flexion.

Strapping
To hold the wrist in the required amount of radial deviation, a metacarpal strap is necessary. If ulnar drift is present in the metacarpophalangeal joints, this strap is essential to control the deformity in addition to controlling the wrist.

Modifying the paddle splint for the spastic hand
Splinting, is, as yet, a highly debatable matter where spasticity is concerned. There are many schools of thought on this subject, some of which consider splinting to be absolutely contraindicated. In general, splinting is used at Farnham Park for those patients whose spasticity is found to be increasing. The paddle splint is used between sessions, and when the patient is resting or relaxing, to maintain the required position of the wrist and hand and to assist in the prevention of contracture.

The splint is positioned so as to put all joints in as much extension as possible. No undue force is applied to the hand since this could result in an overstrained position. Abduction of the fingers and thumb is considered important in splinting spasticity but we have not used this form of positioning for long enough to say whether the results are significantly better. A very simple splint as described by Hurd (1975) to abduct the fingers, made from 12 mm thick Plastazote, is sometimes used in conjunction with this type of paddle splint.

Modifying the paddle splint for individual finger control

A plain paddle splint will not suit every case, and a common problem is encountered with the patient who requires more individual positioning of each finger. To achieve very accurate control and correction a Farnham Park modular splint (*see* page 294) can be used but for many patients a split-finger paddle splint is adequate. This is merely an ordinary paddle splint which is divided between any or each of the fingers. Saw-cuts are made longitudinally in the splint between each finger, so that each strip of the plastic can be moulded individually.

WRIST EXTENSION SPLINT

This splint (*Figure 8.37*) is usually made in a rigid, hard-wearing material, that is, Darvic/Formasplint, so that it may be used to control the wrist in the required position (usually in extension and a little ulnar deviation) whilst the patient is working. Occasionally it is used as a night splint in preference to a paddle splint for patients who only require splinting of the wrist, as it allows all other joints to be left free.

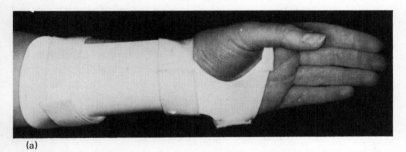

(a)

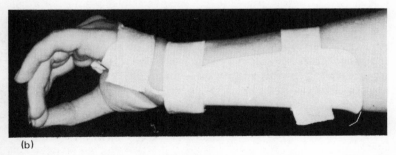

(b)

Figure 8.37. – Wrist extension splint, made from Darvic. (a) Palmar view. (b) Ulnar view

Indications for use

1. To maintain a functional position of the wrist where there is weakness or paralysis of the wrist extensors or ulnar deviators.
2. To assist in gradually increasing extension or ulnar deviation, that is, as a serial splint.
3. To provide stability in cases where the wrist joint requires protection and support, for example, in rheumatoid arthritis. It has also been found useful for carpal tunnel syndrome.

Design and materials

These are dependent upon the amount of support required. If the patient has reasonable hand function, the palmar area of the splint need only be small (*Figure 8.38*). It should be in such a position that it does not obstruct flexion at the metacarpophalangeal joints or opposition of the thumb. The less bulky the splint is the more acceptable it will be to the patient, as it will allow good grasp of implements in the palm and cover as little of the sensory area as possible.

When the patient requires greater support, for instance with paralysis or weakness, the splint can curve round the hypothenar eminence and have a strap round the back of the hand (*see Figure 8.37b*). Care should be taken to mould the splint in a concave curve, to maintain the shape of the metacarpal arch, or the palm may become flattened and cause loss of function of the hypothenar eminence. This supportive splint can be reshaped and remoulded in the palm as the patient gains in strength and control. It is important not to over-support or unnecessarily immobilize.

If the splint is to be made in Orthoplast instead of Darvic, the wrist area should be made much wider, and not waisted. The edges can be folded (*see* Materials, page 276), to provide greater rigidity, or a reinforcement strip of the same material can be added over the wrist. When considering such a reinforcement, it must be remembered that too much bulkiness or thickness on the anterior of the wrist may prevent the patient from being able to write correctly, as his hand is raised too far off the paper. This is especially true if the wrist is being held in considerable extension.

Construction

Great care is taken to place the splint in precisely the required position on the hand. It must not cover the transverse palmar crease or prevent full opposition of the thumb. One of the easiest ways to avoid mistakes

323

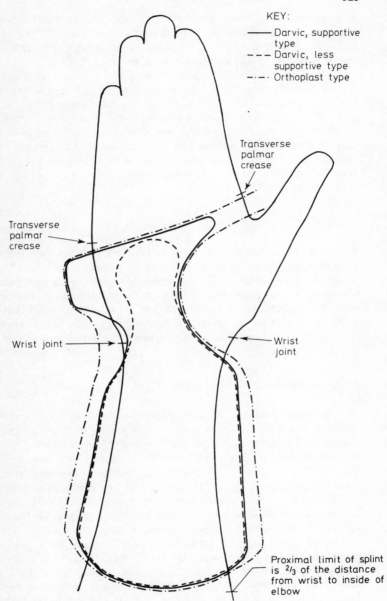

KEY:
—— Darvic, supportive type
– – – Darvic, less supportive type
–·–· Orthoplast type

Transverse palmar crease

Transverse palmar crease

Wrist joint

Wrist joint

Proximal limit of splint is ²/₃ of the distance from wrist to inside of elbow

Figure 8.38. – Patterns for the wrist extension splint

in positioning is to make a pair of small lines, in two places, across the border of the splint and continue them on to the patient's skin. This is best done just before heating the splint, then during moulding the lines can be matched up and accuracy will be assured.

The palmar area of the splint is heated and softened first, and then placed accurately on the hand and moulded so that it fits snugly into the palm, in a concave shape to fit the natural curve of the metacarpal arch. When the palmar area has set, the rest of the splint is heated and moulded over the wrist and forearm, checking that the wrist is in the desired amount of extension and ulnar deviation. The forearm part is smoothed against the patient to form a gutter shape, and the proximal edge is lipped outwards to prevent it from digging in, especially when the elbow is flexed.

Strapping

Cotton webbing, 24 mm wide, is suitable for straps unless the splint is to be worn long-term or during dirty or wet activities, when Corfam or synthetic leather would be preferable. The metacarpal strap is narrowed or rolled (*see Figure 8.15,* page 291) to make it comfortable against the skin-fold of the thumb web. It is usually attached to the palm of the splint by sewing. If Orthoplast or San-Splint is used, a self-strap can be formed and rolled when the material is moulded over the thumb web.

Modifying the wrist extension splint

The majority of patients are comfortable in an ordinary wrist extension splint but one man, with a severe crush injury affecting all the soft tissues of his wrist and palm, complained of great discomfort from excessive sweating. This was a result of the trauma and was so profuse that small perforations in the splint were insufficient to provide adequate ventilation. Since it was a Darvic splint it was strong enough to have 'windows' cut into it. Three large pieces were therefore removed by drilling and fretsawing, removing one triangular piece from the centre of the palm and two rectangular pieces from the forearm part. A border of about 10 mm of Darvic was left round the edges of the splint and the wrist area was also kept intact, so that the strength of the splint was only minimally reduced. The patient found this a great relief, not only because of the much increased ventilation but also because he could wipe the moisture from the exposed skin whenever he wished, without removing the splint.

OPPENHEIMER SPLINT (LIVELY EXTENSION SPLINT)

The design of this splint originates from Boyes (1970); and additional guidelines for construction can be found in Barr (1975). The Oppenheimer is a lively wire splint generally used for radial nerve palsy. It acts on the hand as a substitute for the paralysed extensor muscles, or to assist these muscles if they are weak, thus maintaining normal patterns of prehension.

Indications for use

The splint is worn for all functional activity but for night wear the patient may prefer a paddle splint. Two basic designs are used, depending on the distribution of paralysis:

1. For a severe radial nerve lesion in the early stages of treatment, where there is loss of extension of the wrist and also loss of extension of the thumb and of the metacarpophalangeal joints, the transverse bar is positioned over the proximal finger creases (*not* over the transverse palmar crease) and an outrigger is added to hold the thumb in extension (*Figure 8.39a*).

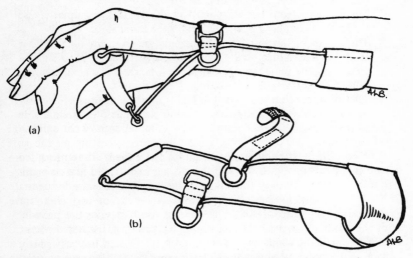

Figure 8.39. – Oppenheimer splint. (a) Showing the splint when used for a more severe radial palsy. The thumb is held in extension by an outrigger which is joined to the rest of the splint just distal to the point where the wire is crossed and coiled at the wrist joint. It is attached by winding with fine wire and then brazing. The transverse bar of the splint supports the fingers by lying across the proximal finger crease. (b) Showing the splint without the outrigger, for a patient who only requires assistance for extension of the wrist

2. For a less severe radial nerve lesion, or as a second stage in treatment when correction of wrist drop alone is required, the palmar bar of the splint must lie on the transverse palmar crease (*Figure 8.39b*).

It is essential to good treatment that the more supportive type of this splint, (1) above, should not be used when voluntary extension of the metacarpophalangeal joints and thumb have recovered. The wrist extension version, (2) above, is then sufficient.

Construction

A pattern can be made by outlining the hand on paper with the wrist in slight ulnar deviation. Careful measurements are taken of the following:

1. The distance from the wrist joint to the transverse palmar crease on the radial side. If the splint is to be used to provide extension of the metacarpophalangeal joints in addition to the wrist, then this measurement must be taken to the proximal finger creases (*not* to the transverse palmar crease).
2. The distance from the wrist joint to the transverse palmar crease (or to the proximal finger creases) on the ulnar side.
3. The length of the transverse palmar crease from the ulnar border to the radial border of the palm. Again, if the splint is to be used to extend the metacarpophalangeal joints, then this measurement must be taken across the proximal finger creases.
4. The distance from the wrist joint to a point two-thirds of the way up the radial side of the forearm, and the same on the ulnar side of the forearm. These determine the proximal limit of the splint.

This pattern must be carefully fitted on the patient whilst the hand is held in a functional position and the wrist is maintained in extension. Without practice, it is easy for this to be inaccurate and some therapists find the following method more simple. A length of soft wire, for example floristry wire or soldering wire, is used to take the pattern. With the hand and wrist held in a functional position, the wire is fitted to the hand in the same way as the final splint would be. It is gently bent into the required angles until it fits correctly, taking care that the patient's metacarpal arch is held in a slight curve. This pattern is then copied in spring wire to make the final splint. The coils at either side of the wrist joint can be most simply made by forming the wire round a piece of wood dowel, 12 mm in diameter. The cross of the wire should be made exactly at the wrist joint, on either side.

Where the wire lies across the palm or fingers it should be neatly covered with very thin, resilient padding, such as Velvotex or Formatex, for comfort. To improve the appearance of the splint, the whole of the wire can be covered with white plastic tubing, the wire being threaded through the tubing before it is bent into the desired shape.

The thumb outrigger may require a lighter gauge of wire than the rest of the splint. It is attached to the splint at the radial side of the wrist joint by binding it tightly on with fine wire. At the other end it is bent into a small loop to act as an attachment for the thumb cuff, which should encircle the proximal phalanx of the thumb. This is made by cutting a small strip of soft leather or Corfam, 60–80 mm long by 10–20 mm wide. The two ends are joined by a leatherwork eye, which is threaded on to the loop of the outrigger.

The arm cuff is made from a curved strip of aluminium sheet, or from a moulded piece of Darvic/Formasplint, 2.5 mm thick, folded and glued round the two free ends of the wire. Alternatively two layers of Vitrathene, 2.5 mm thick, can be used and the ends of the wire sandwiched between them.

The wrist strap must have only one loose end, or the patient will have difficulty in fastening it. The other end should be fitted closely to the splint to make it stable. Therefore, a cinch-type Velcro strap is the most suitable (*see Figure 8.16,* page 293). Alternatively a cuff or strap with no opening can be fitted to lie on the dorsum of the wrist. This is made in the same way as the more proximal cuff but is useful only if the patient is able to slide his hand into the splint.

Materials

Body of splint: Spring wire is used. This is sometimes called piano wire. The following gauges have been found suitable:

14 s.w.g. or 15 s.w.g. for men
16 s.w.g. to 18 s.w.g. for women
18 s.w.g. to 20 s.w.g. for children

Forearm cuff: Darvic/Formasplint 2.5 mm thick; or Vitrathene 2.5 mm thick; or aluminium sheet 1 mm to 1.5 mm thick.

Wrist strap: Cotton webbing 25 mm wide (1 in). For long-term use, Corfam or other synthetic leather is preferable.

Cosmetic covering for the wire: White plastic tubing as used for crafts, approximately 2.0 mm outside diameter.

ULNAR WRIST SUPPORT

This is taken from the design used at Moss Rehabilitation Hospital, Philadelphia.

Indications for use

1. To provide support and protection for the wrist in rheumatoid arthritis, in preference to a gauntlet splint which tends to be uncomfortably warm and may be difficult to put on and take off.
2. To correct or prevent radial deviation of the wrist where rheumatoid arthritis is affecting the ulnar styloid.

The splint (*Figure 8.40*) is worn for work, especially during heavier activities.

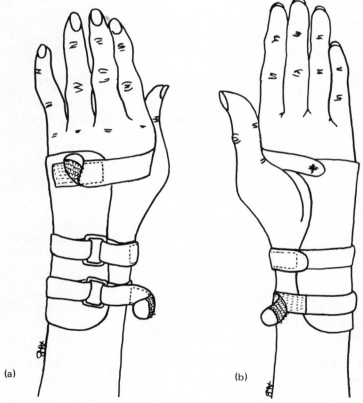

(a)

(b)

*Figure 8.40. – Ulnar wrist support, made from Orthoplast. (a) Dorsal view.
(b) Palmar view*

Construction

The splint is moulded round the ulnar side of the forearm and hand, extending from approximately 90 mm proximal to the wrist to the transverse palmar crease. The wrist should be in slight ulnar deviation if possible, without forcing the joint, and in approximately 20 degrees of extension. The splint should not obstruct flexion of the metacarpophalangeal joints or opposition of the thumb.

Materials

Orthoplast or San-Splint, 3 mm thick. The straps are made of cotton webbing or Corfam, with Velcro fastenings.

THUMB SPLINTS

The selection of splints given in this chapter includes a number which act upon the thumb to improve pinch. This is a vital aim at Farnham Park since most patients will require prehension in order to return to full independence. Choosing the correct splint at the appropriate stage of treatment is important. It should be supportive but not over-supportive, and must be altered or replaced as the patient improves.

The thumb stabilizer is one of the more supportive of this group of splints. It is chosen where there is gross weakness and instability in the thumb, or when contractures make it necessary to grip the thumb very firmly in a splint. It is often the wisest choice for a patient whose skin is frail, since pressure will be diminished by wider distribution than is possible with the rigid opponens splint.

The rigid opponens splint efficiently positions the thumb in opposition, while leaving the maximum area of palmar skin uncovered and so allowing good sensory function of the palm. Although the material used (Darvic) allows some movement, the splint is a largely immobilizing one. This is necessary for a patient whose muscles are too strong or whose joints are too contracted to be controlled by a softer splint.

The Chessington median nerve splint is suitable for a patient who has paralysis without contractures and who needs to build up power in the thumb. It has the great advantage of allowing voluntary extension and adduction of the thumb, and should be used in preference to the rigid opponens splint whenever the force it can provide is sufficient to bring the thumb into opposition.

The soft opponens splint is almost as immobilizing as more rigid splints, due to its enveloping construction. It is primarily used when a rigid material is found to be too hard for the patient's skin, either for comfort or to prevent breakdown when there is loss of sensation.

The Farnham Park median glove gives the most control of all the softer thumb splints, provided that it fits well. It is therefore used for more severely paralysed and contracted thumbs. It limits sensation, because it covers so much of the hand, but has the advantage of spreading pressure all round the hand. This makes it suitable for patients with frail skin, or where muscles are very atrophied. It provides more support than the soft opponens and is gentler on the skin than the thumb stabilizer.

RIGID OPPONENS SPLINT

Indications for use

1. Paralysis or weakness of abductor pollicis brevis.
2. Paralysis or weakness of opponens pollicis.
3. Correction of adduction of the thumb.
4. Correction of contractures.

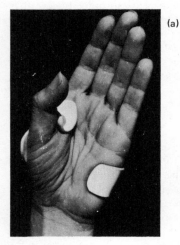

(a)

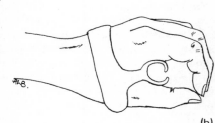

(b)

Figure 8.41. – Rigid opponens splint. (a) Palmar view. This splint leaves most of the palmar surface of the hand free for sensation and prehension, whilst achieving its prime aim of abduction and opposition of the thumb. (b) Radial view

This splint (*Figure 8.41*) has been found useful for selected patients with the following conditions:

Partial paralysis and/or weakness of the hand following a cerebrovascular accident.
Residual paralysis following a brachial plexus lesion.
Median nerve lesion.
After surgery affecting opponens pollicis.

This splint is not used on any patient for whom a less rigid splint would suffice. It is replaced by a less rigid type of splint, such as the Chessington median nerve splint or the soft opponens splint, as the patient's voluntary control of pinch action improves, thus achieving the correct grading of treatment.

Materials

Darvic/Formasplint, 2.5 mm thick, or any rigid material which can be moulded accurately, is used. It must be sufficiently rigid to control the position of the thumb.

Orthoplast is not suitable for this shape of pattern as it is insufficiently rigid. It would be effective, however, if made in a wider and more enveloping shape, similar to the thumb stabilizer (*see Figure 8.47*, page 337).

Construction

This can be a deceptively difficult splint to make since it has to be accurately moulded to the interesting but complex contours present when the hand is held in the pinch position. An accurate fit is essential for comfort and for the effective use of the splint. Success is dependent on both careful pattern-making and skilful moulding.

Pattern-making

The easiest and most accurate method is to cut three strips of paper to approximately the same shape as those shown in *Figure 8.42*, making them a little longer or shorter, roughly to suit the size of the patient. Then, holding the patient's hand in pinch, ensure that the wrist is in 20–30 degrees of extension and that the metacarpal arch is well curved. The three strips of paper are stuck on to the patient, using tiny dabs of Copydex latex adhesive, in the following way.

The metacarpal strip (*see* strip (1) *Figure 8.42*) is positioned from the centre of the 1st metacarpal, closely over the dorsum of the hand and round the hypothenar eminence, to tuck into the palm just proximal to the transverse palmar crease and well clear of the thenar eminence. The strip must lie over the centre of the 1st metacarpal and not over the 1st metacarpophalangeal joint. It is allowed to protrude a little at the thumb end to provide extra support and to allow for final trimming of the finished splint.

The C-bar strip (*see* strip (2) on the diagram) is stuck on next. It should lie along the thumb web and extend from the middle of the proximal phalanx of the thumb to the middle of the proximal phalanx of the index finger. The strip should be long enough to curl inwards a

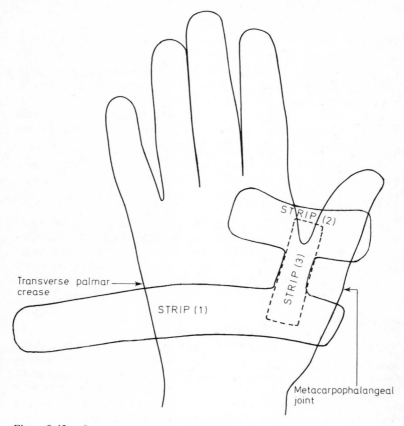

Transverse palmar crease

STRIP (1)

STRIP (2)

STRIP (3)

Metacarpophalangeal joint

Figure 8.42. – Pattern for the rigid opponens splint. The pattern is constructed on the patient's hand by joining the three strips of paper at the correct angles

little at either end, and it must not be so wide that it protrudes into the palm, as this will prevent grasp of objects which should be held in the palmar space.

The neck strip (*see* strip (3) on the diagram) is then stuck on to join the C-bar and the metacarpal piece. It should be placed on the middle of the thumb web and lie at a right angle to the metacarpal piece. It is essential that it is narrow. If not, it will prevent the C-bar from being moulded to a sufficiently deep curve.

When the adhesive has set, the final outline of the pattern is marked on the paper, which is neatened and trimmed, peeled off the patient's skin and transferred to the splint material.

Before moulding is begun, the C-bar on the splint material should be checked, to ensure that the angles where the C-bar joins have been cut sufficiently acutely. If they are too rounded they will pull the C-bar out of shape as it is moulded.

Moulding

Moulding is done in the following sequence.

The patient's hand is again held in the pinch position, with the wrist in extension. The C-bar and the neck area are heated and softened first; the rest of the splint is left cool at this stage. The C-bar is pinched at either end and moulded firmly down into the thumb web. The ends themselves are curled inwards to prevent them digging in and to allow for widening if the patient's abduction is to be increased at a later stage. Holding the C-bar firmly in place, the neck is bent at a right angle to the C-bar.

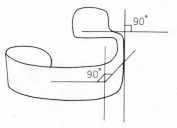

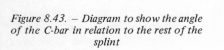

Figure 8.43. – Diagram to show the angle of the C-bar in relation to the rest of the splint

When this has set, the metacarpal part is heated until it is very pliable. The C-bar is fitted back into the thumb web and the metacarpal bar is moulded. Its thenar area is first moulded flat against the thumb metacarpal. Then, holding this area down with one hand, the therapist draws the rest of the metacarpal bar firmly over the dorsum of the hand and round the hypothenar eminence, where it is squeezed into a curve proximal to the transverse palmar crease. It is important to note that the splint should not be pressed down with the fingers over the bony dorsum of the 2nd, 3rd and 4th metacarpals. This would make it uncomfortable, as it would apply too much pressure and the therapist's fingers would form irregularities in the moulding. A firm but gentle pulling action must be used. The splint should only apply pressure over the 1st metacarpal and round the fleshy hypothenar eminence. Correct angulation of the splint (*Figures 8.43* and *8.44*) must be very carefully observed throughout the moulding.

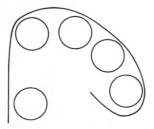

Figure 8.44. – Diagram of a sagittal section of the metacarpals to show the angulation of the splint which is required to allow good pinch

Finally, the therapist must check that the patient has full flexion of the ring and little fingers, that the splint is not blocking this movement and that functional pinch is correct and comfortable.

Modification to the rigid opponens splint

An unusual application of the rigid opponens splint was for a typist suffering from rheumatoid arthritis. Her problem was pain in the metacarpophalangeal joints of both thumbs and, at the time that she asked for help, she was about to give up her secretarial job, feeling that she could no longer tolerate the discomfort when typing and writing. Bilateral opponens splints were made for her from Darvic. They were cut rather narrower than usual as she did not require very strong support. The C-bar was flattened a little so that abduction of the thumb was not forced; in addition to this the thumb was further stabilized by a narrow strut of Darvic which curled from the C-bar round the palmar and radial aspects of the proximal phalanx of the thumb. Thus the metacarpophalangeal joint was held in extension below by the metacarpal bar of the splint and above by the strut to prevent anteroposterior movement. The C-bar and the strut prevented lateral movements. This almost complete immobilization relieved the pain, and the shape of the splint allowed the patient to continue typing and writing.

SOFT OPPONENS SPLINT

Indications for use

1. For a median nerve lesion where there is already some recovery of abduction of the thumb.
2. For traumatic or neurological conditions affecting opposition of the thumb, for example, following a cerebrovascular accident, it may be useful in assisting with hand function in writing.

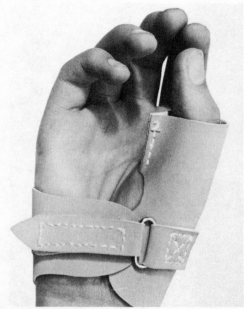

Figure 8.45. – Soft opponens splint. Made in Corfam or synthetic leather, with a cinch-type strap which adjusts to draw the thumb into the required amount of pinch

3. In preference to a more supportive type of splint in cases where the patient's skin condition or scars will tolerate only a softer splinting material.
4. For patients with contractures following paralysis, it holds the thumb in opposition but it is only suitable for those who have some abduction of the thumb.

For patients with strong contractures or very strong voluntary extension of the thumb, a rigid opponens or a thumb stabilizer splint will be necessary (*see* pages 330–334 and 336–339).

Construction

A paper pattern (*Figure 8.46*) is made and fitted to the patient with the hand held in pinch. The splint material is cut out and a seam made on the ulnar border of the thumb, taking care that it is not too tight.

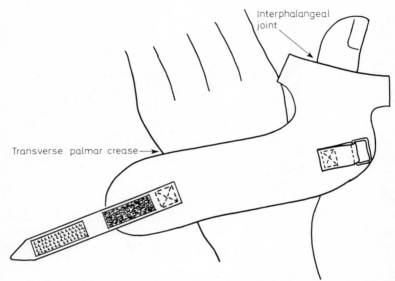

Figure 8.46. – Pattern for the soft opponens splint with Velcro fastening

A cinch-type strap is attached. This allows the thumb to be drawn fairly strongly into opposition and for adjustment to be made easily.

Materials

Corfam, synthetic leather or leather (if not required for wet or messy activities), with Velcro fastenings.

THUMB STABILIZER

This splint may be constructed in two ways: either around the palm of the hand (*Figure 8.47a* and *b*) or around the dorsum (*Figure 8.47c*).

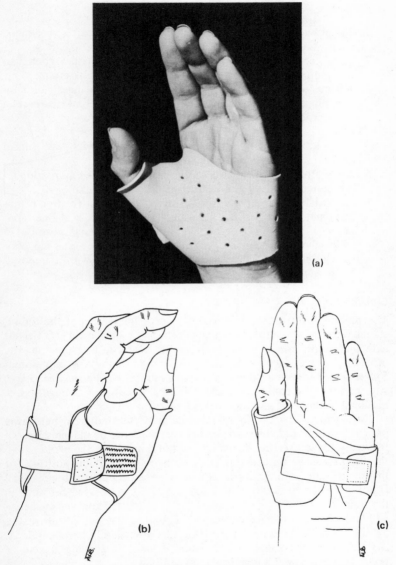

Figure 8.47. – Thumb stabilizer, made in Orthoplast or San-Splint. (a) This version is moulded to the palm. (b) Dorsal view of (a) to show the webbing and Velcro fastening, and method of moulding the splint over the thumb web. (c) Alternative version, moulded to the dorsum of the hand

Indications for use

1. To provide stability of the thumb where there is weakness, paralysis or pain.
2. To protect the carpometacarpal joint and/or the metacarpophalangeal joint where there is osteoarthritis or ligamentous strain.
3. To encourage active movement of the interphalangeal joint by blocking the compensatory movements of the carpometacarpal and metacarpophalangeal joints, for example, after repair of the flexor pollicis longus tendon or following pollicization.
4. To hold the thumb joints in a position which is less painful during function, for example, in osteoarthritis.
5. As an alternative to the rigid opponens splint when more support is required, or to avoid pressure on certain skin areas.
6. As a trial before surgery. This is useful if surgical fixation of the carpometacarpal or metacarpophalangeal joint is being considered, firstly to determine a suitable functional position in which the thumb should be surgically immobilized, and secondly to demonstrate to the patient what limitations will be imposed by the surgery.

Construction

The preliminary pattern (*Figure 8.48*) for a splint such as the thumb stabilizer, which has to fit so many contours of the hand, is difficult and inaccurate when made with paper. Instead, children's plastic modelling putty, such as Aloplast, rolled fairly thinly, or aluminium foil is wrapped round the hand and trimmed to the desired shape. Alternatively the splint material itself can be cut into a rough shape, moulded to the hand and then trimmed.

During moulding the splint material is stretched firmly round the patient's thumb and then wrapped round the back of the hand. A join is usually made over the dorsal area of the thumb web. To avoid a join, the thumb can be pushed through a hole cut in a suitable position but this may result in difficulty in obtaining an accurate fit if the material is not stretched carefully. Care must also be taken to avoid constricting the thumb.

Flexion at the metacarpophalangeal joints must not be obstructed by the splint in the palm, the metacarpal arch should be maintained, and the splint must end just proximal to the interphalangeal joint of the thumb to allow full mobility and good pinch.

Materials

Orthoplast or San-Splint, 3 mm thick.

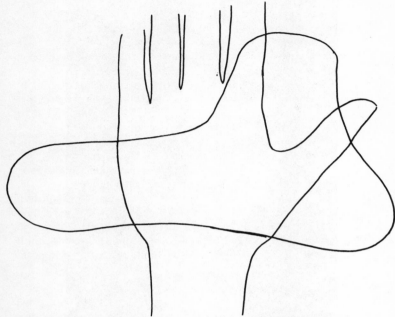

Figure 8.48. – Preliminary rough pattern for a thumb stabilizer

CHESSINGTON MEDIAN NERVE SPLINT

This splint is fully described by Wynn Parry (1973) and Barr (1975).
We have constructed the splint (*Figure 8.49*), however, in different
materials from those described. The wrist cuff is moulded in Orthoplast;
this prevents the tendency of the cuff to swivel round the wrist. The
thumb strap is constructed of wet-suit rubber (obtainable from water-
sports dealers). This has a high degree of cling and, therefore, grips well
round the thumb *metacarpal*, which is essential to obtain the rotational
movement necessary for correct opposition.

Indications for use

    1. Median nerve lesion.
    2. Paralysis of the thenar eminence occurring in hemiplegia.
    3. Post-operatively, for opponens transplant.

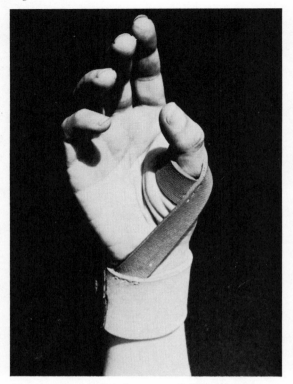

Figure 8.49. – Chessington median nerve splint. To achieve true opposition, it is important that the loop sits well down round the thumb metacarpal

The splint is only suitable for patients who have reasonable passive abduction of the thumb. If this is not present, another type of opponens splint may be more suitable (*see* page 329).

FARNHAM PARK MEDIAN GLOVE

This splint (*Figure 8.50*) was designed and described by Jones (1952).

Indications for use

This is used to obtain good pinch and function in a median nerve lesion which cannot be controlled satisfactorily by either the rigid opponens

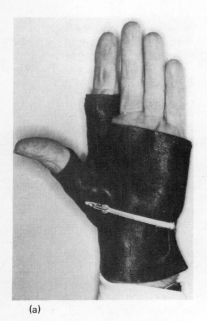

(a)

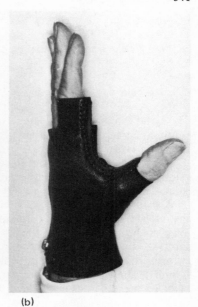

(b)

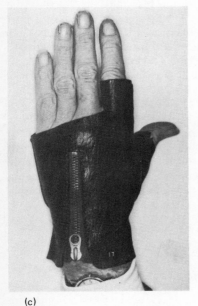

(c)

Figure 8.50. – Farnham Park median glove, made from leather. (a) The elastic is hooked to an eye sewn to the thumb of the glove. This draws the patient's thumb into opposition. (b) Abduction is achieved by a spring stiffener fitted along the thumb web. (c) A strong zip is let into the dorsum of the glove

or the soft opponens splint. It is, therefore, used only on a very strong or contracted hand. A less supportive splint should be substituted as recovery takes place, for example, the Chessington median nerve splint.

Construction

The splint can be made in leather, using a glove pattern, but it is simpler to purchase an ordinary leather glove which fits the patient firmly, and then adapt it.

The middle, ring and little fingers of the glove should be completely removed, and the index finger cut off at the proximal interphalangeal joint. The thumb should be cut off at the interphalangeal joint.

A strip of leather, approximately 10 mm to 15 mm wide, is sewn on the outside of the glove and extending from the proximal interphalangeal joint of the index finger to the interphalangeal joint of the thumb. This forms the pocket for a strip of spring steel or strong plastic, for example, corsetry boning, which will provide abduction of the thumb. The thumb is drawn into opposition by a strong piece of elastic. This is sewn to the ulnar seam of the glove, approximately midway between the wrist joint and the transverse palmar crease. At its free end, a strong dressmaker's hook is sewn. An eye for this is sewn to the thumb of the glove, just proximal to the metacarpophalangeal joint.

The glove should fit closely round the wrist to provide a stable fixing for the elastic. A strong zip is let into the dorsum of the glove to make this possible, and to allow the patient to put it on more easily.

THUMB WEB SPREADER

This is a very simple little splint (*Figure 8.51*) which can easily be altered when required as a serial splint. Provided the strap is fastened firmly, the splint will sit snugly into the thumb web and thus apply leverage to the thumb metacarpal without putting unwanted force on the proximal phalanx, which could cause deformity at the metacarpophalangeal joint of the thumb.

Indications for use

1. To increase the web space of the thumb.
2. To prevent or correct contracture of the thumb web caused by scarring, paralysis or prolonged immobilization.

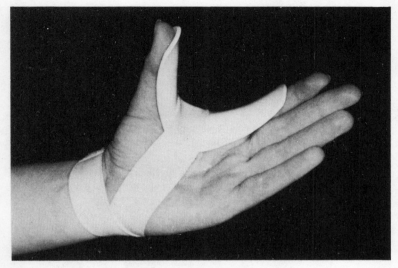

Figure 8.51. – Thumb web spreader

The splint may be worn at night and between treatments, and should be altered as often as necessary to hold the thumb in maximum extension.

Design and construction

It has been found best to draw the shape of the splint directly on the patient's skin. A pattern can then be traced on to flimsy paper held on to the skin. The splint should be wide enough to be gutter-shaped, and should extend from the tip of the thumb to the proximal inter-phalangeal joint of the index finger. It should not hyperextend the 2nd metacarpophalangeal joint. The splint is moulded directly on the patient's hand.

Materials

Darvic/Formasplint, or any rigid material which can easily be altered to provide increase in the thumb web space, is used.

For the straps, white cotton webbing is used with a cinch-type Velcro fastening (*see Figure 8.16,* page 293). It is wound in a figure-of-eight round the hand and wrist. This form of strapping holds the splint well down into the thumb web.

FINGER BANDS

These are very simple little splints, which are used, wherever possible, in preference to finger stalls which always inhibit sensation and therefore discourage good function.

Indications for use

Finger bands can control two or three fingers at a time. They have not been found suitable for use on the little finger, due to the difference in alignment with the other finger joints. The three-finger model can

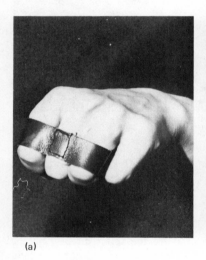

(a)

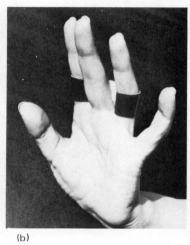

(b)

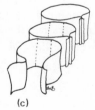

(c)

Figure 8.52. – Finger bands. (a) and (b) Finger band designed to provide flexion of the middle finger. Made of leather with a thin pad of white wool felt where pressure is applied. (c) Diagram to show sewing method for a treble finger band. A double row of stitching is made between each finger for maximum firmness. The closure seams are worn on the dorsum of the fingers

have the middle finger only half-enclosed, either on the dorsum or the palm. Thus flexion or extension can be assisted by the other two fingers or allowed to be voluntary (*Figure 8.52*).

A finger band may be used in the treatment of stiffness of a metacarpophalangeal or a proximal interphalangeal joint, and may also be suitable where there is weakness of one finger, especially if a patient is habitually holding that finger out of the way, for example, following amputation of the finger-tip.

Construction and materials

Finger bands can be made from firm, thin leather or from a synthetic leather if they are to be used for wet or messy activities.

A pattern is made using narrow strips of paper. The splint material is sewn in two places between the fingers to achieve the closest proximity possible (*Figure 8.52c*). If only one line of sewing is used, the splint will have less control. If the fingers are not swollen or painful, the finger band can be put on without a fastening but a Velcro opening may be necessary in other cases. Where a finger is half-enclosed by the splint, a little thin padding may be added.

DRIVING SPLINT FOR A QUADRIPLEGIC

This splint was designed for two purposes: firstly to attach the two Terry clips firmly to the patient's hand, to give him good control when using them to hold on to the Roehampton ball fitted to his steering wheel; secondly to control the flexion of his thumb and fingers which otherwise became caught in the spring clips (*Figure 8.53*).

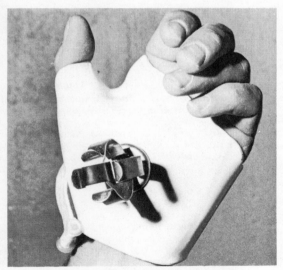

Figure 8.53. – Driving splint for a quadriplegic

Materials

Orthoplast was used to achieve a close fit and to allow the palm to be moulded outwards to provide the correct angulation of the spring clips. A self-hinge was incorporated in the dorsum of the splint to facilitate getting it on and off, and a large plastic rivet was sewn into the free end of the cotton webbing, since the patient used his teeth for fastening and required a hold.

Note: The Roehampton ball was supplied and fitted by an Artificial Limb and Appliance Centre. The two Terry clips, washer and bolt were the inspiration of the patient's father, and can all be obtained from a good ironmonger.

REFERENCES

Ansell, B. M., Williams, J. G. P., Cheshire, L., Lawton, S. and Haines, R. E. (1972). 'Farnham Park modular splint system.' *Rheum. phys. Med.* 11, No. 7, 334

Barr, N. R. (1975). *The Hand. Principles and Techniques of Simple Splint Making in Rehabilitation.* London; Butterworths

Boyes, J. H. (1970). *Bunnell's Surgery of the Hand.* 5th Edition. Philadelphia and Toronto; Lippincott

Hurd, S. (1975). 'Trends in treatment methods and media.' *Br. J. occup. Ther.* 4, 81

James, J. I. P. (1970). 'The assessment and management of the injured hand.' *The Hand.* 2, 97

Jones, M. S. (1952). 'Mechanical aids to treatment.' *Br. J. phys. Med.* p. 115

Larson, D. L. (1973). 'The prevention and correction of burn scar contracture and hypertrophy.' Galveston, Texas; Shriners Burns Institute

Lawton, D. S. (1974). 'Hand splinting in rheumatoid arthritis.' *Occup. Ther.* 12, 219

Malick, M. H. (1974). *Manual on Dynamic Hand Splinting with Thermoplastic Materials.* Pittsburgh, Pennsylvania; Harmarville Rehabilitation Centre

Malick, M. H. (1975). 'Management of the severely burned patient.' *Br. J. Occup. Ther.* 4, 76

Quest, D. and Cordery, J. (1971). 'A functional ulnar deviation cuff for the rheumatoid deformity.' *Am. J. Occup. Ther.* 9, 2

Wynn Parry, C. B. (1973). *Rehabilitation of the Hand,* p. 99. 3rd Edition. London; Butterworths

FURTHER READING

Caldwell, H. (1970). *Progressive Splinting Manual Utilising the Master Template Method.* New Brunswick, New Jersey; Johnson and Johnson

Cheshire, L. (1974). 'Splinting for metacarpophalangeal ulnar drift.' Proceedings of the Sixth International Congress of the World Federation of Occupational Therapists, p. 517. Vancouver

Gilewich, G., Jimenez, J. and Redford, J. B. (1969). *Simple Splints, Principles and Techniques.* Toronto; Mount Sinai Hospital

Houchin, R. and Cheshire, L. (1971). 'Splintage for ulnar deviation.' *Occup. Ther.* **10, 9.** (also reprinted in Swedish (1974) 'Skenor vid ulnardeviation.' *Arbetsterapeuten.* Göteborg, Sweden. No. 9, 569)

Kennedy, J. M. (1974). *Orthopaedic Splints and Appliances.* London; Baillière, Tindall and Cassell

Licht, S. (1966). *Orthotics Etcetera.* Baltimore, Maryland; Waverly Press

Malick, M. H. (1972). *A Manual on Static Hand Splinting.* Pittsburgh, Pennsylvania; Harmarville Rehabilitation Centre

Napier, J. (1956). 'Prehensile movements of the human hand.' *J. Bone Jt Surg.* **38B,** 902

Napier, J. (1968). 'Evolution of the human hand.' *Proc. R. Soc. Med.* **40, 54**

New York University Medical Centre (1971). *Upper Extremity Orthoses.* New York; Institute of Rehabilitation Medicine

Shah, S. K. (1974). 'Upper extremity orthotic systems.' *Br. J. occup. Ther.* **11,** 193

Smith, M. M. (1972). 'Prenyl handsplinting with congenital abnormalities.' *Occup. Ther.* **12,** 941

Willis, B. M. *Splinting the Burn Patient.* New Brunswick, New Jersey; Johnson and Johnson

Willis, B. M. (1969). 'The use of Orthoplast Isoprene splints in the treatment of the acutely burned child: preliminary report.' *Am. J. occup. Ther.* **4,** 3. Reprinted in *Occup. Ther.* **11,** 31

FILMS

Plastazote 16 mm instructional film in colour with sound. Duration: 16 minutes. Available from:

> Technical Information Department,
> Smith and Nephew Ltd,
> Bessemer Road,
> Welwyn Garden City,
> Hertfordshire.

Hand-Splinting – A New Method 16 mm instructional film on Darvic in colour with sound. Duration: 20 minutes. Available from:

> Occupational Therapy Department,
> Farnham Park Rehabilitation Centre,
> Farnham Royal,
> Slough,
> Buckinghamshire.

Films on *Orthoplast* and on *San-Splint,* both made in North America, are also available from the suppliers, but these films are not entirely relevant to hand-splinting.

9

Treatment of Upper and Lower Limb Amputees

The Department of Health and Social Security has set up regional units for treating amputees and for fitting their prostheses. This is specialized work and although occupational therapists can be trained in the techniques of re-education, unless they are treating such patients regularly they will not develop adequate skill to teach patients to make maximum use of an upper limb prosthesis, and they will certainly not be competent to supervise a patient with bilateral upper limb prostheses.

In the past Farnham Park has offered a good range of treatment for post-amputees who were not yet fitted with a permanent prosthesis. There are often considerable delays, however, in the production, fitting and alterations of prostheses. This waiting period not only depresses patients but gives rise to further problems. Stumps can change shape between one fitting and the next.

For both these reasons it is therefore better that amputees should be treated in the specialized units where all the necessary facilities are available and much closer supervision of the patients' progress is possible. However, since such referral is not always feasible, for example for social reasons, techniques of treatment which have been used at Farnham Park and proved valuable are detailed here.

An amputation may occur in trauma or in the surgical treatment of physical disorders which render a part of the body a menace to the existence of the whole. In occupational therapy the aims of treatment include the preparation of the patient for the acceptance and use of a prosthesis. When such an appliance cannot be devised or fitted, the alternative aim is to accustom the patient to make do without the limb or the part of the limb he has lost.

Amputation is a dramatic and tragic incident in the life of anyone. In the early days some of the tragedy is submerged by the stimulation of the sense of drama. It has been noticed that patients who come for rehabilitation soon after amputation are more eager to surmount their difficulties than those who have passed the crest of the wave of drama and plunged into the trough where lies despair.

LOWER LIMB AMPUTEES

Patients with amputations of the lower limb have been of both sexes and widely distributed in age-groups. Neither of these factors has much influenced their treatment in occupational therapy, though the physical build has been of importance in affecting their capacity for general mobility. Those patients with histories of circulatory dysfunction or infective bone disease have shown signs of being accustomed to move about as little as possible, and have been slow to get their balance either on crutches or sitting at work. Nearly all have been middle-aged. The patients with histories of trauma or neoplasm have been various in age. Not only the young show a ready reaction to suggestions for activity. If the suddenness of the catastrophe has interrupted a normal life, the return to such activity is a lively source of hope and stimulus to recovery.

Treatment before a pylon or prosthesis has been supplied

In the early days of occupational therapy amputees of the lower limb could only work seated in a chair at a bench. It was soon found that saddle-stitching in leatherwork entailed contractions of the adductors of the thighs to hold the saddler's clamps steady. A saddler's clamp looks like a gigantic tweezer made from two barrel staves joined together at one end, with sufficient spring in the wood to open the 'jaws' at the other end and insert the leather article to be stitched. By holding the clamps between the knees, the leather is held firmly in place. This is one of the few ways of using static adduction of the hips in occupational therapy. At a later stage woodwork or metalwork was carried out with the patient sitting astride a bicycle stool at a high bench. These activities encouraged development, not only of the adductors, but of all hip and spinal muscles, especially the glutei, to maintain balance and controlled movement. It is particularly important to exercise the glutei in order to avoid getting flexion contracture of the hip. Patients tend to walk with the hip slightly flexed before a prosthesis is fitted, and such contractions can be difficult to correct. These types of work have been continued regularly, but since we developed the temporary working prosthesis, the medical officer can give directions for aims of treatment which directly include development of the muscles of the stump.

Temporary working prostheses for above- and below-knee amputees

Two pieces of apparatus (*Figures 9.1, 9.2* and *9.3*) have been evolved in the occupational therapy workshops at Farnham Park Rehabilitation Centre (Jones, 1952). These enable patients to work on the bicycle saw, foot-power rug loom, or foot-power treadle lathe using the stump of the leg after either an above-knee or below-knee amputation.

A bucket made from firm leather or a suitable synthetic material is made to fit either an above- or below-knee stump. It is split at the back and front to allow for ease of fitting and for adjustment to different sizes of legs. It can be either firmly laced up through eyelets or secured with a Velcro cinch-type fastening (*see* page 293). The bucket is lined with thick felt or Plastazote. For an above-knee stump the bucket may need to be fixed by straps and buckles to a belt round the waist because with a very short stump it may slide forward off the leg. Extra padding on the inner side, as in *Figure 9.3,* may also be necessary. The bucket must fit closely and not slip or rub when worn over the bandaged stump. The bucket is open at the lower end, so there is no risk of pressure on the end of the stump, and two flat pockets are attached, to take the side shafts of the pylon. The bucket is fitted on the stump and the patient can then come on crutches to the bicycle saw, loom or lathe and, sitting on the seat arranged, can slip the shafts of the pylon into the pockets. The lower plate of the pylon should already be screwed up on the pedal of the apparatus on which the patient is to work. With a below-knee pylon it is necessary to have a hinge mechanism at the 'ankle joint' in order to adapt to the changing angle of the foot-plate of the lathe. Otherwise the patient must move the leg forwards and backwards in a compensatory movement. When the pylon is used on a bicycle the pedal remains horizontal and it is therefore immaterial whether there is an 'ankle joint' or not.

It has been found that the actual movement of working the bicycle saw, loom or lathe has been easy, and quickly acquired. In the case of a woman patient who had an above-knee amputation, however, the first reaction was unexpected and very distressing; the phantom pains became exaggerated, so much so that in the early days of experiment the period of treatment had to be limited to a very few minutes. It is suggested that the pattern of movement of bicycling, even though this patient had not been a habitual cyclist, is so closely associated with

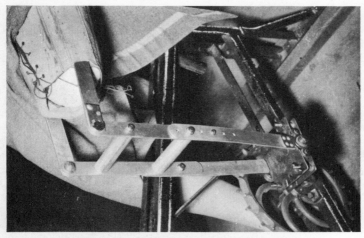

Figure 9.3. – Farnham Park working prosthesis and bucket for above-knee amputee, shown in use on bicycle fretsaw

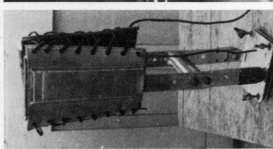

Figure 9.2. – Detail of below-knee working prosthesis

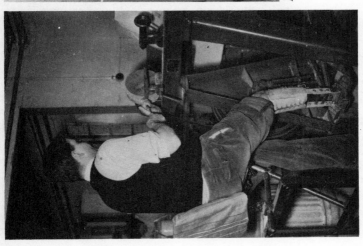

Figure 9.1. – Farnham Park below-knee working prosthesis on the lathe

pressure on the sole of the foot that this is enough to stimulate the nerves of the stump. This woman said that the phantom foot was vividly present and strongly and painfully contorted, but being a woman of sense and courage, she carried on and, as hoped, within a few days the phantom pains began to decrease. Then resistance to the movement was given in the form of sawing plywood. The added interest of following the pattern to make up a wooden toy helped to distract her attention from the phantom pains, and by the end of a fortnight she was able to work for 30 minutes without inconvenience. Later on the patient worked on a foot-power lathe, sanding and polishing a small wooden bowl, which another patient had turned for her.

Another patient, a man who had a below-knee amputation, had no trouble with phantom pains, and he worked on the foot-power lathe and rug loom with considerable force and enthusiasm.

It is obvious that the work which these patients were able to do using their stumps added considerably to the interest of their daily occupational therapy, and the exercise to the hip extensors and the quadriceps was of value. They were both interested also in leather work, and did saddle-stitching, holding their work in saddler's clamps, so that the adductors of the thigh had a share of exercise. In both these cases it was noted that the stumps quickly became firm and well muscled.

It may be of interest to add some details about the manufacture of these working pylons, which was largely carried out by other patients as part of their treatment. For example, a patient, a toolmaker, who had a fractured tibia and fibula, and fractured 5th carpometacarpal joint on the left hand, made joints for the 'knee' and 'ankle' of the pylons. He was not interested in making anything for himself, nor indeed in anything but his own troubles, until the problem of this joint was put to him to solve. After this, he became really interested and co-operative. Much of the filing, sawing and drilling for shaping the bottom plates and shafts of the pylons was done by another patient, who had started an apprenticeship in electrical engineering which was interrupted by an operation for coarctation of the aorta. At first, he was obviously nervous of making any exertion, but the interest in the work encouraged him to make the effort, and shaping up, first $^3/_{16}$ inch duralumin and then mild steel plate, provided the work of gradually increasing physical strain ordered in his treatment.

Much has been made of the patients' part in carrying out these ideas and in designing the details which have made them successful. This has been done not only in fairness and gratitude for their help, but to emphasize the fact that work of this nature should always be available in an occupational therapy workshop, to engage the interest of the skilled patient.

It should be noted that Doris Sym, when working at the Astley Ainslie Hospital in Edinburgh, produced an adaptation of the Farnham Park model made from a wooden axillary crutch instead of metal, and found this satisfactory. The below-knee pylon made in wood has been found as effective as when made in metal, though the 'knee-joint' of the above-knee working pylon has been found less smooth in action when made in wood.

These working pylons have been modified for the use of patients with Syme's amputation of the foot. These patients learnt wood-turning using a working pylon altered for their use by hoops to separate the sides instead of spacing bars. When the surgeon wished the patient to begin weight-bearing a block of wood with a sorbo-rubber pad was inserted under the stump, and he began graduated weight-bearing by treadling the foot-power lathe sitting. Weight-bearing on the stump increased when the patient treadled the lathe standing on the good leg.

Precautions

Patients cannot be allowed to use the working pylons until the operation scars are soundly healed. Though there is no danger of pressure on the tip of the stump, the bucket must grip the leg round the tibial condyles and there is inevitably some stretching of the skin and fascia over the end of the bone. When the scar is healed, this stretching will be of value in preventing adhesions between the layers of skin and fascia around the muscles of the stump.

Further precautions have been observed when the patient has had an amputation as a result of circulatory dysfunction. For some with below-knee amputations we have used an above-knee working pylon so that there was no danger of the bucket pressing on arteries or veins in a vulnerable area. To make it possible to use the above-knee working pylon for these patients the spacing bars were replaced by hoops of metal which were padded inside with rubber. Many of the patients with above-knee or below-knee amputations for circulatory dysfunction could not use a working pylon as the stump was too short. In all such cases, above or below knee, the patient has only been allowed to continue work with the good leg for a short time and under close observation. The appearance of muscular spasm which might possibly be due to poor circulation has brought the session of work to a close until its occurrence can be reported to the medical officer in charge. Often this type of treatment has been discontinued when there is any danger that the exertion might throw too heavy a load on a circulation which is already impaired.

Working in a pylon or prosthesis

When patients with either a temporary pylon or a permanent prosthesis come for treatment, some device is needed to hold the 'foot' on the lathe foot-plate or bicycle pedal. Both the adaptations shown here can be used for either a pylon or a prosthesis. It may be necessary to arrange the straps in a different way for different appliances. Straps are always made long enough to allow for this.

The adaptation for a Union lathe which has a slatted treadle consists of a piece of plywood with slots cut in to take two leather straps (*Figure 9.4*). These are glued to the underside of the wood. The wood

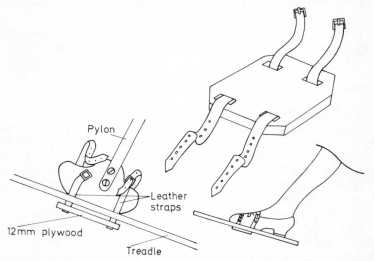

Figure 9.4. – Adaptation to attach either a temporary walking pylon or a lower limb prosthesis to the treadle of a Union lathe

is positioned under the treadle and the straps are passed up through the bars in the treadle. The pylon or prosthesis can then be anchored to the treadle by buckling the straps.

The adaptation for a bicycle fretsaw is a box which fits over the pedal (*Figure 9.5*). The box is made from 12 mm (½ in) plywood and the lid is attached with two 25 mm (1 in) brass butts. The small plywood wedges and the foam rubber on the lid keep the adaptation fixed to the pedal. The lid is held closed by a catch made from a small piece of plywood attached by a large screw. The leather straps which go through the box buckle over the pylon or prosthesis.

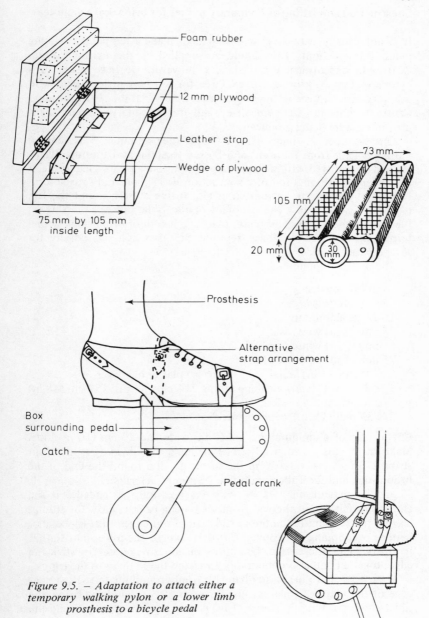

Foam rubber

12 mm plywood

Leather strap

Wedge of plywood

75 mm by 105 mm
inside length

73 mm

105 mm

20 mm 30 mm

Prosthesis

Alternative
strap arrangement

Box
surrounding pedal

Catch

Pedal crank

*Figure 9.5. — Adaptation to attach either a
temporary walking pylon or a lower limb
prosthesis to a bicycle pedal*

Construction and fitting of temporary pylons for below-knee amputees

It is not usually necessary or desirable to make a temporary walking pylon for a patient. This should be supplied by the Artificial Limb Centre. In exceptional circumstances, however, we have made such pylons in the workshops, for example for a young male patient who was very eager to get walking again at a time when the Artificial Limb Centre technicians were on strike and no temporary or permanent prostheses were being produced.

One summer a young man, a below-knee amputee, was sent to Farnham Park from the Kent and Sussex Hospital at Tunbridge Wells. He had been fitted with a temporary pylon, like a pirate's leg, made at that hospital. Its method of construction was simple and satisfactory. A plaster-of-Paris cup had been made, fitting closely round the leg, reaching to just below the condyles of the tibia, but not pressing on the end of the stump, and incorporating a length of broomstick with a ferrule on the end. We have reproduced this pylon successfully for several patients since.

The materials required are:

1 ash broomstick
1 crutch ferrule
16-gauge aluminium
25 mm (1 in) wire nails
5 mm ($^1/_5$ in) white wool felt
25 mm (1 in) adhesive plaster
1 × 25 mm (1 in) and 4 × 15 cm (6 in) plaster bandages
3 × 37 mm (1½ in) webbing straps 214 cm (84 in), 122 cm (48 in)
    and 60 cm (24 in) long
2 × 37 mm (1½ in) webbing buckles

Cut a strip of aluminium 7.5 cm (3 in) wide and 26 cm (10 in) long. Make three cuts down it 23 cm (9 in) long, thus dividing it into four strips 2 cm (¾ in) wide. Wrap the uncut portion round the end of the broomstick and fix it there with two 25 mm (1 in) nails.

Sit the patient on a table, with his legs fully extended. Fit the chiropody felt round the leg, from the patella to just below the stump, leaving the stiff muslin on the outside. The front edges must fit exactly, neither overlapping nor gaping. Cut darts out of the lower part so that it tapers to fit the stump. Use strips of adhesive plaster to stick the edges together and also temporarily to secure the felt cup to the leg.

Wrap a 15 cm (6 in) plaster bandage firmly round the felt. The upper edge of the plaster bandages must fit very snugly around and below the tibial condyles. Wrap a 25 mm (1 in) plaster bandage spirally round the aluminium strips. An assistant must then hold the broomstick and aluminium strips in position around the felt. Great care must be taken to ensure that the broomstick is in vertical and horizontal alignment with the stump. Use a second 15 cm (6 in) plaster bandage to secure the aluminium strips to the felt and to strengthen the region where the cup joins the peg. Take two long pieces of webbing and place them on either side of the plaster cup (the longer on the lateral side) projecting about 15 cm (6 in) below. Wrap half of the third 15 cm (6 in) plaster bandage round these, turn them up for extra security and wrap the rest of the bandage round. If necessary use a further 15 cm (6 in) plaster bandage to improve the shape of the cup, but this will of course increase the weight. Leave the peg-leg to dry for 48 hours.

The webbing straps from either side of the knee loop over the opposite shoulder and buckle over the chest. They are held in place by a second webbing strap sewn on just above the knee and buckled in front.

Finally fit the pylon, mark its length against the other leg, allowing a further 1.3 cm (½ in) for the stump to sink in on standing. Saw off and tip with the ferrule. A coat of paint improves the appearance and prevents plaster flaking off on to clothes. The patient's gait is improved by fitting a rocker (*see Figure 9.7*) instead of the crutch ferrule.

At a later date we experimented further using an old-fashioned wooden shoe last that fitted the patient's shoe (*Figure 9.6*). A beech bar 5 cm (2 in) square was used instead of a broomstick. The shoe last was drilled through at what would have been the ankle joint, and this hole was bushed with a length of brass tubing. A pair of old calipers were sawn off, drilled and screwed to the beech bar and the angle irons slipped into the brass tubing; two cup hooks were screwed on the front and back of the beech bar, just below the plaster cup; two more were screwed to the heel and instep of the shoe last. A pair of 15 cm (6 in) springs were hooked on to control the movement in the pseudo ankle-joint. Strong tension springs such as those fitted to short calipers for toe-raising are very suitable.

The patient for whom this was made was an agile and active young man. He soon discarded sticks and even played cricket, bowling and batting, wearing this temporary aid. It was found necessary to give him a spare spring to keep in his pocket. His activities made considerable demands on the springs and he broke two on different occasions.

The original peg-leg with crutch rubber ferrule allowed great agility and was good on uneven ground, but threw a considerable strain on the knee joint and a patient with poor quadriceps felt very unstable. The improved shoe version is more stable, but considerably heavier and more complicated, making it only suitable for a young, active and determined patient. The other version incorporates a rocker (*Figure 9.7*). This is very stable, simple and light. There is a slight tendency to jar the knee when walking on uneven ground, but this improves as the quadriceps develop. We find this rocker design is the most suitable for the average patient.

These below-knee pylons are simple to make and save much time in rehabilitation. Several patients have returned to work wearing them whilst awaiting the manufacture of the permanent prosthesis. Also, they are cheap to produce. It has been found advisable to allow the patient to wear the pylon for only part of the day, to give opportunity for close bandaging to play its part in shaping the stump.

Until the patient's quadriceps are really well developed he must use sticks, especially out-of-doors on rough ground. These below-knee pylons do not control the sideways play in the knee joint. The permanent prosthesis is usually fitted with metal hinge joints which are fixed in a thigh gaiter laced up closely to give the necessary support.

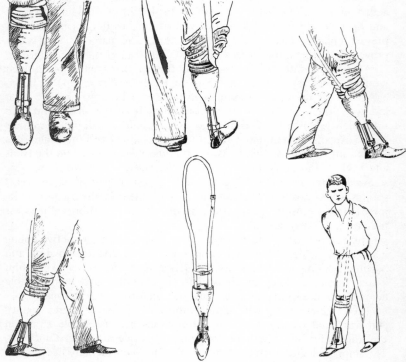

Figure 9.6. – Temporary walking pylon for a below-knee amputee

359

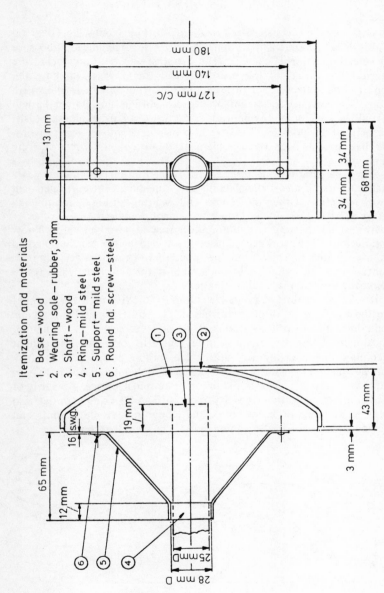

Itemization and materials

1. Base – wood
2. Wearing sole – rubber, 3 mm
3. Shaft – wood
4. Ring – mild steel
5. Support – mild steel
6. Round hd. screw – steel

180 mm
140 mm
127 mm C/C
13 mm
34 mm | 34 mm
68 mm

43 mm
3 mm
19 mm
16 s.w.g.
65 mm
12 mm
25 mm D
28 mm D

Figure 9.7. – Rocker foot, itemization and materials for use with peg-leg described on page 358

UPPER LIMB AMPUTEES

Patients who have been fitted with a prosthesis following either an above- or below-knee amputation may come for rehabilitation because they need vocational guidance. The therapist will well understand the physical limitations of the prosthesis and the patient will have the opportunity of trying out different items of equipment in the work-shops. The normal assessment procedures outlined in Chapter 13 will be followed including, as appropriate, the use of psychological tests, the help of the local Skill Centre in providing a wider range of work, and liaison with both the Disablement Resettlement Officer and the employer.

Some patients will be referred for rehabilitation because they are unable to attend an Artificial Limb and Appliance Centre, for personal or other reasons. Others will come while waiting for the stump to heal, before going to be trained to use a permanent prosthesis.

Almost all the upper limb amputees treated have had below-elbow amputations. The working gauntlets described below can be adapted for use on the upper arm but the scope of work will be very limited. Painting with an extended brush is one of the few practical ways of exercising the shoulder in this situation.

It takes some time to prepare a stump for the fitting of a permanent prosthesis. There is often a further delay whilst this is being made. Sometimes the prosthesis does not fit and has to be sent away for adjustment. Using a working gauntlet will help to prevent the patient becoming 'one-hand minded' during the waiting period, with the risk that he might be inclined to use only a dress hand and not bother to learn the use of a split hook or other terminal device provided, or discard these once their novelty wore off. A working gauntlet also helps to mobilize or keep mobile the elbow and shoulder joints and provide exercise for the remaining muscles in the upper limb.

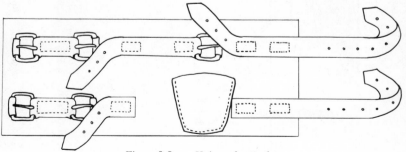

Figure 9.8a. – Universal gauntlet

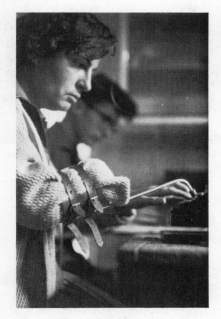

Figure 9.8b. – Typing peg

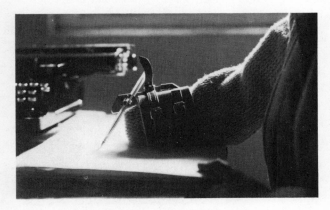

Figure 9.8c. – Writing attachment

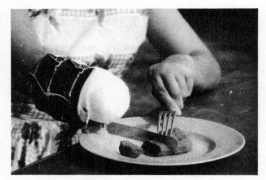

Figure 9.8d. – Practising cutting up plasticine

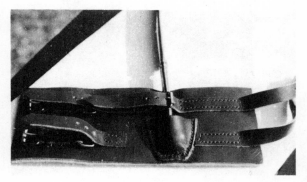

Figure 9.8e. – Knife firmly in position

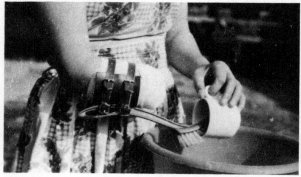

Figure 9.8f. – Washing-up brush strapped in place

A universal gauntlet is shown in *Figure 9.8a*. This can be used with a variety of attachments: a knife and fork, pen or typing attachment or washing-up brush. It is mainly used for ADL activities when little strength or force is required. The typing peg in *Figure 9.8b* is made from a metal rod with a rubber thimble at the end and is the same length as the tips of the fingers of the other hand, since typing is a bilateral activity. With the other attachments, holding the tool nearer to the elbow than normal does not matter, and may be an advantage. The writing aid has a short lever arm and is more easily controlled than if it were the length of the typing peg. The writing attachment is made from a piece of plywood with two small tool clips screwed to it to hold the pen at the correct angle (*Figure 9.8c*). When using the pocket to hold a knife (*Figure 9.8d*) or writing aid, stuffing the sides of the pocket with wedge-shaped plywood or plastic foam will prevent the tool being pushed on to its side (*Figure 9.8e*). The pocket is useful when the tool presses against the gauntlet as when cutting up food with the knife. The two straps are used to hold larger or longer-handled tools such as the washing-up brush in *Figure 9.8f*.

The gauntlet illustrated here was made of leather and fastened with straps. It could equally be made from Corfam or other synthetic leather which has the advantage of being washable as well as cheaper, and could be fastened with Velcro. It is a neat gauntlet which can be put in a pocket and brought out when needed.

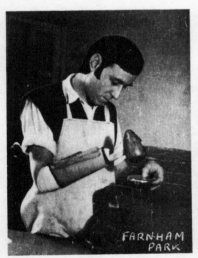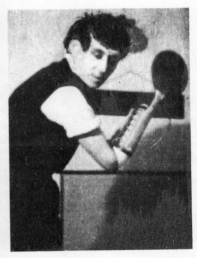

Figure 9.9. – *Gauntlet to hold hammer, mallet, table tennis bat, wood-turning tools or paint brushes*

To use the arm more strongly, a rigid gauntlet can be moulded to fit the individual patient. This is close fitting and made from Orthoplast, a firm material, so that more pressure can be applied to any tool fitted to it. If the stump is short below the elbow, a separate cuff may be made for the upper arm. Elastic straps between the two parts keep the working gauntlet in place on the forearm stump. If it is found, because Orthoplast is so rigid, that the gauntlet does not open sufficiently wide to encompass the forearm, it may be hinged along its length by grooving the inner and outer surfaces to make a thin flexible line or self-hinge (*see* Chapter 8, page 277).

A table tennis bat, hammer, mallet, knife, fork, putter for clock golf or, possibly, a wood-turning chisel or gouge can all be fitted to the gauntlet. A tool can be fixed by bolts through holes drilled in the handle and fastened with wing nuts. Alternatively the tool can be held by jubilee clips (adjustable clips used to fix pipes in car engines) lined with rubber sheeting for extra grip. Some tools will be easier to use if fitted with an extension handle, like the table tennis bat in *Figure 9.9*. This earlier working gauntlet was made from hide, with long side pockets to hold tools and other implements, and was fastened with laces.

REFERENCE

Jones, Mary S. (1952). 'Mechanical aids to treatment'. *Br. J. phys. Med.* **15**, 153

10

Hemiplegia

Unlike as in most occupational therapy departments throughout the country, only a small proportion of the patients treated at Farnham Park are suffering from hemiplegia. There are several reasons for this. Many hemiplegics are too old or too medically unfit to manage the rigorous programme of full day treatment, even with a rest period. Sessional treatment is unsatisfactory. A patient who attends just for those classes that are suitable and then goes home is blocking a place for someone who would benefit from a full day's treatment. Another reason is that if the patient comes from too far away, even if he has reached his maximum level of function when discharged, he is less likely to find a job than a local patient with all the Centre's contacts and expertise to back him up; he may do better if treated nearer home. It has also been observed that too large a number of hemiplegics treated at the same time do not appear to make the same progress as a few working together with patients suffering from other disabilities. We therefore limit the number of hemiplegics to not more than 10 per cent of our total intake. This makes a group of sufficient size so that any individual does not feel conspicuously more disabled than other patients. It also means that there are not too many patients requiring individual attention and slowing down the programme of the rest of their group.

Those hemiplegic patients who benefit most by treatment at Farnham Park are in the younger age group. They appreciate the dynamic atmosphere, the feeling of recovery among the other patients and, perhaps most important of all, they avoid the demoralization of being treated along with geriatric hemiplegics and the consequent feeling that they have no future.

Two observations may be made about the admittedly atypical group of hemiplegic patients treated over the years. Many completely right-sided hemiplegics with little recovery in this hand have learnt very easily to write with the left hand and have had no speech defect. Many of the left-sided hemiplegics have been particularly unco-operative and difficult, even when they have had no evident perceptual defect. This may be associated with organic involvement of the frontal lobes. These patients do not appear to try to overcome their difficulties in the same way as the right-sided hemiplegics.

It has been established that better functional results are achieved more quickly when patients are treated as soon as possible after the onset of any disability. This is especially true for those who have suffered acute injury, onset of disease or incident which changes the whole plan of their lives. The episode may appear to be an overwhelming calamity but in its very suddenness there lies a challenge. The shock may bring to the fore capacities for courage which have lain dormant and undiscovered in ordinary circumstances. With adequate directions for effort the patients will learn new tricks of living. If they are not given time to lose hope, they will the more quickly adapt themselves to overcoming their disability. The needs of these patients in occupational therapy can be met by teaching the development of the residual capacity and adaptation to residual disability, and by quickly instilling hope and belief in the recovery of function. These aims will be more easily carried out while the impetus of the first reaction of courage is still lively and fresh.

Some of the treatment detailed in this chapter would be too rigorous for the older and more disabled patients who are treated in hospital. An outline of more general treatment will be found in Macdonald (1976).

PERCEPTUAL DEFECTS

Areas of perceptual dysfunction must be identified because they may be interfering with the patient's ability to carry out simple activities, such as putting a lid on a saucepan, as well as more complex activities, such as dressing. Perceptual defects may well prevent a patient from returning to work. Perceptual testing is not an end in itself, but the test results will give guidance to the therapist in planning treatment.

Perceptual disorders may occur in both right and left hemiplegia. A patient with the non-dominant side affected is likely to have parietal lobe damage resulting in perceptual defects; a patient with the dominant side affected may also have speech defects.

A patient's inability to perform a simple test may be due to a deficit in any one of a number of basic processes underlying perception. If a patient fails to respond when he is asked to complete a jigsaw puzzle, it may be because he does not see the pieces (visual defect), was not listening when he was told what to do (attention defect), does

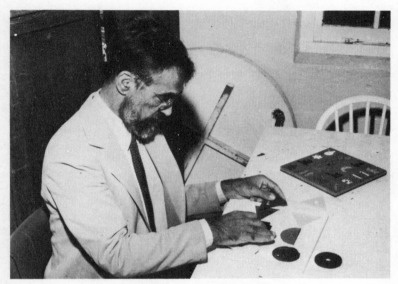

Figure 10.1. – Perceptual testing

not know what the pieces are for (organizational defect) or cannot manipulate the pieces (eye–hand co-ordination defect or apraxia). Although our present state of knowledge prevents us from performing assessments which clearly implicate one underlying process rather than another, any therapist working with a hemiplegic patient should be aware of the different defects which may produce the same end-results.

One way of looking at perception is to use a flow-chart which illustrates the different processes involved. This can show how the flow can be broken at different stages between the presentation of information to the patient and his response to it (*see* page 368).

There are some sophisticated psychological tests which attempt to identify areas of perceptual defect, but many of them can only be administered and interpreted by psychologists. Occupational therapists who have been trained to use psychological tests will find Marianne

FLOW CHART ILLUSTRATING PROCESSES INVOLVED IN PERCEPTION

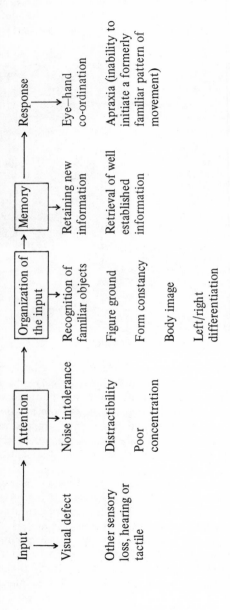

Input ⟶ Attention ⟶ Organization of ⟶ Memory ⟶ Response
                      the input

↓ Visual defect

Attention
↓ Noise intolerance

Organization of the input
↓ Recognition of familiar objects

Memory
↓ Retaining new information

Response
↓ Eye–hand co-ordination

Other sensory loss, hearing or tactile

Distractibility

Poor concentration

Figure ground

Form constancy

Body image

Left/right differentiation

Astereognosis

Understanding of the written word

Retrieval of well established information

Apraxia (inability to initiate a formerly familiar pattern of movement)

Frostig's tests and remedial exercises for visual perception useful, although limited in value because they were devised for children who had difficulty reading and writing. These tests are not, therefore, standardized for hemiplegic adults, nor do they test all areas of perceptual defect. Two other useful sources of information are McFie (1975) and Lezak (1976).

A number of simple diagnostic tests which can be used to identify perceptual disorders are described below. To carry out these tests effectively, simple test kits and printed instructions, giving clear instructions for administering the tests and recording the results, will be needed. Before each test the patient should be sitting comfortably in a fairly quiet situation, wearing spectacles if these are normally used. The therapist should be sitting either opposite or beside the patient on the affected side, to provide maximum stimulation towards the dysfunctioning area.

Once areas of dysfunction have been identified, treatment will be concerned with re-education. Test material should be kept separate for retesting later if required. Practice material of a similar kind to that used for assessment must be compiled to provide reinforcement. Workshop activities can also be planned to help. Putting cups on saucers, for instance, may prove difficult for someone with spatial relationship problems. Perceptual re-education is another area where occupational therapists will find that assessment and treatment are very much inter-related.

Visual defects

Visual defects are the most common forms of sensory loss which will affect the presentation of information to a hemiplegic patient and so interrupt the flow at the input stage.

Poor eyesight often appears to be a problem after a cerebrovascular accident or a head injury, even when there is no major defect such as homonymous hemianopia or diplopia. It is always advisable to find out whether the patient should be wearing spectacles and, if so, to make sure that they are worn. The prescribed lenses may no longer be correct, and a check-up with an optician may be necessary. Making sure, too, that the patient is working in a good light, and positioning him so that his work is at the optimum distance from his eyes, will help to make the best use of his residual vision.

Homonymous hemianopia, the loss of the outer half of the visual field of one eye and inner half of the other, is probably the most common visual defect affecting hemiplegic patients. A right defect is associated with a right hemiplegia, and vice versa. The loss of awareness of everything that would normally be seen to one side of the body inhibits many day-to-day activities. One patient, when laying a table, put down a table mat, a knife and a glass at each plate but omitted to lay forks because she could not see anything to her left. This condition may sometimes be missed in early diagnosis and on occasion has only been discovered by the occupational therapist when a patient had difficulty in carrying out some activity in the workshops. It is, therefore, appropriate to carry out a simple test when the patient is admitted.

To do this, the therapist stands opposite to and about a metre away from the patient, who is told to cover one eye and fix the gaze of the other upon the opposite eye of the therapist. Throughout the test both must keep their heads still and stay facing each other, looking straight ahead. The therapist, holding a test object, brings this inwards from beyond the periphery of her own visual field to a position midway between herself and the patient. This procedure is carried out from above, from below and from either side. In each case the patient is asked to say when he first sees the object, so that the therapist is able to compare the extent of his visual field relative to her own. Both eyes should be tested in the same way and retested as required.

If the patient is suffering from hemianopia, care should be taken in the early stages to place work within his known field of vision. It is possible to teach a patient to compensate by turning his head, but this may disturb his balance. The therapist should sit alongside the patient, on the affected side to provide maximum stimulation. The patient will need to be given plenty of opportunity to practise and improve this technique.

Diplopia means that the patient sees his environment in two completely separate pictures. He is usually given a patch to wear over alternate eyes on alternate days and gradually the two-pictured areas may draw together and overlap. These patients may see more clearly if they are helped to see objects more strongly in three dimensions. The use and value of shadows can be taught to enable them to judge distance and shape. Work must be juggled into a position where shadows are appreciable, sharp in definition and have a definite relationship to each other which is easy to appreciate. Artificial light may be brought in to help but this must be direct lighting, so that it does not throw on to the eye but on to the work.

Some workshop activities require less concentrated use of the eyes than others. Modelling in plasticine or clay has been found useful since it is so dependent on touch and feel, and has been used as a preliminary to wood-shaping with rasps and sandpaper. Wooden spoons are of many patterns to appeal to the housewife, and even roughly-shaped wooden toys have a character of their own. A fine-grained wood such as pear is best for toys, closely followed by cherry and apple.

Attentional defects

Increased distractibility is a problem for many hemiplegics. They may be particularly intolerant to noise which in turn reduces their concentration and may bring on headaches. Any formal testing of patients, for example for other perceptual defects, should be carried out in a setting which minimizes distractibility. A small, relatively bare room, free from external noise should be used. Test for distractibility by getting the patient to perform the same test in a more distracting situation.

Building up noise tolerance will be part of treatment. It is not easy to arrange workshops that have been adapted rather than built for the purpose of therapy so that noise is eliminated or diminished. Perhaps this is not desirable. In treating hemiplegic patients and also post-head injury patients, an aim of treatment has been to accustom them to noise. It is just one of those things that one must first learn to endure and then to forget, unless there is a prospect of retirement to a desert island. When the patient returns home, he must endure if not enjoy the children's playing and the television and radio.

Occupational therapy workshops must be encouraged to be places where patients sing as well as hammer and knock in nails. This may be a rude reception for the patient who has come from hospital. There, life may be quiet during the day even if lifts and trolleys bang about at odd times during the night. It should, however, be possible to arrange therapeutic workshops so that in one part the noises are, so to speak, 'off'. Gradually the patient who hates noise and complains of headache may recover some endurance and then join in the singing and whistling in a distant and plaintive manner. Later on interest in more ambitious projects will lure him into the company of those who make tables and other objects which can only be constructed where there is suitable machinery. Increased interest in activity is observed to accompany less irritability towards noise.

During the summer months many hemiplegics, head injury patients and others who find noise intolerable will be occupied near the workshops in the garden. There they get the noise rather watered down. If they are going to return to indoor work, they must gradually be interested, involved and engaged in some project which requires their attention indoors. If the interest is adequate then it may well be that the attention is distracted from noise to the achievement of the work they have in mind.

Sometimes a patient wants to read, but finds this difficult because of poor concentration. This can be helped by using a piece of card with a slit of suitable size to show one line of type. This helps to concentrate the eyes on the line being read, and can be made for individual books. An alternative is to get large-print books out of the library.

Building up concentration in other areas is similar to building up stamina. The patient can be helped by being given simple tasks which are gradually increased in difficulty; by being given tasks which reflect his particular interest; and by working initially in a non-distracting environment, building up to settings where there are more distractions, helping him to increase his ability to ignore irrelevant perceptual stimuli.

Organizational defects

Once a stimulus has been received, the visual input must be interpreted in a meaningful way. This perceptual organization is very often disrupted after hemiplegia or other brain damage. Patients may be unable to recognize familiar objects or to know when an object is the right way up. There may be body image disturbance which may include unilateral neglect. There may be tactile agnosia (astereognosis), a disturbance in recognition by touch.

Two fundamental organizational processes are figure ground differentiation (eye distractibility) and shape constancy (form constancy). Figure ground discrimination can be assessed by giving the patient a sheet of paper with outline drawings of a square, a circle and a triangle overlapping each other. The patient is asked to draw round the circle to demonstrate that he can perceive an object in relation to its background without being distracted by the other shapes.

Shape constancy can be assessed by giving the patient a sheet of paper covered with a number of complex figures which incorporate circles, ovals, squares, straight and curved lines and other irregular shapes. The patient is then shown a separate picture of a circle and an oval. He is asked to draw round all the circles he can find, at the same time ignoring all the ovals.

Any visual stimulus is seen as differentiated from its background. If this ability is disrupted it becomes impossible for a patient to read, or even to recognize everyday objects. Similarly if it is not possible to interpret an object in different contexts as being the same object, the world becomes totally chaotic. This is why these two processes are fundamental. (Therapists who are trained to use Frostig will find the tests particularly useful in this context.)

Position in space, as it relates to reading and writing, can be assessed by using tests with rows of shapes of everyday articles drawn on a sheet of paper. In each sequence one item is shown in the correct position while the other four are shown with one among them either upside down or facing in the wrong direction. In each case this 'odd man out' must be identified by the patient.

Spatial judgement or spatial orientation, the ability to assess spatial relationships, to recognize shapes and sizes, may be assessed by using a board with cut-out shapes which must be replaced in the correct holes. A simple test could consist of a square, a circle, a semicircle and a triangle. If this proves too easy, a second board with more complex shapes such as a fir tree and a bottle could be used. A child's posting box with differently shaped holes on each side, through which matching shapes must be 'posted', provides a three-dimensional test as a further progression (*see Figure 10.1*, page 367).

Loss of body image may be assessed by asking the patient to draw a picutre of himself. He can also be asked to assemble a cut-out figure consisting of a head, a trunk, two arms and two legs. Another test would be to assemble cut-out pieces comprising a face shape, two eyes, two ears, a nose, mouth and hair. He can also be asked to hold each piece against the equivalent part of his own body.

A verticality test has also been found useful. The therapist, holding a walking stick, faces the patient. The stick is held up vertically and then turned sideways into the horizontal plane. It is put into the patient's unaffected hand and he is asked to turn it back again to vertical. If his conception of vertical is distorted the stick will be turned to an angle which relates to his conception of the world around him.

These distortions of spatial judgement and body image can affect the ability to dress and also account for the patient who leans sideways when sitting or walks in a diagonal direction. Misjudgement of height, width and distance may also occur.

Stereognosis and sensation are closely associated. To test for astereognosis, put the test object into the unaffected hand. An object put into the affected hand may be unrecognized because of astereognosis, but there may also be gross sensory loss or paralysis which affects the results of the test (*see also* page 221).

Memory defect

Loss of recent memory occurs quite frequently after hemiplegia. This can be tested by digit span. Make up beforehand a random sequence of single numbers such as 3, 5, 9. Say these three numbers to the patient, pausing for one second between each number, and get him to repeat them back. Then do it all over again with four different numbers, and then with five. Go on until he fails to repeat them correctly. The average person should manage a sequence of six to eight. Someone who is brain-damaged or elderly will manage far less.

Retrieval of well established information can be assessed by using the Mill Hill Vocabulary scale (which is available to occupational therapists who have been trained to use psychological tests). It can also be assessed by asking simple questions for which the answers can be readily checked, such as the patient's address and his wife's name.

Response defect

A patient may well be able to attend to a stimulus and interpret it correctly but be unable to respond appropriately because of defects in eye—hand co-ordination.

Visual motor perception may be assessed by drawing a line through a simple maze, progressing to a more complex maze. If the pencil must be held in the non-dominant hand, this may affect the result.

The Frostig test may also be useful in testing eye—hand co-ordination. The patient is presented with a series of tasks requiring him to draw a line between two points from 2 to 8 inches apart. The tasks increase in complexity. In the simplest task the patient is asked to draw a straight line 8 inches long inside a boundary of ¾ inch. In later tasks, no boundary lines are given to guide the patient and the shape of the line is made more demanding.

INITIAL ASSESSMENT

On admission the therapist begins assessing the patient's degree of disability and the areas of malfunction in order to plan treatment. Assessment of visual and perceptual defects has already been discussed and this must be carried out before any other area of function is assessed, since these defects adversely affect so many other areas of function. Speech defects and other disorders of communication must also be assessed but this is done by the speech therapist. She will then ask the occupational therapist to plan treatment in the workshops to reinforce speech therapy (*see* page 391).

ADL assessment may reveal that the patient cannot dress himself at all, or it may just highlight common difficulties such as the inability to do up the top shirt button, or the shirt cuff on the affected arm, or it may indicate the need for a Nelson knife to cut up food. It should be

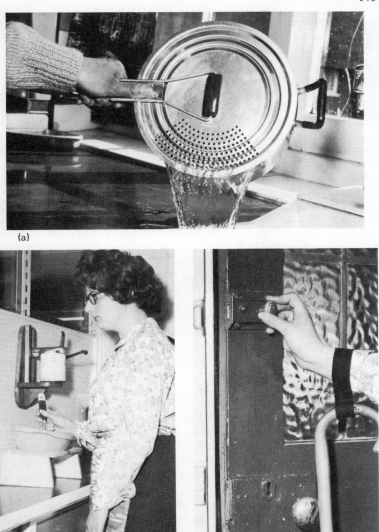

(a)

(b)   (c)

Figure 10.2. − ADL techniques using only one hand. (a) A strainer lid, available from hardware stores. The pivoted handle can be used with left or right hand. (b) Using a one-handed egg whisk and a portable bowl-holder to stabilize the mixing bowl. (c) A loop of wide elastic stitched so that it grips the stick makes opening doors easier

emphasized that with controlled movement of the upper limb, anxiety and the memory of past failures may inhibit the effort or cause movements, due to spasm, far different from those desired. The writer recollected a left hemiplegic whom she was attempting to re-educate in the use of knife and fork at table. A lump of plasticine, representing food, was firmly attached by smacking it on to a workshop table. The mere sight of a knife and fork (even when made strange with built-up Perspex handles) was enough to make the patient jib. 'You can't make me try that one again', he exploded. On inquiry it came out that when in hospital he had been given a fried egg and tomato (both slippery in nature) on a plate on a polished bed-table. He made his effort and jabbed the fork into the tomato, which exploded. His pyjamas and bed, and worst of all the pretty nurse's clean uniform, had been bespattered with tomato juice. It took some considerable time for the therapist to convince him that a lump of plasticine might react differently. He also needed assurance that eating in public would not be expected until he himself was confident of adequate control. Even then he preferred to make his first effort with real food at home one weekend, with his wife as the only observer.

When there is some return of function in the paralysed hand, a general assessment of hand function, as used with other hand injuries, is carried out. This will include pinch, opposition, grip, sensation and an observation of circulation to the limb.

If the patient is clearly going to have resettlement problems, an early assessment of intellectual ability may be indicated. The Standard Progressive Matrices test is useful for screening.

The importance of early assessment cannot be over-emphasized. One patient, with a right-sided hemiplegia, made rapid progress with his physical disabilities. He never had any difficulty in appreciating words but, being strongly right-handed, he had to learn to control his fingers to write with them. Unfortunately we did not test his appreciation of numerals at an early date. His discharge to his own job as a quantity surveyor was being discussed when we found that he could neither add nor subtract even the simplest sums with accuracy. The discovery of this loss came as a great shock, all the worse because he had been accustomed to juggling with long lines of figures when estimating for materials for building.

LOWER LIMB RE-EDUCATION

The recovery of controlled activity in the lower limb is commonly accepted as being both more rapid and complete than that in the upper limb. Leg movements once learnt are usually simple in pattern and are therefore easier to relearn sufficiently to achieve mobility. Although hand and arm movements are also learnt early in life, practice develops more skill and the movements become infinitely more complicated and therefore more difficult to relearn.

Before learning to walk again the patient should have good standing balance and be able to transfer weight from one foot to the other. The physiotherapist will assess this and if necessary include it in her treatment before gait training begins.

Returning mobility, though it may be effective in a limited area, shows certain characteristics. It develops into a habit of movement which is lop-sided. It includes a dragging of the foot on the affected side, in an attempt to catch up with the step of the foot on the unaffected side. This dragging appears to originate in paralysis of the dorsiflexors, making the foot too heavy to lift. In some patients there is spasm of the plantar flexors and resistance to passive dorsiflexion cannot be overcome. In either case the patient will attempt to counteract the nuisance by a lift of the whole leg carried out by lumbar flexion. Without instruction and supervision, hip and knee flexion will not be called into play to help lift the foot. Hip extension spasm also makes it more difficult to achieve a normal gait.

To aid walking, an ankle-foot orthosis may be provided. In treating those patients with spastic plantar flexion the position of contact requires consideration. This should be proximal to the metatarsophalangeal joints; if it is not, it has been observed that spasm is increased. In the area of these joints, particularly on the outer border, the plantar reflex may most easily be elicited. It is therefore, appropriate that the foot-raising appliance provided for the spastic hemiplegic should act as far back towards the subtaloid and mid-tarsal joints as possible, and be placed under the heel of the shoe. It has also been observed that an appliance in maximal contact with the sole of the foot tends to reduce spasm.

Sometimes the occupational therapist may be asked for a temporary ankle-foot orthosis, either to assess whether this will help the patient's pattern of walking or because delivery of the permanent orthosis is delayed. We now supply a Jousto toe-raising appliance (*Figure 10.3*), in preference to the strap and spring type which attached to the toe of the shoe and which was formerly made in the workshops. These Jousto appliances, made by Remploy, are stocked in various sizes and are suitable for most patients; they are also reusable. Such commercially available equipment can be financially justified by the saving of the therapist's time. There is one criticism of this appliance: the top band rests against the calf but if it were longer and reached to just below the knee, it would be more comfortable. There are also other temporary

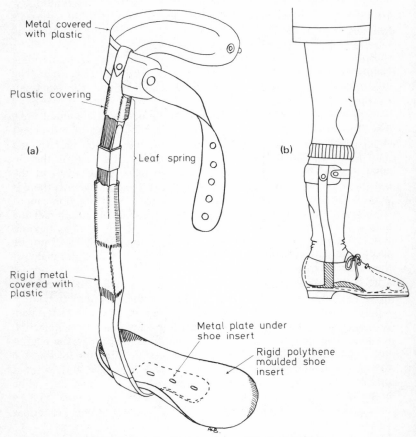

Metal covered
with plastic

Plastic covering

(a)

Leaf spring

(b)

Rigid metal
covered with
plastic

Metal plate under
shoe insert

Rigid polythene
moulded shoe
insert

Figure 10.3. – Jousto temporary ankle-foot orthosis

ankle-foot orthoses on the market, some of which are described by
Murdoch (1976).

It has been estimated that of every 100 patients who survive a
stroke, 90 will be able to walk again but only 10 will recover useful
function in the affected hand. In planning treatment, therefore, good
gait should be one of the first things for a patient to relearn.

He should, of course be taught this by a physiotherapist, but it is all
too easy for such a treatment to become an incident in the day's
programme, with stool-seating or what have you as another incident
carried out in a different department. There he will come in hobbledehoy,

no matter what he has been taught previously in a gymnasium or ward; his destination is a chair in the workshops and he will want to get there and fall into it. An occupational therapist should find out from the physiotherapist exactly what technique has been used for the patient's early lessons and insist that this should be practised. There are many techniques of teaching walking. The writer was taught one method as a physiotherapy student, which she recommends. The patient is taught to stand on the affected leg with the support of the stick in the 'good' hand. He then swings the unaffected leg through, taking a step lasting no longer than the affected leg can easily support bodyweight. The next step is taken standing on the good leg and moving the stick in company with the bad leg. The temptation is to step off when standing on the good leg, so that too long a step is taken for the bad leg to catch up the distance, and it is only brought up level. There will probably be a drag towards the end of the step because of the difficulty of the 'carry over' when standing on the bad leg. There are two maxims which may help the patient because of their simplicity. One is the necessity to 'put the best foot forward' and the other that he must think of 'long and short' as a nice embroidery stitch but not one to be used in walking – these are sufficiently simple for him to remember while putting his attention to walking nicely. Some therapists insist on the patient's swinging the arms alternately, but the writer has found that this injunction distracts the attention too much in the beginning. It is usually sufficient to walk beside the patient, holding the arm and swinging it for him. The art of walking may be slow in developing in the beginning but if and when a therapist has time to insist on it, the occupational therapy workshops provide an ideal environment. There is continual opportunity for the practice of short walks to fetch tools or materials. Some account has been given of the layout of the workshops at Farnham Park and how it has been planned to provide such opportunities. The closest co-operation is needed with the physiotherapy staff if the teaching and practice of walking are intended to encourage a willing and confident pupil. It is not one person's job.

Solidity and stability of chairs and tables are also necessities for the practice of 'good landing'. The patient must have confidence in getting on and off a chair. In most cases it is advantageous to provide chairs with arms, certainly in the earlier stages.

When the patient is fit to undertake leg activities in the workshops, the bicycle machines have been found invaluable (*see* Chapter 2). It is easy to remove the seat and allow the patient to walk up to the machine while holding on to a handlebar. The therapist can then slide the seat in behind him in a comfortable position. The pedal cranks must be adjusted initially so that both suit the range of movement of the affected leg.

The cranks may be gradually extended day by day, or week by week, as the range of movement improves. It has been found necessary to provide toe straps to keep the affected foot on the bicycle pedal (*see* *Figure 9.5*, page 355). It is essential that the patient get his balance right and be taught a smooth and even movement if his treatment is to be of value. This smooth rhythmic movement is found to assist relaxation. There is some challenge to the achievement of balance of the hips which the patient can appreciate, when it is pointed out, by the even distribution of his weight on the tuberosities of the ischia on the bicycle saddle. In some patients the affected leg is too flaccid for treatment on the bicycle. Even with the foot attached to the pedal, the knee may fall outwards, due to poor control, and cause over-stretching of the joint.

The therapist will find that the spastic hemiplegic cannot unclench his hand to hold on to the handlebar. She should help him very gently and slowly to open the hand and then allow the spasm to provide grip again. The writer cannot suggest an explanation for what she has quite often observed — that using a spasm in this way helps to relieve it. At first the affected hand may slip off the handlebar. Then the patient will suddenly notice for himself that the hand is not slipping in spasm but in relaxation, and slowly the day may come when it can be lifted by the patient himself and he can grip and relax at will.

When bicycling, the patient must grip the handlebars and thrust forward with the arms to counterbalance the leg action and stabilize the trunk. This is the pattern of movement used in proprioceptive neuromuscular facilitation to stimulate the extensors of the upper limb.

At first the hemiplegic patient cannot steer his own work against file or saw because the unaffected hand is too much occupied in holding on to the handlebar. Then another patient may help: one who has begun to master finger extension but needs to practise it by pressing down the fingers and moving them and the wrists together. This may be another hemiplegic or a patient with a hand injury with sutured tendons needing extension exercise. The co-operation and conversation between the patients and the therapist are an aid to friendliness and the relaxation that is so essential to hemiplegics with spasm.

UPPER LIMB RE-EDUCATION

It has already been observed that the recovery in the upper limb is slower and less complete than in the lower limb. Although it is right and proper that the affected arm should be used vigorously when there are signs of recovery, there may come a time when this is wasted effort. Some patients become so preoccupied with their affected arm that they are not interested in improving their overall level of function. The therapist will need to persuade them to compensate with the other hand and arm in order to achieve maximum independence in the meantime, and 'in case' the affected limb does not recover.

One of our patients was a deeply religious woman. She was convinced that if she only had sufficient faith in God He would restore her paralysed arm. Any suggestion of learning to compensate with her other arm, even for the time being, was rejected since such a step would imply lack of faith on her part.

Sometimes there is a different problem. When the affected arm hangs uselessly by the patient's side he may ignore it and seldom even be sure where it is without looking at it. This is likely to be due to loss of body awareness due, in turn, to perceptual dysfunction, although in some patients there may be an element of wilfulness in forgetting the responsibility for a limb that has ceased to be a faithful servant. In treating these patients the writer has observed that recognition of possession of the hand and its position will be much encouraged by keeping the hand within range of vision. Even when it is too useless to help in work the hand must be kept in sight; its spasm can be used as an anchorage, a weight or a vice in which the work is fixed. Interlinking all the fingers of the good hand between those of the affected hand will make possible various bilateral activities. An example would be picking up pegs or large bottles which are then placed into holes to play a game of draughts. These bilateral activities are particularly appropriate when the symmetrical approach to the treatment of hemiplegia is being used (Bobath, 1973).

Working one-handed or with a second hand which is clumsy and ineffectual is frustrating. A programme of activity aims to be interesting enough to stimulate the patient to persevere. It may be best to divide the time so that part is spent on activities the patient most wants to do, and part on those the therapist feels will be of particular benefit.

The use of an overhead arm support can sometimes assist relaxation of the affected limb. By its buoyancy this has been found to encourage small movements of extension and abduction in the shoulder, and extension of elbow and wrist. The support also has the great advantage of positioning the affected hand where it can be seen. The old adage 'out of sight, out of mind' is very true.

Stool-seating, with the stool clamped to a table if necessary, can be done with one hand, the affected hand giving minimal assistance. If hand function improves, the clamp can be removed. The finished stool is likely to win praise from friends and relations, which breeds confidence and ambition, both of which are commonly lacking in the patients' mental outlook.

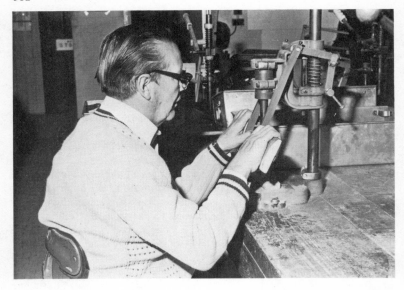

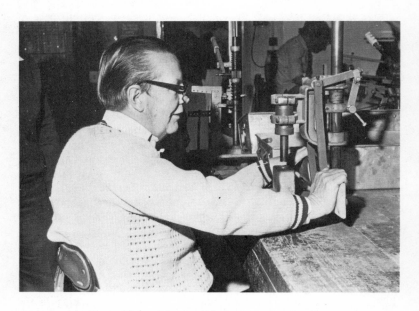

Figure 10.4. – 'Hemi-push' adaptation to a hand-press

Clay modelling and remedial games help to re-educate hand function. The upright rug loom requires co-ordination of all four limbs. Using the electric sewing machine will be of interest to some women, and so will practising cooking and laundrywork.

Printing, using both hands on the machine, the unaffected one slightly covering the other, is a good bilateral activity encouraging extension of the elbows to press down the handle. When this can be done standing it helps to develop better balance. Otherwise the patient can be perched on a bicycle stool to bring him up to the correct height.

An adaptation of the hand-press used for industrial outwork has been made specially for hemiplegic patients (*Figure 10.4*). It has been designed to follow the Bobath method of treatment which utilizes movements which are opposite to the spastic pattern in the upper limb. This 'hemi-push' adaptation requires protraction of the shoulder, extension of the elbow, hyperextension of the wrist and extension of the fingers.

Gardening is another popular activity. There are several one-handed tools, such as a hedge-clipper and lawn-edger (*Figure 10.5a* and *b*). There are also ways of making a flower bed more accessible, such as by using large pipe sections stacked on end (*Figure 10.5c*). Many other ideas are suggested in the book *The Easy Path to Gardening* (1972).

For those who like heavier activities in the workshops, wrought iron work has proved suitable. This is a good masculine activity but not too heavy. We have also had patients with hemiplegia working in the engineering section. One from Wales showed an aptitude for welding. We took him to the local Skill Centre to demonstrate his ability and they were impressed enough to train him. His paralysed arm prevented him from using a hand-held protective mask but this problem was solved by giving him a helmet to wear (*Figure 10.6*). This had a protective section which he could push up or down with one hand, or which could be adjusted by a jerk of the head. When he went to his first job his employer had some doubts, not about his welding ability but whether he would be able to move quickly enough to avoid injury if some of the metal he was welding accidentally fell to the floor. He got the job and did well.

Woodwork provides opportunity to exercise the hemiplegic hand and arm. Special apparatus has been devised, mainly for use in sanding but also for sawing, planing and filing. Someone with a particular interest in woodwork may be able to produce a finished article but many patients will manage no more than sanding and polishing. It is possible to buy kits for making rustic stools and bookshelves. These are big enough to provide plenty of sanding work and can be assembled and polished or varnished very easily, so that the patient will have the satisfaction of having produced a useful finished object.

384

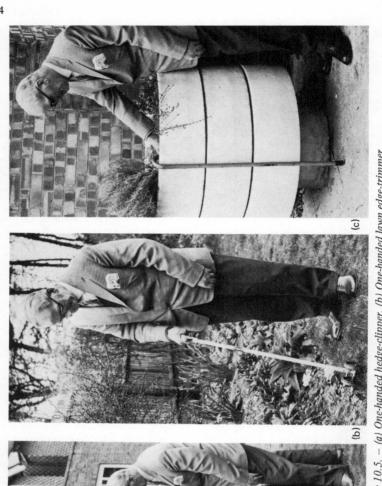

(a)

(b)

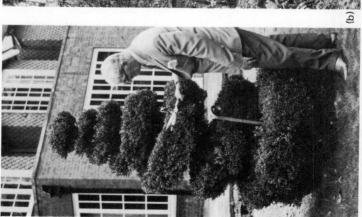

(c)

*Figure 10.5. – (a) One-handed hedge-clipper. (b) One-handed lawn edge-trimmer.
(c) Raised garden bed made from stacked pipe sections*

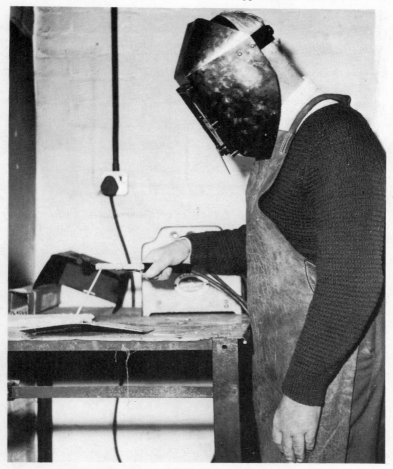

Figure 10.6. – Welding, wearing a protective helmet

The limitation in range of movement for which occupational therapy has least to offer is in extension of the fingers. The power of extension in the fingers is of a weak nature. Boyes (1970) gives a table of the amplitude of excursion of the tendons of extensor communis digitorum. This shows a small pull on the proximal interphalangeal joints and none on the terminal joints of the fingers. The interossei act primarily as adductors and abductors of the fingers, and only secondarily through their attachment to the dorsal expansions of the long extensors, as extensors of the interphalangeal joints (Backhouse, 1968, 1975). Practically speaking, finger extension is only used to extend the fingers as a preparatory movement to the strong gripping action of the flexors. This can easily be proved. A woman with a small left hand can grip the the right fist of a strong man and prevent him from extending the interphalangeal joints. He will even have difficulty in extending the metacarpophalangeal joints without raising the elbow and dorsiflexing the wrist.

Abduction of the fingers is also important for the spastic hemiplegic. The sanding and filing attachments described below work the fingers in abduction as well as extension.

Sanding block

A sanding block was made with the hand print carved about 1.3 cm (½ in) into its surface (Jones, 1950). It was observed that the thumb print should be carved in at least 1.3—2.6 cm (½—1 inch) deeper than the fingers, to encourage thumb opposition as well as extension. A metal

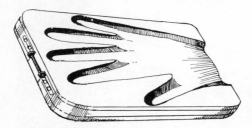

Figure 10.7. — Finger extension sanding block

frame, with screw fixation, such as is used in an embroidery frame, is fitted round the block to hold the sandpaper or the polishing pad in position (*Figure 10.7*).

The activity of sanding to get a fine surface finish will encourage active extension of the whole upper limb. If the sanding block is made to accommodate one hand over the other, with the hand extended, an upper limb which is spastic after a cerebral episode causing hemiplegia will be taken through its full range of movement by the activity of the unaffected limb. The affected side may start its excursions as a passenger, but if there is even a flicker of recovery in cerebral nerve control, the recognized system of reciprocal innervation, when movements are bilateral and similar, will bring the affected side into tune with the other. In fact the 'good' hand will help to teach the 'bad' hand. A recognized picture of position and movement must be re-established before such movement can be instigated or brought under control.

It has been found that if the patient places the good hand over the spastic one and pushes out both hands, stretching out the arms, slowly backwards and forwards, in a rhythmic stroke, a gradual relaxation of the flexors is obtained. In addition to passive extension this may encourage some static extension of the wrist and finger extensors.

Finger extension plane attachment

A finger extension block can be attached to a smoothing plane. This is designed to swivel freely so that the patient can push forward in extension in the forceful part of the movement. The withdrawal to

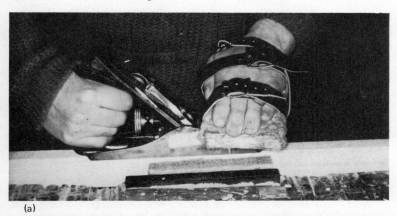

(a)

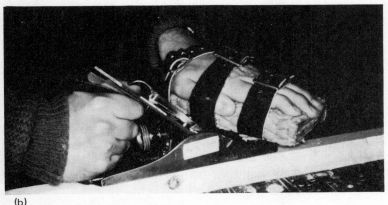

(b)

Figure 10.8. – Finger extension plane attachment. (a) Starting position. (b) The block swivels and the hand turns during the action of planing

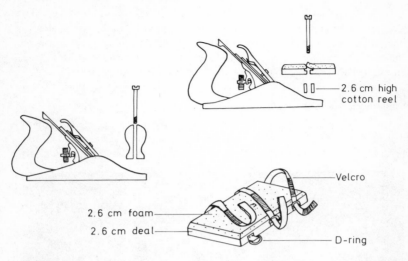

Figure 10.8 (cont.) – (c) Construction and fitting of finger extension plane attachment

flexion of the whole arm is a preparatory movement and does not require the effort or intention involved in the push forward.

The prototype block shown in use in *Figure 10.8a* and *b* has now been modified as shown in *Figure 10.8c*. The block was found to move more freely if raised up slightly from the plane by using a small piece of wood with a hole in it, such as a section of a cotton reel. The straps are now made from 2.6 cm (1 inch) webbing fastened with Velcro. The surface of the block is padded with 2.6 cm (1 inch) thick foam with a small flap cut in the centre to let the screw pass through. When the screw is tightened the foam flap covers the screw head. The hole to take the screw is 0.4 cm ($^3/_{16}$ in) in diameter, countersunk to a depth of 0.6 cm (¼ in).

File holder

Another useful method to encourage extension is a metal plate covered with leather, with an inch-wide (2.6 cm) strap threaded through slots. The fingers are inserted in the loops and the fingers held down in such passive extension as the patient can reasonably stand. The strap is fastened with a buckle so that the patient can relax. The leather covering of the metal plate is opened at one side, to take the end of a long file.

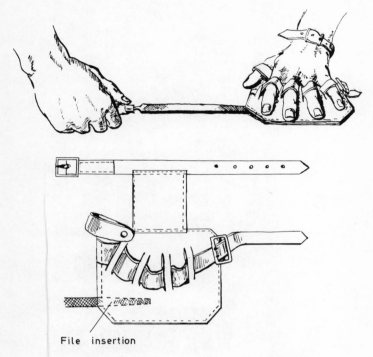

File insertion

Figure 10.9. — File holder to encourage finger extension

The patient is taught to file with long rhythmic strokes with the emphasis on extension. This type of extension splint used as a file holder must be made specifically for right or left hand as needed (*Figure 10.9*).

Bilateral saw handle

This handle can be attached to a panel saw or a tenon saw, and so convert it for two-handed use (*Figure 10.10a*). The handle must be made adjustable. It screws into place at the same angle as the grip of the saw handle so that the hands grip with the wrists in slight ulnar deviation. If necessary the affected hand can be strapped in position. The handle did not originate in the workshops at Farnham Park, but was described by Epprecht (1962). It deserves wide use, and we have therefore included working drawings (*Figure 10.10b*).

390

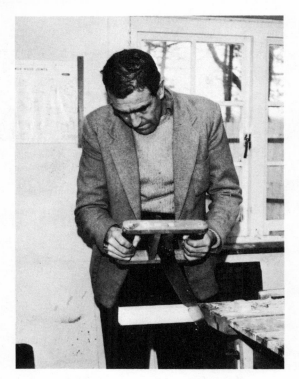

Figure 10.10a. – Bilateral saw handle

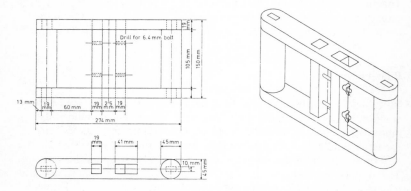

Figure 10.10b. – Detail of bilateral saw handle

Push-pull sanding box

This box works on a similar principle to a cross-cut saw. Sandbags inside grade the resistance. The box must be long enough so that two people working either side of a woodwork bench can reach it easily as

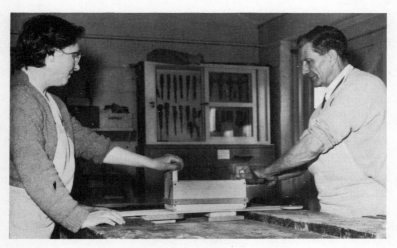

Figure 10.11. – Push-pull sanding box

in *Figure 10.11*. Sanding with this box necessitates a good thrusting movement of the arm. It also has the advantage that two people work together and this can be more stimulating than sanding alone.

SPEECH AND LANGUAGE DISORDERS AND OTHER COMMUNICATION PROBLEMS

A speech therapist is available to patients at Farnham Park, six sessions a week, and works closely with the occupational therapists. She provides a detailed assessment of the level of function in all areas of communication, and advises on ways of reinforcing her treatment while patients are in the workshops. She is also available for consultation. Therapists from all disciplines must be aware of the degree of language impairment and the level of recovery the patient has reached; for example, if he understands only simple sentences, instructions must be given at this level.

This giving of advice is not one-sided and the speech therapist expects the occupational therapist to help her in other areas of function. Can the patient take off his own jacket or does he need helping? What sort of help should she give? What sort of writing aids should he be using? What activities is he doing in the workshop to reinforce what he is learning with her? If he is practising dressing she will introduce the vocabulary of dressing during her treatment session. If he is going out on a shopping errand she may coach him in handling money. Close liaison between occupational therapist and speech therapist will widen the scope of treatment and give the patient increased opportunity for speech practice. In addition the occupational therapist is often able to insist on a better level of performance from her patient, having been told what he is able to achieve.

There are three types of speech disorder which commonly affect hemiplegic patients. Expressive dysphasia is limitation in expressive speech, with reading and writing similarly affected. Receptive dysphasia is difficulty in understanding the spoken and written word. Dysarthria is slurred speech as a result of weakness and/or inco-ordination of the speech organs. The degree of difficulty depends upon the extent of the damage to brain tissue. Defects occur in varying combinations, so that a detailed assessment is essential. It is possible for a receptive loss to be combined with some form of hearing defect, and it is a wise precaution to screen all patients with apparent receptive loss for deafness.

Speech practice for dysphasic patients

Aphasia is a complete loss and dysphasia a partial loss of language. In the workshops patients with these defects are particularly encouraged to try to communicate with other patients working nearby. Sometimes it is possible to ask a responsible patient to give individual help, though more usually a student will be given this to do as a special task. Patients with limited expressive speech are at a great disadvantage socially and often lack confidence.

The speech therapist will give guidance about the patient's level of comprehension. Someone who answers 'yes' or 'no' quite readily may not be giving the appropriate response. It is quite common to say 'yes' to sugar in tea when meaning 'no'. Once the patient can indicate yes or no meaningfully, the speech therapist will suggest the introduction of questions requiring other single words in answer. A question such as 'Do you like tea or coffee?' allows the patient to reply with a word he has just heard. The next step would be to ask questions requiring several words in the answer. Asking questions at the right level gives the patient a much better chance to communicate.

Talking to the patient while he is carrying out an activity also helps to reinforce his vocabulary. The therapist can say, 'Now lift up your arm; now put your hand into the sleeve' and get the patient to join in and say what he is doing. As comprehension improves, more sophisticated instructions can be given, such as the double order, 'Lift up your arm and put it into your sleeve'. Information can be fed to him, by telling him 'This is a cup' and then asking him what it is, and not just asking him 'What is this?'. The therapist can then build up to giving and asking for the names of several objects together.

Serial speech should be utilized. The patient may not be able to answer directly 'What day is it today?' but he may be able to manage 'Monday, Tuesday, Wednesday, *Thursday*'. Similarly, to 'How long have you been at Farnham Park?' he may reply with 'one, two, three, four, *five* days'. Automatic response can also be used such as 'cup and . . .', 'knife and . . .'.

Joining in singing during a party or social evening may not be really helping a speech defect but, even if it is only 'la-la-la', it does give confidence and helps to relieve the frustration of not being able to use the voice. Songs like 'Daisy, Daisy' may be sung automatically, rather like serial speech. When planning a party with dysphasic patients attending, it may be worth while to include deliberately a selection of familiar songs for this purpose.

Structuring situations where speech is demanded can be useful as the patient improves. If he goes out on a shopping expedition, speaking to a stranger behind the shop counter will need better speech than talking to a therapist. Another example is asking the patient to explain a simple technique to another patient.

Speech practice for dysarthric patients

Dysarthria is difficulty in articulating sounds, due to neuromuscular weakness or inco-ordination. Patients with this condition may also have problems with eating and drinking. This is also something with which the speech therapist may help.

Patients doing exercises in speech therapy in a quiet room without distraction may achieve a much higher level of function than in a noisy workshop. If the occupational therapist knows this level of achievement she will be better able to monitor speech in the workshops. Projects such as visiting shops will provide opportunities for realistic speech practice. It should be remembered that sometimes both speech and eating are made more difficult by ill-fitting dentures and that these may need checking.

Reading

Hemiplegic patients, even those without language disorders, frequently have great difficulty in concentrating for any length of time. This is often apparent where reading is concerned and a previously avid reader may not manage more than five or ten minutes. The fact that a patient can read two or three sentences without difficulty may not mean that he can read a newspaper. Building up reading tolerance may be achieved by gradually increasing the length of each reading session.

When a patient has a reading deficit, the speech therapist will assess the level of reading comprehension and oral reading. Practice reading material must be at the appropriate level and close liaison between the two therapists is therefore essential. Suitable material for reading practice must be adult in content even if simple in vocabulary. The speech therapist may be able to lend books, and also games, from her department, and the *Readers Digest* series of books, *Improve Your Reading*, is also of a suitable level. Games, such as matching sentences to pictures or, at a more advanced stage, Scrabble, can be played with another patient or with a student.

The patient's understanding of words may be increased by bombarding him on all fronts with similar vocabulary. For example, when cooking lunch in the ADL unit, he or she can be asked to read out the recipes and also to write down a shopping list of the ingredients required. If the speech therapist is forewarned, she can structure her next session with the patient to include the same subject and the same words. Advantage may also be taken of the patient's particular interests. An enthusiastic gardener, for instance, will have more incentive to relearn gardening terms. He might spend part of his workshop time working in the garden, talk with the occupational therapist about the job to be done and at the next speech therapy session read from a gardening book, practising names of plants and gardening tools.

With some patients the written word is a good stimulus for speech and it may be better for them to read instructions rather than to be given them verbally. It will, of course, be necessary to know the standard of reading the patient has reached.

Writing

If a patient is relearning to write with a partially paralysed hand, the speech therapist will need advice on the type of pen or pencil that will be most suitable, particularly if some enlargement of the handle or some other attachment is needed to aid a weak grip. If the good hand is to be used, advice will be needed on the best method of stabilizing the paper, either with the affected hand, a clip board, magnetic writing board or other device, to suit the patient. The occupational therapist will need advice on what the patient should write so that the material is within his capabilities. At the simplest level this could be copying letters and numbers. A progression would be copying words, sentences and then suitable extracts, while at an advanced level there would be spontaneous written work. It would be confusing to the patient to be asked to copy material beyond his reading capability.

Some patients are reluctant to try to write but lined paper may help, since a whole blank page can look daunting. Most people need at least to write their name on a cheque or pension book, and often a relative can bring in a specimen signature which can be copied. This achievement may provide sufficient encouragement to further efforts. Some patients, however, apparently never normally need to write and, if adamant about not wishing to regain this skill, there is no point in trying to insist.

Most reading material is printed mainly in lower case and it is usually better for the patient to start writing in this way, even though capital letters may appear to be easier. If he is allowed to practise in capital letters initially, he may have difficulty in transferring to lower case ones later. Either way he must use the same form with both therapists, not capital letters with one and lower case with the other.

The speech therapist may have books giving suitable material for copying. The series *Writing and Writing Patterns* by Marion Richardson provides good, clear lower case sentences. Copying from newspapers is not satisfactory because, although the content may be interesting, the small type and narrow columns force the eye to keep jumping across the page. When copying from a book, it helps to cover the line both above and below the one being copied. This may be done by using either two short rulers or a piece of card with a slit of suitable size cut in it.

Some patients need to learn to write with the non-dominant hand. Changing over to left-handed writing involves positioning the paper so that the top left corner is farther away from the body than the right. This slope enables the left hand to move in a more natural diagonal line across the body, and also prevents the hand from getting between the eyes and the word being written. Gardner (1958) gives clear directions on this technique.

REFERENCES

Backhouse, K. M. (1968). Functional Anatomy of the Hand. *J. Chart. Soc. Physiother.* **54–4**, 114

Backhouse, K. M. (1975). 'Aspects of hand function and dysfunction.' *J. Soc. Occup. Med.* **25**, 112

Bobath, Berta (1973). *Adult Hemiplegia: Evaluation and Treatment.* London; Heinemann

Boyes, J. H. (1970). *Bunnell's Surgery of the Hand,* p. 14. 5th Edition. Philadelphia and Toronto; Lippincott

Epprecht, Elsbeth (1962). *Gadgets and Aids for the Treatment of the Upper Extremity.* Basel; Milchsuppe, Sozialmedizinsche Abteilung des Bürgerspitals

Gardner, W. H. (1958). *Left Handed Writing Manual.* 19 North Jackson Street, Denville, Illinois; The Interstate

Jones, M. S. (1950). 'Equipment for occupational therapy.' *Br. J. phys. Med.* **13**, 249

Lezak, Muriel Deutsch (1976). *Neuropsychological Assessment.* New York; Oxford University Press

McFie, John (1975). *Assessment of Organic Intellectual Impairment.* London; Academic Press

Macdonald, E. M. (1976). *Occupational Therapy in Rehabilitation.* 4th Edition. London; Baillière Tindall

Murdoch, G. (1976). *The Advance in Orthotics.* London; Edward Arnold

Readers Digest Association in conjunction with the Disabled Living Foundation (1972). *The Easy Path to Gardening*

Richardson, Marion (1935). *Writing and Writing Patterns.* University of London Press

Richardson, N. K. (1959). *Type with One Hand.* New Rochelle, New York; South Western Publishing Co.

11

Pulmonary and Cardiac Disorders

LUNGS AND THORAX

Farnham Park lies on the edge of the Thames Valley. This situation is far from ideal in terms of climate or atmospheric conditions helpful to patients suffering from disabilities affecting the respiratory tract. Nevertheless most patients attending the Centre and going through the regimen of a five day week of graded exercise and work achieve an improved level of function whatever their disability. Someone with a chest condition, whose general level of function has improved during his stay of a month or more at Farnham Park, may find on his return home to a more suitable climatic environment that he has benefited more than it appeared on discharge from the Centre.

All patients have been encouraged to work out-of-doors whenever the weather has been suitable. They have done sedentary work at benches just outside the workshops where there is a stretch of level concrete, partly under trees which give shade on a sunny day. Some have progressed to hoeing in the garden, mowing the lawn and sweeping up fallen leaves. When the weather is cold or damp they work in the workshops. There they can do stool-seating, rug-weaving, light wood-work or industrial outwork on the bilateral hand-press. The aims of treatment have been to improve mobility of the thorax and chest expansion, with much emphasis on good posture. These patients are easily fatigued and soon show signs of this by slouching in a bad position, either sitting or standing. Their progress is slow, and their increase in work tolerance is often set back by slight episodes of respiratory infection. This is largely due to local climatic conditions.

There have been a few patients who have sustained damage to the thoracic wall or the diaphragm in accidents, from congenital weakness of muscle or fibrous tissue or from the growth of cysts. The climatic conditions have not interfered with their programme of rehabilitation.

Patients who have had multiple injuries naturally come for active rehabilitation much later, and fractures of the ribs have usually been the least considerable part of their injuries. But the long period in bed while fractures of legs or pelvis have been treated in immobilization, or the long unconsciousness from concussion, produces considerable stiffness of thoracic joints. Patients who have had haemopneumothorax show very marked loss of elasticity, and poor chest expansion. One woman, aged 24 years, developed empyema after fracture of three ribs in the left upper thoracic region. She had to undergo an operation for decortication of the lungs and came for rehabilitation 14 months after the accident. She had limited chest expansion and there was limitation of shoulder movement. She was apprehensive of using her left arm and unwilling to move it away from her side. To use her left hand at bench level she bent her elbow, and to move higher shrugged her shoulders to her ears, bending sideways in her left lumbar region. This is the usual pattern of movement observed in a patient who has a frozen shoulder. She was given a chair with a swing arm support, the sling held up by a 15-pound spring. The buoyancy of the spring gave her some confidence, and helped to improve her balance. She began to sit better and to use the arm and hand more freely. Her progress was soon interrupted by a feverish cold, and she had to return to hospital for two weeks. On readmission here she did rug-weaving on an upright loom. The spring arm support was decreased and then discarded. She then returned to Alaska, where her husband lived, a climate that must make considerable demands on physical fitness and thoracic expansion. Her shoulder movement was then fairly free and her chest expansion improving. Her general condition was satisfactory. She has written since that she is doing well.

Another patient was a housewife aged 38 years. She had two years' history of increasing dyspnoea. She had no pain but when first seen at hospital was cyanotic. Investigation showed that the left side of the thorax was occupied by a large cyst. Thoracotomy was performed, the cyst was found to be pedunculated and was excised. The left lung was noted as appearing otherwise normal. Seven weeks after operation the patient was sent for rehabilitation; she then had no dyspnoea but there was still some limitation of expansion of the base of the left lung. She easily became tired and had to rest for an hour after the midday meal. In occupational therapy she started by learning to net, sitting with her work attached to a frame 91 cm (3 ft) from the ground. This interested her, as her husband had a small farm plagued by rabbits. In about 10 days she started weaving on an upright rug loom with spring resistance of 25 pounds on each side of the beater. After a month she showed considerable improvement in chest expansion. She stopped having to rest after lunch. In the workshops she had finished weaving a 183 cm (6 ft) rug, and started woodwork. She made a clothes-horse, and a folding ironing-table, the latter to her own design, broad enough to take her husband's shirts without continuously moving them around, and high enough for her to work without stooping. She worked at a bench about 91 cm (3 ft) high, being herself 165 cm (5 ft 5 in) when standing. Her weight went up steadily from 51 kg (8 stone) on admission to 56 kg (8 stone 11 pounds) on discharge after a 10 week stay. Her vital capacity had improved from 2800 ml to 3500 ml before discharge. She went home to a heavy job of looking after five children between the ages of 13 years and 18 months and helping her husband with their small farm. Some home help was arranged for her.

Occasionally patients with diaphragmatic hernia have been accepted for rehabilitation. Two of these had histories of trauma. A man aged 31 years had had a gunshot wound through the chest, and a man aged 20 years had been injured by a bus. They were both repaired by operation some years later by which time considerable portions of their viscera had herniated into the thorax. Both these patients were keen to do woodwork right from the day of admission. With some slight caution they were allowed to start on this by making small articles such as a toy wheelbarrow, and a model ship. They both stayed for about six weeks. The younger man returned to his own job as an apprentice electrician, and the older man, who had been working in timber hauling, found himself a job in helping his father-in-law as a pest control officer — which lofty title betokened rat-catching.

CARDIAC CONDITIONS

Although cardiac patients have come for rehabilitation in different age-groups and for varying reasons, they have all shown one characteristic in common. They are very frightened people. They show confidence in the doctor or surgeon, but regard him as a miracle-worker, as no doubt he is compared with his compeers of a generation ago. The patient's attitude towards his past experiences of unpleasant sensations of bumpy rhythm, or acute pain in his heart, is one of real terror. It would appear that though the miracle has occurred to save, salvation is not entirely accepted. This may be understandable and may in fact be true with many heart conditions. It is also true that anxieties and fears will bring on symptoms which are reminiscent of previous experiences, without necessarily being a truthful forerunner of repetition of these experiences.

If these patients are to return to a reasonable amount of activity outside the hospital, their conscious attention must be diverted from the rhythm of their heartbeat. It is essential that the occupational therapist should keep closely in touch with the doctors and nurses who listen by stethoscope or feel the pulse. These tests should be carried out in their suitable surroundings, clinic or surgery. They should never be done by a therapist in a workshop. There the therapist must learn to watch the colour of the lips or ears, and the rate of breathing, without the patient's appreciating that this is being done.

The common fallacy in differentiation between 'diversional' and 'specific' occupational therapy is never more obvious. It is the diversional attribute which provides the specific value in this treatment. That the diversion should be purposeful goes without argument. The type of work suggested to the patient is of little consequence so long as in the beginning it requires minimal physical effort, and will produce an article with sufficient appeal to catch and hold the patient's interest. The patient who is unnecessarily nervous of increasing the pace of work may be encouraged by the therapist's interest in its rapid completion, and by discussion about something more desirable — and more demanding of exertion — for the future. If, on the other hand, by observation, or by information received, the therapist knows that activities should be curtailed, the converse method may be adopted. Work that is monotonous and of less interest will slow up production. We have found it convenient to keep in the background some work of this nature. The patient will find it hard to refuse if it is to help in the workshops. New tapes on aprons, and running in threads of a badly-woven rug, disentangling skeins of wool left forgotten by a patient, take little effort and are slow work. The therapist must be cunning to whistle the tune fast or slow in accordance with the measure of improvement.

Light work which may be suitable for these patients includes collating and stapling duplicated papers, compositing and electric sewing machining. A progression would be stool-seating, industrial outwork, gardening, light woodwork and light wrought iron work. In the later stages work should be positioned to encourage elevation of the shoulders and chest expansion. With medical approval patients are encouraged to go on to more strenuous activities.

On occasion it has been found that the patient's nervous fears are creating a different danger. The patient has become ashamed of fear and 'dares' himself into doing something too heavy or too quick for his stage of recovery. Warnings against this may come best from the doctor. The casual mention by the therapist that a 'dicky' heart is no more disgrace than a broken leg may be useful. For example, an Irishman who had had a fairly recent valvotomy was supposed to be raking the lawn gently to remove moss. He was observed when he suddenly seized on the roller and started pushing it along. Another elderly man who had had a coronary thrombosis was just checked before he pushed a heavy patient in a wheelchair up a steep ramp. They both muttered the same excuse, that they 'wanted to see if they could do it'.

Few therapists nowadays will have to treat an adult patient with congenital malformation or maldistribution of the circulation in relation to the heart. These are now dealt with at an early age before secondary disabilities interrupt the normal life of an adult. During youth there are so many new experiences to be met day by day, that fears and anxieties about the heartbeat will not be noticed.

12

Peptic Dysfunction

A large number of patients have been sent to Farnham Park for re-habilitation after surgical treatment for peptic dysfunction. The majority have been referred following partial gastrectomy but we have also treated patients who have had vagotomies and pyloroplasties. At one time a local surgeon used to book a bed at Farnham Park before con-firming the date of operation with his patient, in order to ensure continuity of treatment. Patients with peptic dysfunction are pre-dominantly male; we have treated almost 30 men to every one woman. Many of the patients had long histories of dyspepsia and this gradual onset is psychologically as well as physically disabling.

Eating is the simplest and commonest pleasure in life. It is the first enjoyable sensation to be appreciated by the baby at the breast and perhaps one of the last to be enjoyed in old age. The intellectual will develop eating into an art, both in the quality of the chosen food and in the methods of its preparation, and this may be accompanied by a ritual of service which enhances the grace of living. Beautiful china, glass and silver are designed for the purpose of pleasure in eating. Equally, perhaps, those persons of simpler tastes will be appreciative of a quantity of food which provides them with energy for other activities and the 'nice full feeling' that makes for a genial and kindly outlook on the world in general. Eating is, in fact, an occasion for sociability, not only as a public function when the banquet is spread, but as the regular and intimate meeting of family or friends.

With the gradual loss of pleasure in eating, the chronic dyspeptic tends to lose his place in social life. He cannot eat what others can; special dishes must be cooked for him. The sufferer soon begins to look upon himself as being different from his fellow men. Even with care in choosing food, pain is expected after eating. Courage is said to be an expendable quality. There are few people who can stand up to pain which is incessantly and inevitably repeated. Vitality and energy are sapped by the inability to digest adequate nourishment. With these factors as the side-effects of peptic dysfunction it is easy to envisage a general disintegration of personality, a lowering of morale and a lack of confidence. These are the mental characteristics commonly noted in the patient with a long history of dyspepsia; they require special consideration in a rehabilitation programme planned to make permanently effective medical or surgical treatment undertaken to eliminate the original cause.

In studying records of patients it has been observed that many have very long histories of symptoms. For example, 20 male patients, all under the age of 30 years, had an average history of duodenal symptoms of five years before the operation for partial gastrectomy. Of these, 16 had dyspepsia for eight to nine years. Patients in higher age-groups frequently laid claim to 20 years. Many had previous medical treatment in hospital and probably had tried unorthodox panaceas without success. It would appear advantageous in such cases that a period of rehabilitation should be spent away from home and without the habitual consideration and sympathy of the family. The diet arranged for them with a graduated approach to ordinary food is of the first importance. Correct breathing and general exercises will help to mobilize the thorax and develop the abdominal muscles. The place of the occupational therapist is to provide and suggest work that they can carry on in a good position and to watch and remind them to maintain it. The work must be arranged to make gradually increasing demands for expenditure of energy. This will arouse the appetite for food. The work must be sufficiently interesting to keep the conscious mind thoroughly occupied and so divert the thoughts from symptoms of abdominal discomfort.

Occupational therapy for all patients with abdominal disorders has aimed to provide a 'general tonic' in addition to improving the tone of the abdominal muscles. The work that has been found suitable is much the same as for those patients who have had disabilities affecting the spine. In early stages they must avoid heavy lifting or working in a stooping position. The work has been planned to encourage small turning movements of the body with a view to developing the abdominal muscles, preventing contractions of an abdominal scar if there has been an operation, loosening up the joints of the thorax and improving chest expansion when sitting or standing. Considerable attention has been paid to maintaining the angle of pelvic tilt so that the abdominal muscles work in the inner range of contraction and the weight of the intestines is supported in the basin of the pelvis and not dragging on the mesentery where it is attached to the posterior abdominal wall. These are all aims of treatment and precautions which have been previously discussed in sections considering the re-education of the postural reflex and the details of treatment of spinal conditions.

Treatment of patients who have undergone partial gastrectomy has now become standardized and this plan is used as a basis for treating all other patients with peptic dysfunction. Treatment normally lasts three to four weeks. In the remedial gymnasium and in the physiotherapy department the patients are given graduated exercises, and in the occupational therapy workshops graduated work. Whenever possible they are treated out-of-doors. In the dining room they are gradually encouraged to return to a normal diet. This team approach enables the patient to regain confidence in his physical ability, and in his ability to eat normally again, in a very short period of time. Patients who are not given this intensive treatment post-operatively are inclined to return home to their previous invalid existence because they cannot believe that their condition has been cured.

The occupational therapist will be aiming at providing work to rebuild the power of the abdominal muscles, to promote healing by increasing the circulation in the area of the scar and to build up physical fitness, at the same time stimulating the appetite. It will also be necessary to improve the patient's psychological state and feeling of well-being. This can be done by getting the patient interested and involved in the work that he is undertaking. Such involvement helps to give a maximum sense of security and empathy, and leaves no time to dwell morbidly on his symptoms.

Work in the garden is ideal for these patients, starting with light activities, such as hoeing or sweeping up leaves, which require slight flexion of the abdomen but no real bending. In the early stages of treatment the patient should work within easy reach of a lavatory. The work should be graded to include more bending and heavier tasks, building up to digging or cross-cut sawing before discharge.

Some patients are not interested in working out-of-doors, and sometimes the weather is inclement. Woodwork and metalwork can be used to provide rhythmical movements to stimulate contraction of the abdominal muscles, and both activities can be upgraded. Wood-turning is useful in the later stages of treatment. Painting and decorating are other suitable later-stage activities, although the smell may contra-indicate them for some people.

Some authorities suggest that it is possible to find a relationship between the individual's attitude towards his job and the condition of peptic dysfunction. It may be found interesting to make some assessment of a patient's normal occupation and the satisfaction found therein. There are patients who will talk more freely over their work than they will when sitting on a chair in an office. The information gleaned by the therapist may be of interest to those in charge of social welfare. It is obvious that in the social report there may be information that does not tally with the patient's opinion of the trials and tribulations he suffers in the outside world. Domestic responsibilities, housing problems and rates of pay come into the picture as much as the job of work. Neither the doctor, social worker nor therapist can dictate to alter another's chosen pattern of life. It may be possible to recognize that certain factors in the pattern could be deleterious, but the interdependence of circumstances and characters may be too involved to justify interference without risk of making bad worse.

Monotony of work is sometimes cited as being a possible factor in developing a tendency to peptic dysfunction. If this is true, then the encouragement of a satisfactory hobby for leisure hours should help in treatment, but it is not always possible to ensure the practicality of this solution.

On one occasion a skilled toolmaker confided that most of his workmates had symptoms of peptic dysfunction and that he had more or less drawn out of the hat the role of the 'guinea-pig' who would face a partial gastrectomy for the alleviation of his symptoms.

He was a well-paid man, but his job, though requiring skill, was monotonous. He was about 32 years of age, married, with two children and unwilling to change his job to one which, though more interesting, might not have enabled his family and himself to continue the standard of living which he and his wife felt desirable. Instead of employing him in metalwork and fitting it was therefore suggested that he should take up woodwork, which he might continue as a home hobby. He learnt the technique well and was able to take away with him several nice small pieces, a coffee table and a corner cupboard. He was obviously not anxious to speed his return to work, and his rehabilitation took seven and a half weeks, which is almost double the average time needed after a partial gastrectomy. The replies to follow-up enquiries have, however, gradually improved in tone and the last one, 15 months after discharge, stated that he had completely recovered.

Another patient, a very pretty young girl with a two year history of peptic dysfunction, worked in the same bank as her father and travelled to and fro in his company. She led a restricted social life and, despite a charming, light singing voice and some capacity for dramatic mimicry, had not joined any of the choral or dramatic societies for which the bank was justly famous. Her rehabilitation was not successful, her symptoms recurred, and it was only when she changed her job to become a tapestry saleswoman in a needlework shop that she reported a full recovery. Subsequently she married a man she had met at Farnham Park and now leads a busy domestic and social life with no untoward symptoms. Escaping from the eagle eye of her father and making social contacts outside the family did more for her than any medical rehabilitation.

Another man had records of both an injury to his back three years earlier and partial gastrectomy for a duodenal ulcer. He was aged 40 years when he was sent for rehabilitation. His work history ranged over boxing trainer, poultry man, engraver and long-distance lorry driver. In the occupational therapy workshops he started with leatherwork and quickly progressed to woodwork. He showed considerable capacity for accuracy and careful work, but he had found the job of engraving nameplates for instrument panels in aeroplanes a monotonous and boring job. He continued to complain of his back, though some medical authorities questioned whether there was much physical cause for his symptoms. After a rather prolonged 12-week period of rehabilitation he made up his mind to train as an instrument-maker at the local Skill Centre. He returned several times just to pay a visit to the workshops, and his complaints and his symptoms seemed to disappear gradually but steadily.

A man of 39 years had complained of epigastric pain after food for 10 years. This pain, in his own mind at any rate, was associated with times of worry. Between the ages of 15 and 39 years he had been in 10 jobs, the longest-lasting being his apprenticeship as a toolmaker for five years, and as a chief engine-room artificer for five years. He had only once actually been off work on account of the epigastric pain and that was during his naval service. He had a partial gastrectomy and was then sent direct to us for treatment. In the workshops he showed interest and co-operation. He was at first keen to try woodwork and started to make a pelmet for a window in his own home. Then another patient was admitted who had lost his right hand and forearm just below the elbow and the tips of the fingers of his left hand in an accident at work. This young man was badly incapacitated and we had the idea of making for him a temporary prosthesis to fit over the still-bandaged right stump. The engineer—toolmaker showed great interest and sympathy. He made a most useful gadget which fitted into a leather gauntlet laced up over the bandages. He found great satisfaction in seeing the young man, an unskilled machine operator, learning to use an oxy-acetylene torch held in the temporary prosthesis. He also made him other tools, including a table knife which fitted into the clamp of the prosthesis. This skilled man mentioned on several occasions how much more pleasurable it was to be doing that sort of work than working with machines for man's destruction. After he had finished the prosthesis, he returned to his woodwork and finished his pelmet for the furnishing of his own home. After four weeks' stay in the Centre he returned to his own job, which at that time consisted of travelling up and down the country inspecting machinery. The follow-up reports after three and then 15 months were satisfactory.

Case histories of patients who have had partial gastrectomy for peptic dysfunction appear incomplete without mention of the three brothers F. The first treated, D. F., at the age of 47 years had a history of 14 years of dyspepsia. A duodenal ulcer had been diagnosed radiologically and treated medically 10 years before partial gastrectomy. He was a gardener at Farnham Park and did not fancy the idea of coming as a patient after operation. Five months later he had acute abdominal pain which necessitated further operations for peritonitis and appendicitis. About six weeks after the last episode he came as an out-patient for the full day's programme of exercise, work and graduated diet. In occupational therapy he started doing sedentary work but soon went on to woodwork and metalwork. He was discharged as fit for his own work after eight weeks. Since then he has been doing his full day's work, and in his spare time he serves as a special constable as well as lending a helping hand with hay-making, setting posts and fencing, and clipping hedges for his neighbours and friends, among whom the writer is pleased to include herself.

His brothers, P. F., aged 55 years, and C. F., aged 43 years, followed him. They made uninterrupted recoveries and went back to their own jobs, which included strenuous work, after between five and six weeks of rehabilitation. Their regular social visits have given assurance of their continuing health and activity. These three brothers came from different hospitals, and their operations were performed by different surgeons. The writer's longstanding knowledge of their continued well-being makes them memorable.

The follow-up reports quoted after three months may give a picture that is unduly rosy. These have been chosen as the most informative because so many patients get careless about replying time and again to inquiries at longer intervals. We may not know with any certainty what has happened later on. At any rate the results as quoted show an immediate improvement in health and return to work after a comparatively short period in hospital and rehabilitation centre. This must be of some comfort to the patient who has endured many years of most trying and disabling symptoms.

Those patients who have recurrent symptoms (sometimes diagnosed specifically as 'post-gastrectomy syndrome') well established before being sent for rehabilitation show a much less satisfactory result. Fifteen patients of this type were treated over a five year period. Only eight of these patients returned to work in three months, three went back to hospital for further treatment, one was retrained at a Skill Centre, three did not reply to any of the inquiries sent to them. This is a rather depressing story after much longer periods of rehabilitation than is customary for patients sent directly after surgical treatment.

This group of patients who have recurrent symptoms presents, of course, a difficult problem. They have lost confidence in themselves and in others, lost interest in work and play and indeed in everything but their own symptoms. They need a great deal of individual attention and encouragement, yet if this is too openly displayed they sometimes react with exaggerated symptoms, hoping for more attention. It is understandable that people suffering from such long-standing disabilities should be doubtful, if not suspicious, of treatment. They have tried many panaceas, both orthodox and unorthodox, and still they suffer from pain and nausea after food.

It would appear that the only course left open to the therapist is to encourage the patient to relegate the unpleasant sensations to a compartment of the unconsciousness to which little attention is given. If the habit can be formed of keeping the attention fixed on the job in hand, it may help to distract the conscious attention from the symptoms. If the work is of a type that demands both attention and exertion the worker will inevitably get hungry and so go to a meal with some appetite.

Perhaps if the individual realizes that others may suffer from the same symptoms he will feel a little comforted, less different, less outcast from the pleasures of normal people. There are many who suffer from nausea before an important examination or having to speak in public. Some may outgrow this with practice or when repeated success in the event breeds self-confidence. Others will say, resignedly, that they always get 'butterflies in the tummy' before an ordeal and that it is just one of those things they have got used to. Such a habit of thought takes time to become established.

13

Assessment for Return to Work

The majority of patients attending Farnham Park have had no difficulty in returning to their original work. About 10 per cent have needed help, so that we have been able to spend a substantial time tailoring assessment to the needs of individual patients.

When formal assessment was first started we needed material with which to work. The considerable resources of the workshops and the rest of the Rehabilitation Centre were at our disposal but there was little to help in assessing ability in English, mathematics or clerical work. It was decided to devise some form of test battery and we made this a project, the occupational therapy staff giving up one evening a week to work on it. We were fortunate in having the help of a retired headmistress who designed some of the papers for us. The final result was a basic battery of exercises and scoring and interpretation systems of different levels suitable for adults, some of which are still in use today.

Parts of the workshops were rearranged because somewhere quiet was needed where patients could work through paper and pencil tests without interruption. The storeroom was turned into the new assessment room, the stores were moved into the students' cloakroom and a room in the main building was found for the students.

More recently the British Psychological Society has agreed that occupational therapists may be trained to use certain categories of psychological tests. Members of the staff at Farnham Park have attended the courses and have learned to use a number of standardized tests which provide much greater accuracy of assessment in certain areas. They have also learned the importance of administering each test in a consistent way and of keeping careful records of test results in order to build up a file of knowledge about the performance of patients. More realistic conclusions from the test results of any individual can then be reached by comparing them with the results of other patients as well as the test standardization groups. A psychological test is, however, basically another tool and the main criterion of assessment is the way in which a patient functions overall in the nearest equivalent to a work situation.

The use of psychological tests by occupational therapists does not mean that we no longer need the help of a psychologist in assessing some of our patients; indeed, the reverse is true. We now have a better understanding of the contribution of psychologists and therefore know when to enlist their help. There can be a very good partnership between the two professions, the psychologist making a prediction about the patient's future performance and the occupational therapist assessing the extent to which this prediction worked out in a practical situation.

We have found that on the whole an assessment based on the use of realistic work available in the workshops is of more value than one based on artificial work samples or formal paper and pencil tests. A job that is being done for a purpose offers more stimulus than one being done as a test piece. This is especially true for patients with a secondary modern or technical school background who have not been brought up on competitive examinations.

Another factor is that when time is available, a much more realistic assessment can be gained, even accepting that a trial of this kind will not be as stringent as the real job situation. In New York, psychologists have devised the Tower system of assessment. They have taken a number of jobs, typical of local industry where many of their patients work, such as jewellery-making, machine-sewing, welding, shorthand and typing, and have analysed the basics of what the jobs involve. The shorthand and typing section requires the patient to go through a considerably shortened version of a shorthand and typing course. The welding assessment requires the patient to take various measurements, as if preparing a job, and to make the types of movement used in welding, with a pencil attached to the welding torch. Professor W. Usdane, one of the psychologists concerned with devising the Tower system, visited Farnham Park. We asked whether, in his opinion, we should stop assessing patients on actual welding or typing and give them the more formalized Tower assessment instead. He was horrified and explained that the only reason for the existence of the Tower system was that no workshop facilities like those at Farnham Park were available in New York.

Work-related activities at Farnham Park have included painting, pointing, bricklaying, labouring, gardening, centre lathe turning, milling, welding, industrial outwork assembly, drawing plans or diagrams, woodwork, clerical work and also using the telephone switchboard and doing housework.

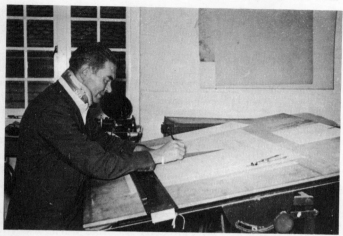

Figure 13.1. – Assessing a draughtsman's ability to return to work. This drawing board, made in the workshops, is adjustable in height and angle. A sliding ruler, working on cords at the sides, has a set square attached. This makes the board also suitable for the patient with only one hand

There is a popular misconception that work assessment is only concerned with finding out what work the patient can manage. It is equally important to assess whether he can do any work at all since even a negative result supplies useful information.

Work assessment carried out by an occupational therapist will inevitably be somewhat subjective. There are two ways of making it more objective. One is to include a number of specific tests which produce scores that can be related to the performance of others, for example, psychological tests and the Disablement Resettlement Officer's (DRO's) tests. The other safeguard is to involve more than one therapist in the assessment process, so that at least two opinions are reflected in the final report.

Assessment must be a continuous process. The patient's physical condition should improve and his attitude of mind will often change during his period of rehabilitation. It is vital, therefore, that assessment should start early in treatment so that when the patient is ready for discharge, provision has already been made for his future. It is wrong to delay the patient's return to work by postponing his assessment until he has completed his treatment.

Dr C. J. S. O'Malley, who started the Rehabilitation Centres at Garston Manor, Watford, and at Camden Road, London, based on his experience in rehabilitation in the RAF, had a motto for his patients: 'Rehabilitation always, resettlement sometimes, and retraining as infrequently as possible'. There is still a great deal of wisdom in this adage. If a patient has already established himself in a career and has built up a good relationship with an employer, he is much more likely to get sympathetic treatment on returning to his old place of employment. If, handicapped by his disability, he goes to a new employer or, more difficult still, to a new employer and a new, untried form of work, he may not succeed. This is particularly a problem for someone who, due to his disability, may require time off work for further treatment, or where there is a poor prognosis.

Patients who are being assessed for return to work fall broadly into three groups:

those who cannot travel to work but could work if they got there;

those who can travel to work but could not work when they arrived;

those who would have difficulty with both travelling and working.

Once the patient's most pressing problem has been identified, the treatment at the Centre will be directed towards his particular needs. The remedial gymnast will play a bigger part if the problem is lack of mobility, the occupational therapist if there is a work problem; either way, they will supplement each other's treatment.

Mobility

Mobility will affect not only a patient's ability to get to work but also his ability to manage once he has arrived. Driving to a local firm in an invalid tricycle may be easy enough but can he get from the car park to the place where he works? What about entrance steps or stairs? Is there a lift and can he manage it? Perhaps as a concession he may use a goods lift but are the doors too heavy for him to open? Where are the lavatory facilities and where is the canteen? Can he get to them? Many of the questions will only be resolved by a personal visit to the place of work.

Farnham Park has good facilities for assessing patients' mobility. Patients are taken out on graduated walks, especially in the summer, by the physiotherapists and remedial gymnasts. They can be asked to go on errands to the village, less than a mile away, either with an occupational therapy student or alone. They can be sent on a bus trip into the nearby town, Slough, and back again, accompanied by a student and with a pause for tea in the middle. Expeditions requiring greater mobility can be arranged by giving the patient a shopping list which entails visits to different shops in different parts of the town, as well as two bus trips. Once we sent a young hemiplegic into town by himself with a 6.3 kg (14 lb) sledge hammer which needed repair. Rush hour travel may also be included.

Assessment of a patient's ability to drive is carried out by a co-operative local driving school in their dual control car. The instructor advises the patient on his best course of action, whether, because of his handicap, he will be required to retake the driving test, whether he needs adaptations to his car or should get one with an automatic drive, whether he should apply for an invalid tricycle, or whether he will need further practice. The instructor also reports his findings to the occupational therapist. This service is paid for by the patient if he can afford it; if not, from special funds.

The law requires anyone who holds a driving licence to notify the Driver and Vehicle Licensing Centre if he becomes aware at any time that he has any medical or physical condition which may affect (either immediately or in the future) his ability to drive safely. Only temporary conditions, not expected to last more than three months, are excluded. The duty to report such a condition rests with the patient.

Activities of daily living (ADL)

Patients will be unlikely to think of returning to work until they are able to be personally independent. This may sound obvious but there have been cases of patients who were prevented from returning to work because of an inability to get dressed in the morning. In other words, dressing proved a more complex activity than work.

One patient, a young man who had suffered a hemiplegia with residual paralysis of both arm and leg, had a job supervising female clerks in an office. He could manage the job, he had no speech defect, he could cope with public transport and could even play golf. He could not, however, pull up his trousers when he went to the lavatory. It was not until the occupational therapist had made extensive adaptations to his trousers that he was able to return to work.

A proportion of women patients will be going back to being housewives and need assessing to see whether they can manage this work. Others may be going out to work in a domestic capacity and some men may be assessed for such jobs as sweeping up or valeting.

Assessment and training in activities of daily living are discussed on pages 92–95.

DIFFERENT TYPES OF ASSESSMENT

Assessment for the patient who expects to return to a particular job

The therapist will first find out from the patient exactly what the job entails, in considerable detail. Sometimes, for example if the patient has had a head injury, it may be necessary to get this information from someone else such as the employer or Disablement Resettlement Officer. This will give a baseline for assessing the patient's ability and stamina. A well-equipped workshop may make it possible to simulate the patient's own job, although it is rarely possible to produce conditions that are as stringent as the real thing.

One of our patients was a hairdresser who was recovering from a severe episode of low back pain. In view of all that he was capable of doing in woodwork and in remedial gymnastics, we felt he could manage his own work, but he lacked confidence. We borrowed all the necessary equipment from the Centre's visiting hairdresser, and one afternoon he shampooed, set and combed out all five of the occupational therapy students' hair in the ADL unit. (We could not ask for volunteer patients because this would have taken trade from the visiting hairdresser.) He managed this trial with no difficulty, his back felt no ill effects and he was satisfied, although this one afternoon was far less demanding than his normal full-time employment, and went back to work.

Another patient was a steeplejack who had had a lower limb fracture. He was able to manage the wall bars and the scaffolding in the gymnasium but he was worried about having the stamina to climb tall chimneys. Near the workshops there is a two-storey old barn, used as a store, with a 4.5 m (15 ft) iron ladder up one wall. We worked out how many times he would have to climb this ladder to equal the height of a tall chimney. Every morning for a week he climbed up and down the ladder non-stop, watched by an occupational therapist who counted the trips for him, to give the equivalent of going both up and down his chimney without even pausing at the top. He was discharged feeling quite sure he could manage his job.

An elderly man, who had had his leg amputated above the knee, was a builder's labourer. He wanted to return to his original job, and this was open to him if he could manage the work. We were dubious because, although he walked well in his prosthesis, he was elderly and walking constantly on uneven ground could be hazardous. In the grounds at Farnham Park there was an old air-raid shelter, partly hidden by rhododendron bushes. We persuaded the Administrative Officer that this could be a hazard to patients and should be filled in with hard core, of which there was plenty in the old kitchen garden on the other side of the Centre. During his two or three daily sessions in the workshops, the patient loaded up a wheelbarrow, pushed it over gravel paths, an asphalt road and finally through a flower bed to tip the hard core into the shelter before going back for more. He did the job so quickly and effectively that we were convinced that he could manage to work as a builder's labourer.

Assessment for resettlement in an alternative type of work

When a patient cannot go back to his original job he may well need help to find an alternative. His interests and aptitudes, his previous experience, his physical limitations and the location of his home in relation to work opportunities must all be considered. Sometimes it may be possible to try out jobs in the workshops, in the engineering section or in the clerical section, to assess whether the patient has an interest or an aptitude for a particular type of work. Sometimes the DRO may suggest some job that is available and which can be simulated in the workshops.

An Irishman was admitted to Farnham Park, at the request of the DRO for work assessment. He had suffered from schizophrenia and spent many years in an institution in Ireland but had recently responded to a new drug and been discharged to go to live with his sister in Slough, some two miles from the Centre. Understandably he did not want to go away again, so he came to us instead of to an Employment Rehabilitation Centre. After a period of time spent in trying him out on various simple tasks, encouraging him to mix with other patients and attempting to build up his confidence, we heard that the DRO had a possible job for him, as a tea boy on a building site. Most of the men working there were also Irish and it was hoped that they would be sympathetic — but could he manage the job? We practised with him until he was able to go alone to the local shops to buy a designated amount of tea and sugar, and to bring back the correct change. We did not suggest that he fetch milk because it was a half mile walk to the shops. We got him making tea and bringing it to the staff in their office, and he also practised pouring water from a teapot into cups on a tray and carrying this tray up and down the workshop. We were able to report that it seemed likely he would manage the job of tea boy.

Another patient was a bricklayer with osteoarthritis of the hips. Although he improved with treatment, he still had a limited range of movement and walked with a stick. We tried him laying bricks (there is usually some wall at Farnham Park that needs repairing), which he managed, but he had difficulty in getting down to the lower section of the wall. He would certainly have had difficulty in climbing a ladder and working on scaffold boards. Some form of clerical work seemed the only possibility for him but he had left school at the age of 14 many, many years before and had always worked out-of-doors. He went into our clerical section with some reluctance and worked on a variety of different tasks. He showed an aptitude for figures and confessed that arithmetic had been one of his best subjects at school. During the three months or so that he was with us he came to accept that perhaps he did have sufficient ability to take a clerical job. He was fortunate in finding work with a builder's merchant where he could combine his previous knowledge of building materials with a largely sedentary job.

A young hemiplegic man had been a bus conductor and this was the job he wanted to go back to more than anything else. He loved the buses but he was almost entirely aphasic and showed no signs of recovery, so that a return to his old job was out of the question. He was unrealistic about his condition and required a great deal of convincing. His potential was so severely limited that a sweeping-up job seemed to be about all he could manage. We gave him the responsibility of sweeping up the woodwork section at the end of each afternoon which he did with some lack of enthusiasm. Then the DRO came up with a sweeping-up job at a local factory and we arranged for him to go to the interview with an occupational therapist to speak on his behalf. He was given the job but we felt that this was due more to the effect of the occupational therapist's enthusiasm on the personnel officer than to the personnel officer's assessment of the patient's ability.

Assessment for resettlement with no particular job in mind

It is easy to forget that many people drifted quite at random into their original employment and are happy to do so again provided they are earning. Some patients are so minimally employable that assessment for work is mainly concerned with finding anything at all that they can do which may be of use to a prospective employer.

The patient's personality may be one of his most important assets. If he is friendly, co-operative, relates well to others, is reliable, punctual, sensible and of good appearance, these qualities may compensate for weaknesses in other areas (*see* check list on personal assessment, page 420). Any such attributes should be included when writing an assessment report.

The following basic check list for the practical assessment of unskilled patients may be useful:

Reading, e.g. simple signs and notices, newspapers.

Writing, e.g. own name, simple lists or forms (speed and accuracy only slightly important).

Handling money — giving change.

Walking — how far?

Use of public transport.

Shopping, with money and list of commissions.

Messenger jobs — taking letters or messages to selected members of staff who will report back later.

Cleaning, sweeping up, washing windows, dusting.

Tea-making.

Lifting and carrying.

Industrial outwork.

Gardening — including reliability when unsupervised, and ability to return tools.

Climbing stairs, scaffolding, ladders.

Supervising parking of cars.

As may be seen, this is general observable information which may require the creation of deliberate test situations but which is not readily amenable to systematic comparison or evaluation.

Some of these assessments take careful planning, however. We once wanted to assess a young man's ability to supervise the parking of cars. There is a small car park behind the workshops taking five cars. We arranged that three staff members would drive up in turn to be parked, drive away again and return to park a second time but not in too rapid succession. The result of the assessment was a failure. The patient was quite unable to position himself in relation to a car and was in imminent danger, most of the time, of being run over. He was also quite incapable of deciding whether a car should go off to one side or the other.

Assessment for retraining

There is only a limited number of training courses available in Skill Centres, colleges for the disabled and local training colleges. Usually the DRO will be able to supply information on both the physical and educational requirements for such courses. On occasion we have sent a patient to spend a day at the local Skill Centre to see for himself what courses were available and which of these might interest him.

Physical requirements are not always obvious. A television engineer must normally be able to carry television sets for delivery to customers, unless he has already been guaranteed a bench job. A motor mechanic must have sufficient knee bend to get into and drive most makes of car. A watch and clock repairer or an instrument maker must not have sweaty hands, otherwise his work will rust.

Most training courses require the patient to have a certain educational level in mathematics and perhaps in English; this is where accurate testing, scoring and result analysis need to be carried out. A welder will have to measure accurately and understand decimals; a centre lathe turner will require a higher level of both decimals and fractions; while a clerical worker will need good basic English and the ability to add up figures. The DRO will be able to give information about the minimal educational requirements. Some examples of the mathematical levels required are given on page 427. Many of our patients have needed considerable practice to bring them up to the level they were at when they left school, or even beyond it, before they were eligible to start a training course. We have found it helpful to give the patient the opportunity to practise the skill in which he hopes to train whenever this is possible. One such patient, who eventually trained as a welder, is described on page 52.

Two other patients who were successfully trained illustrate the process of assessment. A man aged 34 years with Friedreich's ataxia was admitted to Farnham Park for work assessment soon after being made redundant. He was intelligent and as a boy had passed for entry to a grammar school but the weakness of his intrinsic muscles made it difficult to hold a pencil and write, so he was not able to take up his place. At the age of 18 he had been trained in leatherwork at a college for the disabled. Later he developed bilateral nystagmus and was trained at a workshop for the blind to make chimney sweeps' brushes, which he then did for 10 years. Latterly he had worked as a driller in a local factory. In addition to the weakness and wasting of all the small muscles, there was sensory loss in both hands. He had a high-stepping gait and found stair-climbing difficult. He used an invalid tricycle.

We agreed that his greatest asset was his intelligence and that, in view of his disabilities and the fact that he had a progressive illness, some form of clerical work would be most appropriate. So we set out to find some way of helping him to write. We explored all the reference books and tried a variety of writing aids without success. Then we made him a Chessington median nerve splint to bring his thumb into a functional position. A rubber band linked his thumb, index finger and the pencil together, thus compensating for his weakened first dorsal interosseous muscle — and he could write. He needed practice to improve his speed and we found him various writing jobs in the workshops. On assessment, his mathematical ability was above average and his English and spelling proved satisfactory.

The DRO suggested that he might be trained as a telephone order clerk and he was sent to Queen Elizabeth Training College, Leatherhead, for assessment. They thought more highly of him and recommended a six months' book-keeping course. While he was on the waiting list for this we continued with his writing practice, working on exercises similar to those in the first part of his course. We felt that this extra coaching would help him to keep up with others since his writing was still not quite up to normal speed.

On completion of the book-keeping course he got a good job, and later tried to study for accountancy examinations. He could probably have managed these without too much difficulty when younger but, with his increasing disability and the years of unstimulating work behind him, it did not prove possible.

The second patient was a tall, obese young man aged 28 years who had had infantile left hemiplegia. His father had died when he was 14 years of age and he had helped his mother to carry on the family butcher's shop. Eventually this had got to be too much for his mother, who was aged 62 years when he was admitted to Farnham Park, and the business had been sold. Our patient had done various decorating jobs at home and for relatives, and had been seeing the DRO regularly for 18 months without being successfully placed.

This patient's major problem was a lack of confidence in his own abilities. Being tall and fat, with little useful function in his left arm and hand, he felt conspicuous. He walked well but needed a stick. He had led a sheltered life, had been educated privately, was not really used to mixing with people, and was very shy.

We tried him on a variety of activities to prove to him as much to ourselves that he had ability. He did some simple woodwork, using his affected hand when encouraged to do so. He did some painting and decorating which he enjoyed, and although ladders were a problem initially he progressed to using scaffolding and worked to a good standard. Then he went into the printing section where he showed considerable perseverance but not great accuracy. He joined in social evenings with the other patients and was even persuaded to dance. He helped to run the hospital shop, which is open at lunch time, and showed enthusiasm for this. His confidence improved.

We assessed his intelligence which was average, his mathematical ability which was reasonably good, and his English which was poor and a subject he disliked. We also asked a psychologist to see him and her findings agreed with ours.

Since he had some facility for figures and clearly needed a sedentary job, we decided that training in general office routine or even, possibly, book-keeping would be appropriate. He was trained, after some delay, in the former and on his return home he obtained a job as a clerk. In his follow-up report he told us that he was earning a reasonable wage, that his general health had improved and that he was content.

TECHNIQUES AND AREAS OF ASSESSMENT

As has been shown so far, work assessment should be a continuous process, producing a mixture of complementary information, to the level of resettlement envisaged and incorporating the following:

Social and personal considerations.
Physical capabilities, both observed and tested.
Specific areas of work, tested accurately with results interpreted realistically.
General observation of work done during treatment.

A summary can then be made of the conclusions drawn and the options which seem appropriate for the patient. More details of how to obtain the information are given below.

Assessment of the patient as a person

When a patient is first admitted for treatment it is usually already evident if he is likely to have resettlement problems. An indirect assessment can be started immediately, with the therapist observing him doing remedial work in the early stages of treatment. Further information will be available in reports from other members of the treatment team at case conferences. Assessment has been defined as informed and organized observation (Macdonald, 1976), and this is what it should be.

A check list for assessment as a person should include:

Interests, aptitudes and hobbies.
Personality and confidence.
Initiative, perseverance and reliability.
Punctuality, neatness and good appearance.
Motivation.
Attitudes towards employment and towards disability.
Relationship with Centre staff and with other patients.
Ability to follow written and verbal instructions.
General standard of work; speed, accuracy and care of tools.

This assessment can take the form of a general introduction to a report of work assessed, like the practical assessment for unskilled work (*see* page 417), or of comments relating to specific assessment areas such as 'perseveres more in physical activities than in intellectual work'.

Psychological tests

A number of these tests are now used by suitably trained occupational therapists in the workshops, mainly as a screening process and to get some basic data about a patient at the beginning of his formal assessment. To enhance their value the therapist collects statistics of patients' test results, both successes and failures, to provide normative data against which to compare future test results.

Standard Progressive Matrices and Mill Hill Vocabulary Scale

The former uses non-verbal items to measure a person's present capacity for intellectual activity. The latter uses vocabulary questions to assess the fund of information he has acquired. When these tests are used together they show the psychological significance of any discrepancies between the two.

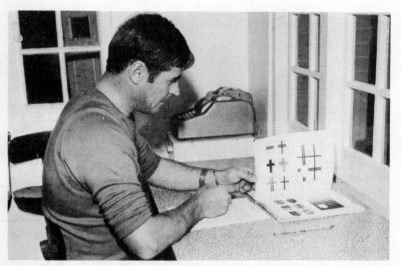

Figure 13.2. — Patient working through the Standard Progressive Matrices in the quiet of the assessment room

The matrices can be given to people with a broad range of ability levels, and the test is especially useful with those whose language skills are limited. It can be made more difficult for more able people by applying it with a time limit, for example 20 minutes.

It should be understood however, that this is not a totally 'culture free' test because it assumes familiarity with geometric shapes; and some people and some cultural groups do not have this knowledge.

AH4 and AH5 intelligence tests

These are progressively more demanding tests. The former is a test of general intelligence and the latter of high-grade intelligence. Both include items having a verbal or numerical bias followed by items of a diagrammatic character. The AH4 is more often used than the AH5 which is usually kept as a reserve test to enable the therapist to assess the occasional patient of high-grade intelligence with resettlement problems.

General clerical test

This tests clerical speed and accuracy, numerical ability and verbal facility. It is usually administered as part of our clerical assessment, which is described later. It does not supersede the more practical tests commonly used by occupational therapists but it can complement them. The total score for the test gives a measure of a general aptitude weighted in favour of the person who possesses clerical aptitude or skills. This means that when interpreting the test results, the patient's performance can be compared with that of clerical staff in industry and commerce, and of people with similar levels of education. There is a speed factor in this test and it may cause results which are inconsistent with those obtained from untimed practical tests.

Marianne Frostig Developmental Test of Visual Perception

It is hoped to include this test in the near future at Farnham Park. Although devised as an aid for evaluating the perceptual skills of young children, it can be used to give an indication of the areas of perceptual defect in brain-damaged patients. This test covers five different perceptual areas, eye motor co-ordination, figure ground, consistency of shape, position in space and spatial relationships. (Although this test is not primarily related to work assessment, it seems appropriate to mention it here while discussing psychological tests.)

One of the difficulties that we have found in carrying out assessments is to relate the standard achieved by a patient to the average performance of the general population. Most of the patients we assess are of below average ability, so that when one performs at a much better level than other patients it is easy for the therapist to over-estimate his level of functioning. Psychological tests have the great advantage of comparing performance with normative data from other sections of the population, but these norm groups may not always provide a relevant comparison.

The development of local data on the relationship between test results and performance in response to therapy and ultimate placement would be useful as a guide to what might be expected of any particular patient. However, because of the individual characteristics of each patient and of each disability, the information collected most probably would need to be grouped generally and used as a broad guide to 'employability' or 'treatability'. Over a period of time it may be possible to make the groupings, and therefore the predictions, more precise.

Specialized tests

If it is necessary to test a specific attribute which may be needed in a particular type of job, some of these attributes may be assessed by the psychological tests already described, or by the assessment of hand function detailed in Chapter 7. In some cases, however, it may be necessary to devise a suitable test.

Care must be taken to make sure that the specific attribute or area of function, and only that one, is being assessed. If the task chosen is too complex, it may involve the use of several attributes and if the results are poor it will not be clear where the difficulty lies. If the patient is badly positioned, an additional handicap such as poor eyesight or limited shoulder movement may prevent him performing well with his hands. Some examples of single aim tests are as follows:

Colour discrimination

This is important for electricians, TV repairers and Post Office linesmen. Dr. Ishihara's Tests for Colour-blindness (Ishihara, 1976) are most useful but, as a simple 'homemade' test, a design made with pegs of different colours and different shades on a peg board can be copied with similar pegs on a second board. To give this test validity, levels of acceptable and unacceptable performances must be worked out.

Spatial relationships

The ability to recognize spatial relationships is important for some engineering jobs, while a major deficit will affect most areas of potential employment. The test is also used for screening perceptual dysfunction. A shape board is made from plywood, with a wide variety of different shapes cut out which must be fitted back into position. A board with irregular shapes with only slight differences can be used as a progression from a simple board with easily identifiable shapes (*see also* page 373).

Reaction time span

A reasonably quick reaction time is important for the patient who is going to drive. A simple test can be constructed with the therapist switching on a light, the patient reacting by pressing a bell and the time lag being recorded. To make this test relevant it is necessary to try it on a sufficient number of drivers, in order to provide data on an acceptable time lag.

Hand–eye co-ordination

This is important in assembly jobs where speed is vital. It can be assessed on industrial outwork, putting circlips on nylon sockets, provided there is no physical defect, such as weakness of the arm pulling down the lever handle, which could affect the result. This test, again, would only be useful if data on the normal speed of operation had been obtained previously (*see also* page 374).

Handling money

This is a basic skill which can be assessed and practised very easily. A graded assessment can include the following:

Handling money from pocket or purse and identifying specific change, such as 10p, 25p, 13½p.

Checking the contents of the occupational therapy department cash box; adding up the receipts for purchases and checking the total against the money in the box.

Going on errands to the local shops and on return giving an account of the money spent.

Running or helping to run the shop in the Centre which is open twice daily and sells basic commodities such as cigarettes, sweets and tissues. (The shop is serviced from a local cash and carry store, and a volunteer patient runs it.)

Reading and writing

It is not unusual to find illiterate patients. Illiteracy may be discovered when a patient has difficulty in following the time-table he has been given for his programme of treatment.

Assessing whether a patient can read presents few problems but needs to be handled tactfully. People who are illiterate, or semiliterate, are often ashamed of this and also show great skill in concealing their problem, sometimes from their own families. Such an assessment should be done privately. A text with large type may be easier than small print, especially if the patient has defective eyesight. Childish content should be avoided as this may upset the patient. Some tabloid newspapers are suitable since they tend to avoid unfamiliar words. Books designed for adult illiteracy classes will provide good practice material but if there is a major resettlement problem, or if the patient can be persuaded that it is not too late to learn to read, skilled help should be sought. There are many adult illiteracy programmes running throughout the country.

A patient who had been evacuated during the war had left one school before learning to read and arrived at the next to join a class that could already read. He spent his schooldays at the back of the class, concealing his handicap. He grew up to work on the railways and became foreman of a maintenance gang but one day, while working a particularly noisy machine, he was run down by a train and suffered multiple injuries. The railway was prepared to take him back in lighter work but stipulated that he must be able to read simple notices. We arranged for the pre-preparatory training bureau of the British Council for Rehabilitation of the Disabled* to send a teacher to give him lessons while he was still undergoing treatment. This gave him a good start to joining an adult literacy scheme.

Writing assessment is usually concerned with finding out whether a patient can record simple messages as part of a job. In practice this may involve making notes, for example about a telephone conversation. The level of achievement may be graded as follows:

1. Making notes of instructions for immediate personal action.
2. Making notes for personal reference for action later in the day.
3. Making memos of simple information to be passed on to others.
4. Making more structured reports for other people.

Such an assessment will cover not only the ability to write legibly but also the ability to phrase instructions in writing.

*Now amalgamated into the Royal Association for Disability and Rehabilitation

English

When assessing a patient either for returning to some type of office job or for changing over to that work, we normally do an English assessment. We devised several test papers of increasing difficulty, the hardest being about O level standard, because we could not find any in textbooks that met our needs. We also produced a clear marking guide for each paper to ensure comparability of results.

Our questions include comprehension, first extracting answers from the text and in later papers doing this from memory; putting specified words into sentences to show their meaning; giving opposites of words; describing some action such as washing a shirt; writing a letter to a friend describing Farnham Park; summarizing a printed extract; explaining the meaning of more complex phrases or terms. We tried to make the questions adult and interesting in content. In addition to the marking guide, which gives answers and maximum marks carried by each question, we produced suggestions of points to look for when marking English papers:

Handwriting; neatness, legibility, appearance, form.

Spelling: especially of everyday words. Note if words are wrongly copied.

Intelligibility: whether the reader is able to understand what the writer is trying to tell him. Does he try to pad.

Grammar: reasonably correct English is necessary for any job involving letter-writing or bookwork. The finer points of grammar are less important but the use of correct tense and person is important.

Fluency: does the writer express himself with ease and good style or does he appear to be struggling to find the right words?

Following instructions: very important. The instructions in the test are all clearly and simply given.

Punctuation: evidence of ability to write intelligibly; note especially the use of full stops and capital letters.

Speed: of writing and answering questions. If candidate answers well but slowly, he is obviously accurate but slow. Alternatively, if he gets through the paper but leaves out questions or answers them wrongly or badly, his standard may be low or he may be slapdash.

Essays should fill at least half of a foolscap page.

Standard English tests are available from DROs at the levels required for different training schemes. Although we have some reservations about the validity of these tests, it is useful to know exactly what the Department of Employment is expecting the patient to achieve to be accepted for entry to a particular course.

Mathematics

Facility with figures is very important in many types of work and some ability is required for all training schemes at Skill Centres. All patients who are likely to be recommended for training or skilled resettlement should be given a relevant mathematics test and, if necessary, some tuition to refresh their memories for certain mathematical processes.

Apart from assessment for work, mathematics may also be useful in treating patients with hemiplegia, head injuries or various neurological conditions, even if their future employment is not in doubt or if they are unlikely to return to any sort of work. Concentration and attentiveness can be assessed and built up using mathematics. The *Teach Yourselves* books on Arithmetic and Algebra provide good practice material with minimal supervision, and may also be used to assess the level the patient has reached.

Vernon's Graded Arithmetic and Mathematics Test

This test covers most basic mathematical processes, which are arranged with increasing difficulty. The patient's score reflects the level of his attainment. This test is used by some of the training colleges for the disabled to screen entrants. We were asked not to use the exact test with patients because previous use might help them to achieve an artificially high score if assessed by a college. So we devised our own parallel version.

The local DRO has an arithmetic test designed for use with entrants to Skill Centres. This is very easy to administer and to mark, taking only 10 minutes. Data is available for the level of achievement required for all the different training courses offered. This ranges from nine marks out of a possible 30 for the least demanding courses, such as plastering, spray-painting or hairdressing, to 27 marks for training as an engineering draughtsman or in industrial electronics. We have made up a parallel test which can be used at an earlier stage in the patient's assessment to give an indication of the revision in arithmetic that may be necessary.

Clerical testing

Many different jobs may be associated with clerical work and the following is only a guide to some of the tasks and tests used at Farnham Park in assessing patients. Some are very simple basic jobs, and it should be realized that the fact that a patient can carry them out does not necessarily indicate that he is suited for a job in an office; office work nowadays may be highly skilled and fast moving, and the more basic jobs tend to be done by juniors. Most of the patients we assess for clerical work are older people who can no longer do manual work. They could not live on a junior's pay and must therefore be able to do work of a higher standard. Jobs in industry which are classified as 'clerical' tend also to require the worker to be able to carry out several types of work. As an example, a storeman, as well as looking after the books in the store, needs to be able to climb ladders and carry heavy weights. It is essential to consider all aspects of the work.

General clerical test

This may be used as a general screening test for anyone who is being assessed for clerical work (*see* page 422).

General considerations including physical ability

Ability to read and write. Neatness and accuracy. Speed of working. Concentration. Ability to learn; to plan and organize own work; to mix with others; to take responsibility; to move around in the office; to take files from all parts of a large filing cabinet; to carry papers or files; to manipulate a card index system.

Use of simple office procedures

Any office worker should be able to use or do accurately the following:

Stapler — and put in refills.
Guillotine.
Hole puncher.
Sellotape stand.
Tie labels and wrap up parcels.
Tear postage stamps and attach them.

Repetitive office work

Jobs from the general office are sometimes available. These are useful for patients who have sufficient ability to do them to an acceptable standard. Two examples are:

Using a rubber stamp on the Farnham Park prospectus and crossing out an incorrect passage. The patient's approach to the job and his speed are noted.

Writing addresses on envelopes, copied from a master book. This is a routine job but one step up from purely repetitive work. The accuracy of copying, neatness and speed are noted.

Filing

We have made a box file test consisting of 50 typed cards which can be filed alphabetically or numerically. A series of questions requires the patient to abstract information from these cards.

Any filing test must be easy to correct, otherwise it will take up too much of the therapist's time. Data to be abstracted from the files can easily be marked against an answer sheet but putting cards into alphabetical or numerical order is more difficult. It thick card is used a coloured pattern can be drawn underneath the cards that will match only when they are in correct order; a different pattern in a different colour is used for each sequence.

Where it is necessary to assess stamina and other attributes required for filing, a practical test, such as non-confidential departmental filing, is used.

Cash analysis

The patient is asked to add up the money in the departmental cash box, add up the receipts for purchases and compare the totals. It is best if the therapist or a student checks the amounts for accuracy before, rather than after, the patient, otherwise a genuine imbalance might be wrongly attributed.

Electronic calculator

This type of machine is routinely used in office work. It is also a useful aid for patients with numeracy problems. Our patients practise totalling the petty cash receipts, adding up the monthly attendance figures, or adding columns of figures and doing multiplication sums taken from our mathematics assessment tests.

Errands

It is often necessary for an office worker to be able to carry out errands efficiently, quickly and accurately. These can vary between going to fetch one particular article or giving a short message, to fulfilling quite complicated instructions. At Farnham Park it is usual for a patient to be sent to the general office to collect stationery, and for the office to be told in advance what he is going to request.

Telephone

An office worker should be able to make a call through an internal switchboard and ask for the person he wishes to speak to, make an outside call, use a public telephone, receive a call and also give information clearly and accurately.

A patient being assessed may take over telephone duty in our workshops for a period, answering the main telephone, taking down messages or going to fetch people as appropriate. The switchboard operator is always told when such a trial is to take place.

Some one-handed patients may manage everything easily, except for taking down messages. It is possible to hold the receiver between shoulder and chin, to use a Telerest or to make a special holder so that the hand is left free for writing.

Switchboard operating

Occasionally it is possible for a patient to operate the general switchboard at Farnham Park. This is useful especially in the case of younger women patients who might have this sort of work to do, but it has only been allowed in suitable cases and for short periods.

Typing

A standard typing instruction book includes specific tests which can be timed in words per minute.

Shorthand

Reading a prepared passage to a patient makes it easy to check her ability to transcribe her shorthand. Counting the number of words and recording the time needed to take them down will give an estimate of speed. However, a therapist who is not used to dictating may not get the best speed from an efficient stenographer.

Using outside resources

Outside help has often been forthcoming for assessment of all kinds. One patient went to a nearby District General Hospital with a bigger switchboard, to be assessed there. On another occasion, we were not sure whether a patient with a back injury would be able to return to milking cows. A local farmer readily agreed to let him practise on his herd and at the end of the day both patient and farmer were satisfied that he could manage the job.

Another patient, a young boy with a severe hand injury, wanted to be an artist. He could hold a brush and paint with it but we did not know if he had sufficient creative ability to train in this field. We sent him to London to be assessed at an art college. When we received their report, regretfully we had to persuade him to choose a different career.

Sometimes it has been possible to arrange for a patient to return to his own firm on a trial basis, to find out if he can manage either his own job or an alternative one that may be more suitable. If the patient's firm is too far away, a local firm providing similar work may be willing to give him a short period of assessment. Trial periods in a work situation may last for a day, a week or even a month. The firm is aware that if the patient is unable to manage, he can return to the Centre where he will be reassessed and helped to find alternative work. The employer is therefore more likely to give the patient this chance to prove himself since, if the trial fails, there will be no question of having to turn him away with no further prospects. In practice we have found that the patients usually survive the trial period and become reinstated in their old jobs.

There is great potential goodwill among employers towards disabled people provided there is not too much financial risk involved. We try to build up contacts with local firms and local people who might help us. Some of the patients, too, who are admitted for treatment may be and, indeed, have become employers of future patients. They also help in other ways: a personnel officer arranged for his firm to give us a milling machine that was no longer required, and an engineer got his firm to overhaul all our elderly wood-turning lathes.

Another source of help in the employment field has been the firm which has supplied us with industrial outwork. On one occasion they took on a blind, euphoric patient with a brachial plexus lesion who had already been assessed by the Royal National Institute for the Blind as suitable only for sheltered employment. He learned to work our hand-presses, was taken by the firm on trial and proved acceptable. His daily journey to and from work included a quarter mile walk partly across a caravan site, and two bus rides; he was not temperamentally suited to have a guide dog.

Many local people may be able to offer help or professional advice. For example, a patient who might work as a petrol pump attendant could be given a trial by a local garage. The filling station manager could even be flattered at being asked to display his expertise in assessment if approached in the right way. It is only by approaching local people that the occupational therapist will find out whether they are prepared to help patients.

Factors which complicate a return to work

Patients respond to situations in different ways. As one of the DROs who worked with us used to say, 'It's not so much what happens to a person as the person to whom it happens.' Some patients are able to take maximum advantage of the treatment facilities offered to them. Others have not the inner reserves to do so. This applies not only to regaining maximum physical competence but also to readjusting to everyday living; if necessary to a changed job situation.

During a period of economic depression many competent people become unemployed. The longer they are out of work the more demoralized they become. During the 1930s men who had been unemployed for long periods were sent to what are now Employment Rehabilitation Centres to help them regain the work habit. Disabled people face similar but greater problems because they may well have less to offer a prospective employer. The longer the time between the onset of disability and a period of intensive treatment, the harder it may be to get the patient back to work. The therapist must not only provide the opportunity the patient needs but may need to help stiffen the resolve of those who are unable to take advantage of such an opportunity unaided. She will not always succeed.

There are other factors. Some patients live in the 'wrong' place. For example, in parts of South Wales most jobs are in heavy industry which makes finding light work difficult for everyone and puts someone with a substantial handicap at a greater disadvantage. Another example is Remploy. It is little use recommending a patient for such sheltered employment if the nearest factory is 50 miles away. On occasion a patient has moved to another part of the country in order to get work.

The patient may come for rehabilitation at an inauspicious time. When there is recession and unemployment throughout the country it is particularly difficult to find suitable work for the disabled. It may be necessary to discharge a patient and readmit him for a further booster period of rehabilitation when the economic climate improves.

Returning to work may create a financial problem. Sometimes a disabled man who wants to return to work can lose money. If he is badly incapacitated the only job he can manage may be worth less than the payments he is receiving from the DHSS. A family man who wants to get out of the house and back to work may feel he is letting down his dependents because of this reduction in income.

Another problem has always been that some of the jobs in industry that would be suitable for disabled men were classified as women's work and carried a lower wage than could reasonably be offered to a man. To avoid creating problems no man could be offered this work. The Sex Discrimination Act, although aimed at correcting such anomalies, does not appear to have provided a complete solution to this problem.

REPORTING

Occupational therapy assessment is almost always carried out as an integral part of the treatment programme and is used to discover the patient's weaknesses and strengths. The therapist then sets out to devise measures to improve the level of function in the weak areas. When writing a work assessment report it is therefore not usually relevant to give details of everything that the patient has been doing in the workshops; this would merely show how hard the therapist has been working. As a rule it is sufficient to give a brief outline, concentrating on areas of achievement and relevant areas of non-achievement that provide contraindications for likely work.

Writing a report on a patient who appears to be unemployable can seem a heavy responsibility. Usually, however, the therapist will not be the only person expressing an opinion; the doctor will also be involved and so the responsibility will be shared. At Farnham Park the therapists are expected to fill in the major part of the practical comments on the DP1 form. Using the phrase 'at this time the patient is unemployable' allows for the possibility of further improvement and reassessment at a later stage.

Reports should be written in clear English with a minimum of medical terminology, and should be concise since a long, rambling report will just not be read. An outline report form developed at the Medical Rehabilitation Centre, Camden Road, London, in collaboration with one of the occupational therapists from Farnham Park, is given below together with, by kind permission of Wenona Keane, two assessments of patients who attended the Centre. This form provides a basic outline of facts to be collected for the final assessment report. When writing reports based on this format, up to half a page is usually sufficient for each of the four sections.

ASSESSMENT REPORT

Name: Age: Date:

Diagnosis:

Former employment:

Period of assessment:

Regularity of attendance:

Personal/Social adjustment

1. Personal appearance
   (*a*) Grooming
   (*b*) Does disability detract from appearance?

2. Relationship with fellow workers
   (*a*) Can he work with others?
   (*b*) What is his attitude towards workmates?

3. Relationship with supervisor
   (*a*) Can he accept criticism and correction?
   (*b*) Does he depend on supervision?
   (*c*) What is his reaction to pressure?

4. Attitude towards work
   (*a*) Does he like to get down to work?
   (*b*) Has he good judgment?
   (*c*) Is he able to make decisions?
   (*d*) Is he responsible and honest?
   (*e*) Does he show initiative?
   (*f*) Is he able to budget time effectively?
   (*g*) Can he concentrate?

5. Adjustment to disability

6. Self-confidence

Physical capacity for work

1. Extent to which disability is a handicap

2. Physical tolerance and ability
   - (a) Standing
   - (b) Sitting
   - (c) Carrying
   - (d) Balance
   - (e) Lifting
   - (f) Stooping
   - (g) Climbing
   - (h) Co-ordination
   - (i) Manual Dexterity
   - (j) Public Transport

Work tested – Work performance

1. Results of the work patient has been tested on

   Areas of work assessment
   - (a) Clerical; Educational
   - (b) Service, e.g. kitchen, janitor etc.
   - (c) Mechanical
   - (d) Manual

2. What type of work does he produce?

3. Does he learn a skill easily and how much practice does he need to develop it?

4. Can he retain and follow instructions?
   - (a) Written
   - (b) Verbal
   - (c) Diagrammatic

5. Has he special vocational interests?

Conclusion

1. Employable: Type of work

2. Trainable: What sphere?

3. Unemployable: Why?

ASSESSMENT REPORT

Name:	Mrs A. B.	Age: 48 years
Diagnosis:	RTA head injury	
Former employment:	Temp. clerical officer	
Period of assessment:	Three months	
Regularity of attendance:	Regular	

Personal/Social adjustment

A. B. is a smart attractive woman who takes great pride in her appearance. She gives a first impression of being co-operative, charming and eager to please. It would be unwise to estimate her probable performance from her behaviour at an interview. In fact, she does not work well with other people. She becomes easily impatient and can be extremely tactless, e.g. she frequently draws attention to other patients' disabilities. For most of the time A. maintains that she has no psychological impairment. However, when she finds herself unable to carry out an activity or feels that she is being criticized, she will claim it is solely due to the effects of her head injury and that her difficulties have not been understood. It is evident that she has a very unrealistic appreciation of her own limitations and that this influences her behaviour in many situations. She becomes agitated and frequently aggressive when she is:

1. pressured to work faster or more accurately;

2. criticized about her work or attitude to it;

3. not given immediate and individual attention when she requests it.

She has shown evidence of disorientation and memory loss which can vary considerably from day to day. She is at present involved in a memory training programme, in which she shows some improvement.

She will work for limited periods of about 20 minutes when given a task but she has never shown any initiative to begin an activity and will always wait for 'step-by-step' direction. She appears unable to make effectual decisions in a work situation.

She shows an attitude of complete detachment from the group situation surrounding her in the department and is intolerant of any change in routine or delay in staff attending to her. She is unaware of the needs of other patients.

Physical capacity for work

A. B. has made very good physical recovery. Her remaining problems are:

1. slightly clumsy gait;
2. difficulty stooping to lift articles without dizziness;
3. poor balance when she moves quickly or when others rush past her.

She manages public transport unaccompanied.

Work tested – Work performance

Writing: Clear and accurate.

English: Fast speed, accurate – good understanding of grammar.

Standard general clerical test: Very poor understanding – needed instructions repeated – when more detailed instruction was refused she became very agitated and aggressive.

General clerical work:
1. Involving filing, recording names and reference numbers, etc.; filling in forms, addressing envelopes, etc. A. did this activity three times – each time she had no recollection of having done it previously. Her pace of work was very slow and she became easily distracted and on the last occasion inaccurate.
2. Collating papers – accurate but very slow pace of work.
3. Filing – this test was given at the beginning and the end of the assessment period. First result: average speed; accurate. Second result: did not grasp the instructions and did not complete the test. Again, no recollection of having done the test before.

Light packaging: Able to concentrate and maintain speed of work for 40 minutes 3 times a day. However, she expressed boredom with this kind of work and seemed ashamed to do it.

Christmas Cards: Sorting/punching/guillotining/packaging. At first she enjoyed this activity but later thought it too menial a task.

Games:
1. *Hand function games* – unable to retain the purpose of the game – became bored.
2. *Social* – became impatient with others, became confused at times.

Conclusions

At present we consider Mrs. A. B. is unemployable due to the following:

1. Her personality problems and erratic behaviour and function indicate that she would not be acceptable in open employment of the type she is used to.

2. The type of work she could cope with, such as packaging or machine operating, would not be acceptable to her.

ASSESSMENT REPORT

Name: Mr C. D.   Age: 44

Diagnosis: Spinal cord compression in the cervical region with resultant slight weakness of the right side

Former employment: Lorry driver

Period of assessment: Two months

Regularity of attendance: Excellent

Personal/Social adjustment

Mr C. D. is a charming, self-effacing man whose disability is very apparent particularly because of a facial palsy. He wears a surgical collar, walks with one stick and wears a right below-knee caliper. He is punctual and reliable and willing to try anything asked of him. He has a pleasant manner and gets on well with staff and patients. He shows intelligence and initiative and is always willing to accept criticism and correction. He is anxious to improve himself and yet has natural doubts about his ability.

He has adjusted very realistically to his disability and accepts that he is unlikely to progress physically due to the irreversible nature of his condition.

Physical capacity for work

He is able to sustain a reasonable level of activity all day but is tired by the end of the day. He can stand, sit, balance, stoop and climb stairs without difficulty. He can walk 1.6–3.2 km (1–2 miles) comfortably. His right hand remains less strong than the left but co-ordination and manual dexterity are nearly normal. Public transport presents no problem.

Work tested – Work performance

Writing: Clear slightly untidy writing of reasonable speed.

Vocabulary: Above average compared with people of similar age and education.

Arithmetic: Worked well and accurately but needs practice in fractions and multiplication.

General intelligence: In tests measuring general ability was above average in comparison with people of similar age and education.

Clerical work: The general clerical test results showed above-average ability compared with people applying for general clerical work in a public utility. A filing exercise was completed in normal time with average accuracy.

Woodwork: Tackles work with enthusiasm and initiative. Use of wood-work tools correct. Standard of work good. However, with prolonged use of tools (sawing, planing) his right arm does become tired and he has to take short rests. Fine finger work he also finds tiring.

Special vocational interests: Would very much like to work for the British Museum, cataloguing pieces, as his chief hobby has always been archaeology and Greek and Roman history.

Conclusions

1. Trainable: This man shows obvious ability and should have no difficulty with clerical training. He is realistic in wanting to pursue clerical work which is sedentary and would give him reasonable job security.

2. Employable: Prior to retraining clerically, it is possible that the British Museum may employ him on a temporary basis as a museum assistant. He has made the appropriate enquiries and is waiting to hear from them.

Note: This patient was trained in clerical work and did eventually obtain employment.

REFERENCES

Ishihara, S. (1976). *Tests for Colour-blindness.* Tokyo; Kanehara Shuppan. London; H. K. Lewis

Macdonald, M (1976). *Occupational Therapy in Rehabilitation,* page 84. 4th Edition. London; Baillière Tindall

Sources of Equipment and Materials for Splint-making

Equipment

Burgess Electric Bandsaw BBS 20 and general-purpose blades for same	Burgess Power Tools Ltd, Sapcote, Leicester
Electric hotplates (preferably paired)	Domestic appliance and hospital catering equipment suppliers
Electric sander, capable of low speed, with stand	Ironmongers, DIY stores
Heatrae oven, and stand for same	Heatrae Ltd, Norwich, Norfolk
Heat guns	Rapmac Ltd, Towerfield Road, Shoeburyness, Southend-on-Sea, Essex
Infrared lamp	Domestic appliance suppliers or Boots Chemists
Stainless steel dish, approximately 40 cm × 30 cm × 9 cm deep (16 in × 12 in × 3½ in)	Hospital catering equipment suppliers
Non-rusting tongs, or pottery tongs	Kitchen equipment stores or craft suppliers
Metal funnel, seamless, approximately 12 cm (5 in) diameter	Ironmongers

Wax pencil, e.g. Chinagraph	Stationers
Engineer's scriber	Ironmongers
Aluminium foil (as used for cookery)	Grocers, hardware stores
Aloplast, children's plastic modelling putty	E. J. Arnold & Son, Ltd, Butterley Street, Leeds
Soldering wire	Hardware and DIY stores
Needle files, half-round, flat, rat-tail	Ironmongers, craft suppliers
Drill bits, 1.5 mm to 5 mm ($^1/_{16}$ in to $^1/_5$ in) (as used for carpentry)	Ironmongers
Revolving punch pliers	Nottingham Handcraft Co, Melton Road, West Bridgford, Nottingham; other craft suppliers
Leather punches and rivets	G. E. Taylor & Sons, Ltd, Wapping Wharf, Cumberland Road, Bristol
Riveting tool	Nottingham Handcraft Co
Silicone-treated release paper	Smith & Nephew Ltd, Alum Rock Road, Birmingham B8 3DY
Dermatological gloves	Seton Products, Ltd, Tubiton House, Medlock Street, Oldham, Lancashire

Materials

Darvic
Formasplint
Orthoplast
San-Splint   *see* Table of materials, page 246
Vitrathene
Plastazote
Plaster-of-Paris

Metals, brass rod, aluminium etc.	Engineers' merchants and suppliers; Tunes Engineering Ltd, Slough; Miller Morris and Brooker Ltd, Slough
Spring wire (piano wire)	Ormiston & Sons, Ltd, Broughton Road, London W13
Plastic cane (tubing)	Homecraft Supplies Ltd, 27 Trinity Road, London SW17
Polystyrene lining (for insulating Darvic) 60 cm (24 in) wide by 0.5 mm thick, 7 m (23 ft) roll	Nottingham Handcraft Co, Melton Road, West Bridgford, Nottingham
Paddings and linings, medical quality, all types except as below	Hinders-Leslies Ltd, Higham Hill Road, London E17
Plastic and rubber foams and sheetings, industrial and domestic quality	Conrad Lewis, 87 High Road, East Finchley, London N2
Formatex padding	Nottingham Handcraft Co
Wet-suit rubber	Water sports suppliers
Stockinette, Tubinette	Seton Products Ltd, Tubiton House, Medlock Street, Oldham, Lancashire
White cotton webbing (strapping)	Nottingham Handcraft Co
Corfam synthetic suede (also known as Polcorfam)	Skorimpex, Lodz, Poland
Velcro touch-and-close fastener, 16 mm and 22 mm wide, 10 m (33 ft) roll	Nottingham Handcraft Co; Selectus Ltd, Biddulph, Stoke-on-Trent, Staffs
Leathers, all types	William R. Pangbourne & Son, 1 and 2 Queen's Parade, Bounds Green Road, London N11

Tubular rivets, nickel-plated, 7 mm   Nottingham Handcraft Co;
Homecraft Supplies Ltd,
27 Trinity Road,
London SW17

Oval and rectangular rings and loops,   Nottingham Handcraft Co;
nickel-plated, various; buckles and   Radcliffe, Son & Crockford,
fastenings, various   14 Trinity Lane,
London EC4

Oval loops, 18 mm X 8 mm,   Selectus Ltd, Biddulph,
nickel-plated (for the MUD splint)   Stoke-on-Trent, Staffs

Plastic rings that stand up (known as: Fred Sammons Inc, Box 32,
Heavy duty 1 inch nylon 'D' rings)   Brookfield, Illinois 60513

Fishing-line, braided, nylon or terylene   Sports stores
approx. 10 kg strength

Adhesives

Copydex adhesive, 112 g (4 oz) jar   Nottingham Handcraft Co;
with brush attached   stationers

Evo-Stik impact adhesive   Hardware and DIY stores

Croid solvent adhesive No. 6143   Croda Polymers Ltd,
153 New Bedford Road,
Luton, Bedfordshire

Adhesive tape, double-sided,   Nottingham Handcraft Co;
pressure-sensitive, 25 mm (1 in) wide   Smith & Nephew, Ltd,
Alum Rock Road,
Birmingham B8 3DY

Dry-cleaning fluid (carbon-   Hardware stores
tetrachloride), e.g. Dab-it-off

Index

445